Advanced Bariatric and Metabolic Surgery
Edited by Chih-Kun Huang

Published by InTech
Janeza Trdine 9, 51000 Rijeka, Croatia

Publishing Process Manager Iva Simcic

Technical Editor Teodora Smiljanic

Cover Designer InTech Design Team

Additional hard copies can be obtained from orders@intechopen.com

Advanced Bariatric and Metabolic Surgery, Edited by Chih-Kun Huang
p. cm.
ISBN 978-953-307-926-4

For EU product safety concerns:
IN TECH d.o.o., Prolaz Marije Krucifikse Kozulić 3, 51000 Rijeka, Croatia,
info@intechopen.com or visit our website at intechopen.com.

Meet the editor

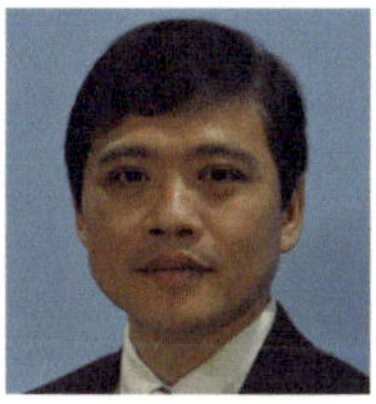

Dr Chih-Kun Huang is the director of the B.M.I. Surgery center and International Minimally Invasive Surgery Training Center of E-Da hospital in Kaohsiung, Taiwan, as well as the president of Taiwan Obesity Support Association (T.O.S.A). Dr Huang has been devoted to minimally invasive surgery and bariatric surgery since 2004. He performed the first single incision trans-umbilical laparoscopic Roux-en-Y gastric bypass in 2008, and the first laparoscopic adjustable gastric banded application in the world in 2009. His center was also designated as the first International Center of Excellence for Bariatric Surgery (I.C.E) in Asia-Pacific area in 2009. Due to his contribution and devotion, he was awarded the Endos Award in Medical Science & Technology in 2010, and the International Award by American Society for Metabolic and Bariatric Surgery (ASMBS) in 2011. Dr Huang is also included in the Marquis Who's Who in Medicine and Healthcare 2011-2012.

Contents

Preface

Obesity was formally recognized as a disease by the World Health Organization (WHO) in 1997, and its prevalence is increasing at epidemic proportions worldwide. The enormous changes in human life regarding labor, exercise and diet habits have largely provoked the development of this multi-factorial disease. It has been confirmed that obesity causes many diseases, including cardiovascular disorders, type 2 diabetes mellitus, obstructive sleep apnea and degenerative joint disease. Even though many kinds of medical treatment are recommended, most therapies have not been successful in keeping sustained weight loss and controlling obesity-related comorbidity, especially in morbid obesity. Until now, only bariatric surgery has proven to be an effective procedure, and in the last 40 years, the number of bariatric procedures has been increasing exponentially in the world. This book provides an overview and updated knowledge of bariatric surgery and patient care. In it, we discussed various procedures, preoperative preparation, perioperative care and postoperative nutrition support, and the brand new, "transformed" bariatric surgery in type 2 diabetes–metabolic surgery and scarless bariatric surgery has also been included. We hope that this book will contribute to the future development of weight loss management.

Chih-Kun Huang
Bariatric & Metabolic International (B.M.I) Surgery Center, E-Da hospital, Taiwan
International Minimally Invasive Surgery Training Center of E-Da hospital, Taiwan
Republic of China

1

Surgical Procedures to Achieve Weight Loss

Roman Grinberg, John N. Afthinos and Karen E. Gibbs
F.A.C.S.,
USA

1. Introduction

Obesity is one of the leading medical problems facing our society today. At least two thirds of the U.S. adult population is considered overweight and approximately one-third of American adults are obese, creating an epidemic of obesity. Clearly, there has been an increase in the number of individuals struggling to lose weight. Additionally, obesity has become increasingly prevalent in the pediatric population and 30% of U.S. children have a BMI greater than the 85th percentile for their age.[1] The relationship of childhood and adolescent obesity to adult obesity is a strong one with 20% of children who are obese at 4 years of age and 80% of adolescents who are obese will be obese as adults.[2] The annual cost of managing obesity in the United States alone amounts to approximately $100 billion, of which $52 billion are direct healthcare costs. Hypertension, sleep apnea, diabetes, stroke, myocardial infarction and malignancy is a short but representative list of problems associated with obesity. Approximately 300,000 U.S. deaths per year are related to obesity.

While medical options such as weight loss programs, diets and drug therapies are ever-present and increasing, only 3-7% of patients with a diagnosis of obesity are able to achieve effective and consistent weight loss. [3] This statistic demonstrates the continued failure of the medical management of obesity. On the other hand, patients undergoing bariatric surgery demonstrate 23% weight loss at 2 years after operative intervention and 16% by 10 years.[4] These patients had dramatic improvement in quality of life scores and validated measures of psychiatric dysfunction compared with only minor and inconsistent improvement in patients undergoing medical treatment for their obesity. After 10 years of follow up the improvement in the surgical group diminished somewhat due to weight regain. Regardless, outcomes of groups of patients undergoing surgical treatment were superior to those treated medically.[5,6] Surgical options for weight loss have been consistently more successful at helping individuals to lose weight and maintain that achievement permanently.[7-9]

Weight loss surgery has been evolving since its inception and the final chapter is yet to be written. Since the 1950's astute minds and dedicated surgeons have tried to find the one operation that would yield the definitive answer to the problem of obesity. As time has progressed, no silver bullet has been identified. It is clear that there is no procedure that is superior to another for every patient.

Each operation that will be discussed here has its own story to tell in terms of patient selection, operative technique, outcomes and complications. Each has an important role to play in the world of weight loss surgery and it behooves those involved in the trenches of bariatric surgery and the subsequent care of these patients to be familiar with the individual nuances of the operations. In this chapter, we will discuss the various common, and not so common, surgical options currently being employed to assist the morbidly obese patient.

1.1 Patient selection

The patient selection criteria consist of a group of objective and variable components. The objective component was set by the National Institutes of Health (NIH) in 1991. In order to be eligible for bariatric surgery the patient must have a body mass index (BMI) of 40kg/m^2 or a BMI of 35 kg/m^2 with associated co-morbidities. These co-morbidities can include medical conditions such as:

1. Hypertension
2. Diabetes
3. Obstructive sleep apnea
4. Hyperlipidemia
5. GERD
6. Degenerative joint disease[4]

Other subjective criteria include:

1. Sustained attempts at weight loss over a period of at least five years
2. Recognition of the effect of morbid obesity on the patient's health
3. Demonstration of a reasonable understanding of the surgical tools available for weight loss with the associated risks and benefits
4. Ability to understand and conform to the postoperative diet and lifestyle changes necessary for success
5. Realistic expectations of the desired surgical procedure.[10,11]

1.2 Weight loss

Weight loss patterns in bariatric surgery are one of the major differences between the various surgical tools available. While most patients are concerned about the absolute weight loss in terms of pounds or kilograms, in order for there to be an objective method of comparing the differences in weight loss between the different procedures other means of measurement have evolved with time. Weight loss is generally measured according to the patient's BMI or a change in the percentage of excess weight lost (%EWL).[12,13]

1.3 Complications

Intimate knowledge of the exact operation is necessary for any clinician to be able to assess and manage post bariatric surgical patients. Some postoperative complications such as infection, pneumonia, urinary tract infections, deep venous thrombosis and pulmonary embolism may be standard concerns after intra-abdominal surgery but other issues such as erosions or slippage of a gastric band, internal hernias, bleeding and anastomotic leakage require a physician to be knowledgeable about the intricacies and variations of weight loss operations, as many complications may be overlooked or missed by the unsuspecting observer. Complications specific to each operation will be discussed with the review of each operation.

2. Laparoscopic vs. Open Approach

All bariatric operations have been performed using the open approach. With increases in knowledge, technology, skill and ingenuity, all of these procedures are now possible via a laparoscopic approach. Over time, laparoscopic surgery has gained wide acceptance and is now more common in primary procedures in bariatric surgery than the open approach.[14-16] Regardless of the method used to perform any particular weight loss procedure the surgical endpoints are the same. All primary bariatric procedures can generally be performed laparoscopically with clinical results comparable to those of an open counterpart. The major reported benefits of the laparoscopic approach include: superior exposure, reduced soft tissue trauma, better postoperative pulmonary function, less postoperative pain, decreased rates of wound infection, decreased rates of abdominal wall hernias, earlier return to physical activities, decreased length of stay, earlier return to work and better cosmetic results. The laparoscopic approach can also serve as a useful diagnostic tool in bariatric patients when imaging studies may be impossible to perform, or when signs and symptoms of an ongoing surgical problem may be vague due to the patient's body habitus. Disadvantages of the laparoscopic approach primarily include higher operative costs, longer operative times, need for specialized training and steep learning curves.

3. Types of Surgery

In general, the bariatric surgical procedures are classified by their mechanism of action. They are subdivided in three types:

1. Restrictive operations are based on decreasing the size of the stomach, limiting portion size, and increasing early satiety. [17,18]
   - Vertical Banded Gastroplasty (VBG)
   - Sleeve Gastrectomy (SG)
   - Adjustable Gastric Banding (AGB)
2. Malabsorptive operations rely on the surgical rearrangement of the gastrointestinal system to decrease the absorption by limiting the exposure of the small bowel to the ingested meal. [17,18]
   - Jejuno-ileal bypass (JIB)
3. Mixed operations are a combination of the restrictive and malabsorptive procedures.[17,18]
   - Roux-en-Y Gastric Bypass (RYGB)
   - Biliopancreatic Bypass with Duodenal Switch (BPD-DS)
   - Laparoscopic Sleeve Gastrectomy with Duodenojejunal Bypass (LSG-DB)
   - Ileal Interposition with Sleeve Gastrectomy (IL-SG)

4. Vertical Banded Gastroplasty

The Vertical Banded Gastroplasty (VGB) is like many other bariatric operations which experienced changes from its initial inception until the accepted version that was performed. The procedure, which was first performed in 1971 by Mason, underwent an evolution. The initial operation included a transverse gastroplasty which served to partition the stomach. The final variation involved the creation of a vertical gastroplasty along the lesser curvature. Operatively, a window is made through the anterior and posterior gastric wall using a circular stapler positioned close to the lesser curvature. A linear non-cutting stapler is then applied through the gastric window, created by the circular stapler, in a vertical fashion directed towards the angle of His. A ring of polypropylene mesh is then placed through the gastric window around the lesser curvature (see Figure 1). This procedure has since been adapted to the laparoscopic approach in which the stomach is generally transected vertically.[17,18,19,20] This anatomic change results in early satiety with reduced meal portions.

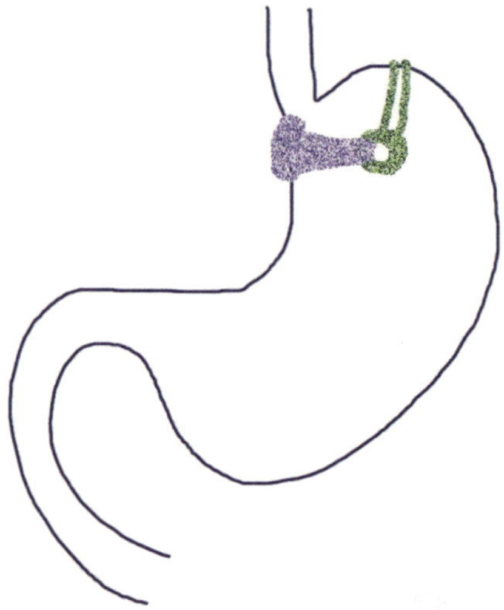

Fig. 1. Vertical Banded Gastroplasty

4.1 Weight loss

This procedure generally was able to effect a 50-60% EWL within two years. The VBG appears to be more dependent on the patient's ability to maintain lifelong alterations of his or her eating habits. These changes include avoiding high-calorie liquids and such calorie-rich foods as cake, cookies, and other junk foods that undergo substantial liquefaction in the mouth and thus arrive in the VBG pouch as a liquid slurry that is not restricted by the outlet. This dependence on patient behavior led to a higher failure rate due to weight regain which in turn has led many to abandon the VBG in preference to other simpler restrictive procedures.[20-22]

4.2 Complications

The majority of problems with the VBG generally surrounded stomal issues. The stoma could be too loose which would lead to little restriction and ultimately poor weight loss. Conversely, the stoma could develop a stricture which could then lead to difficulty with oral intake.

Staple-line dehiscence was also a well known problem. Small dehiscences do not substantially impede the restrictive effects of the operation. A dehiscence larger than 1 cm would generally lead to both weight regain and gastroesophageal reflux disease. This would render the operation ineffective as the restriction would be lost, yield inadequate long-term weight loss and require revision of the initial operation. Sporadic staple-line dehiscence was also seen in postpartum patients—the reason for this association is unknown.[23,24] It is possible to restaple a dehisced staple line; however, reapplying staples to a thickened, scarred stomach wall may be associated with not only another dehiscence, but tearing of the tissue. The success rate in resuming and maintaining weight loss with reapplication of staples is also generally less satisfactory when compared to the degree of weight loss after the initial operation.

Pouch enlargement was another well recognized complication of this procedure leading to gastric stasis and reflux. It primarily occurs due to repetitive vomiting, inclusion of an excessive amount of fundus during the initial procedure or continued overeating. One should be aware of the fact that one of the innate functions of the fundus is to dilate to accommodate ingestion of the food bolus. Thus, inclusion of a significant amount of fundus may promote pouch dilation. To help to avoid this, the initial vertical staple line should be placed precisely at the angle of His. The VBG was quite popular in the 1970's but is much less commonly performed today. [25,26]

5. Sleeve Gastrectomy

The Sleeve Gastrectomy (SG) was initially used as the first part of a two-stage procedure for the super-obese patients who were considered poor surgical candidates and who would not tolerate a prolonged or more involved procedure. The operation was designed to allow the patients an opportunity to achieve some weight loss before being converted to the more complex gastric bypass or biliopancreatic diversion with duodenal switch (BPD-DS).[27] Keen observation noted that the weight loss with the gastric sleeve alone was significant and, in fact, many patients refused further operative intervention to promote continued weight loss. Currently, this procedure is used as a definitive weight loss procedure. Despite the perceived simplicity and efficacy of gastric sleeve, enthusiasm for this procedure is often tempered by the lack of data on long-term outcomes beyond 5 years. It was discovered that SG also produces a decrease in ghrelin levels for up to a year, which may reduce the desire for food.[28,29]

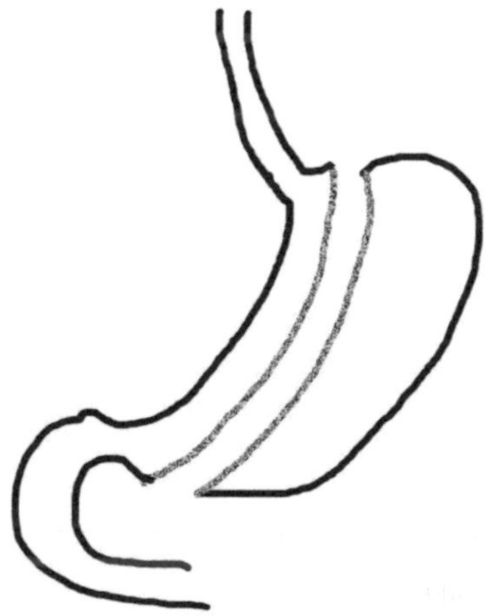

Fig. 2. Sleeve Gastrectomy

The operation involves a vertical gastrectomy performed parallel to the lesser curvature. The more receptive greater curvature is resected and the patient is left with a long tube-like stomach (see Figure 2). The operation consists of releasing the vascular supply of the greater curvature as well as the posterior gastric attachments. A bougie is advanced into the distal stomach or duodenum and the greater curvature of the stomach is resected. The transection of the stomach is begun approximately 4-5cm proximal to the pylorus. With the bougie in place to size the stomach along the lesser curvature, a vertical gastrectomy is created using a linear cutting stapler.[27] Different sized bougies have been used to date, somewhat limiting the comparison of available results. Standardization is still awaited for this procedure that is certainly a valuable addition to the surgical armamentarium.

5.1 Weight loss

While no long term weight loss statistics are available, medium-term results are indeed encouraging with an expected 62% EWL at 12 months and 68% EWL at 24 months.[27,30] Review of current literature also demonstrates that at 6 years, the %EWL is approximately 57.3-72.3%.[24,31]

5.2 Complications

Along with the standard postoperative concerns, the most common complications with the SG have surrounded staple line disruption, leakage from the long staple line and bleeding. The majority of leaks occur in the area of gastroesophageal junction.[32,33] It most likely occurs because this area has diminished blood supply compared to the rest of the stomach. Also the stomach wall in this area is thinner and hence less resistant to ischemia and thermal injuries by energy devices. [32,33] Another common site for a leak is along the antral staple line. Disruption of the staple line in this location is believed to occur due to the relative obstruction caused by the nearby pylorus.

Stenosis and dilatation of this narrow tubular stomach has also been reported.

The gastroesophageal junction and the angularis incisura are the two most common areas where stenosis occurs, and this can be diagnosed by an upper gastrointestinal series. The most common reasons for the development of narrowing or stenosis are over-sewing the staple line, using a bougie that is too small, creating non-parallel staple lines or using non-absorbable suture material.

Even though we mentioned that variable bougie sizes are being used by different surgeons, a 32 to 40 French bougie is most often utilized when SG is performed as a definitive operation. Larger bougie sizes, up to 60 French, can be used when SG is being performed as a part of a staged procedure such as BPD-DS.[32] Management of stenosis primarily consists of endoscopic dilation vs. stent placement. If the area of stenosis is too long, surgical intervention may be necessary with conversion to a gastric stricturoplasty, RYGB or resection with gastrogastrostomy. Management of gastric sleeve stretching is currently controversial. There are multiple reports of successful repeat sleeve gastrectomy as well as conversion of SG to RYGB or BPD-DS.

6. Adjustable Gastric Banding

In 1983, while looking for a safe surgical method to fight obesity, Dr. Lubomyr Kuzmak introduced a Dacron-reinforced silicon band. This original system had no ability to adjust the gastric restriction and was considered a permanent implant. The Adjustable Gastric

Banding System was introduced in 1985 by Dr. Dag Hallberg of Sweden. Laparoscopic adjustable gastric banding (LAGB) was advocated in 1992 by Favretti and Cadiere and made a revolutionary change in the history of bariatric surgery. Over time and with technological improvements, the first laparoscopic adjustable gastric band device was approved by the FDA for use in the United States in 2001.

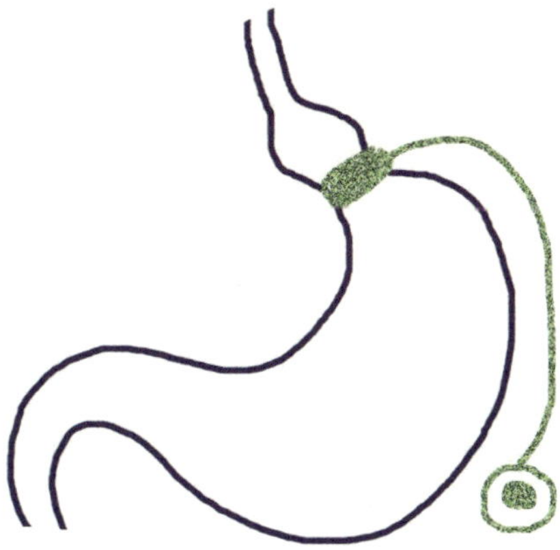

Fig. 3. Adjustable Gastric Banding

Adjustable Gastric Banding (AGB) procedures have now virtually replaced the VBG throughout the world. A number of bands are available on the market, but only two devices are currently FDA approved and available in the United States.

Gastric banding procedures rely on the restriction of enteral intake to achieve weight loss and its maintenance. There is no alteration of the native anatomy and as such the neurohormonal mechanisms involved in weight control are largely left intact.[34,35]

Over a period of time many modifications to the gastric band were created by different manufacturers.

The AGB is commonly placed laparoscopically, generally with a short operative time and limited morbidity. Hospital stay is often one day and, recently, is more commonly being performed as an outpatient procedure. Operatively, the goal is to place the band in a position at the gastric cardia near the gastroesophageal junction that will yield a small gastric pouch with a 20-30 mL capacity. The small pouch provides the restriction needed to assist in weight loss. The optimal technique has changed with time and is now agreed upon to be the pars flaccida technique. The band encircles the upper stomach, and its ultimate position is determined by using a calibration tube as a guide intraoperatively. It is then sutured in place with the use of anterior gastro-gastric sutures for stability, while posteriorly the band is held in place by natural attachments between the posterior stomach and the right diaphragmatic crus.[34,35]

The band system consists of three components (see Figure 3):

1. The band which is placed at the gastric cardia near the gastroesophageal junction and effectively divides the stomach into two segments; an upper smaller pouch and the larger intact stomach.

2. The port which is the access point for adjustments. The port is placed on the abdominal wall, directly attached to the rectus abdominis fascia. An adjustment consists of using a Huber needle to access the subcutaneous port at which point normal saline can be injected or aspirated from the band. The injection or aspiration of fluid changes the tightness of the band around the stomach and can therefore assist with the management of food consumption, appropriate early satiety and subsequent weight loss.
3. The silastic tubing which connects the band to the port.

The major advantages of the gastric band include the minimally invasive nature of the operation, its reversibility, the adjustability of the band and the maintenance of gastrointestinal anatomy.

6.1 Weight loss

The weight loss patterns for the two available AGBs are comparable. The expectations for weight loss are for the patient to obtain a 30-35% EWL in the first year, 50% EWL at the second year and 60% EWL in the third year. Ultimately the goal is to achieve a gradual, effective and durable means to lose weight. These results have been quite variable in the literature and ultimately are still being debated.[34-37]

6.2 Complications

Perioperative complications occur in 1-2% of cases and this safety profile associated with the AGBs make them an attractive choice for many patients and surgeons when compared to the other surgical options available for weight loss. One band-related complication includes stoma obstruction. This occurs most commonly due to inclusion of excess perigastric fat, use of a band of insufficient diameter for the thickness of the tissue, significant tissue edema, band infection, delayed gastric emptying or gastric perforation. The majority of these require surgical management, including band removal or repositioning.

Late band related complications include erosions, slippage or gastric prolapse, port or tubing malfunction, port migration, leakage at the port site, tubing or band, pouch or esophageal dilatation and esophagitis.[35] Slippage is diagnosed when a portion of the stomach below the band has traversed the band and now lies above it. This movement initially creates a large upper gastric pouch which diminishes the restrictive function of the adjustable band. As more of the inferior stomach passes cephalad, it ultimately leads to obstruction of the stoma which will present with persistent nausea and vomiting and inability to tolerate even saliva. This is a scenario which must be diagnosed early as it can lead to gastric necrosis if not identified and treated in a timely fashion. Erosion is an infrequent but serious complication of gastric banding. It often presents with evidence of a port site infection, but there have been reports of gastric outlet obstruction from an intraluminal band. A high index of suspicion is crucial to avoid a delay in diagnosis. The diagnosis of an erosion mandates the removal of the gastric band. This can be done operatively or endoscopically in select cases.

7. Jejunoileal Bypass (JIB)

The jejunoileal bypass (JIB) was first introduced in the 1950s at the University of Minnesota. It was the first most commonly used procedure for the treatment of severe obesity. The operation consisted of creating a jejunoileostomy and shortening the effective length of the small intestine. Observing patients suffering from short gut syndrome spawned the idea of using jejunoileal bypass in order to lose weight. A short length of proximal jejunum (8 to 14 inches from the ligament of Treitz) was connected to the distal ileum (4 to 12 inches proximal to the ileocecal valve) as an end-to-end or end-to-side anastomosis (see Figure 4). Patients with the end-to-end anastomosis, which could achieve a higher degree of weight loss, also required decompression of the bypassed small intestine into the colon via an ileocecostomy. The diminished length of the functional small bowel exposed to food boluses as well as the diminished surface area for absorption was the key to the JIB. It was indeed successful in its objective of weight loss but it later became apparent that the dramatic weight loss was not the only outcome.

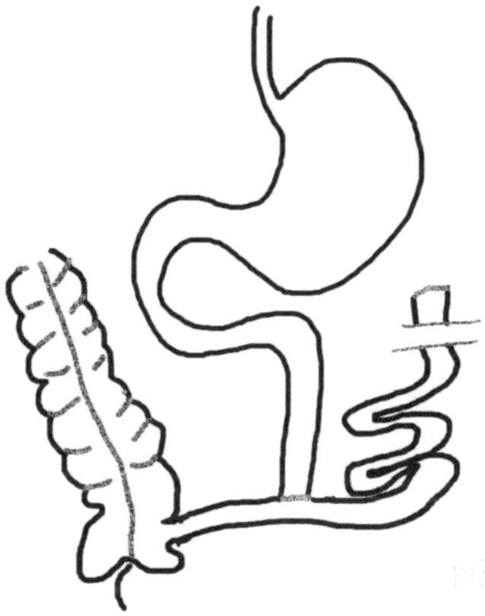

Fig. 4. Jejunoileal Bypass

Approximately 25,000 patients underwent JIB in the United States when it was realized that complications of this procedure were, ultimately, common and would present with significant morbidity and mortality. Complications such as severe diarrhea, electrolyte imbalance, kidney stones, kidney failure, gastro-intestinal tract bacterial overgrowth and liver failure were unexpected problems which ultimately led to the abandonment of this procedure and the reversal of JIB in many patients. Variations of this small bowel bypass were used in the 1960's, but over time these were abandoned as well given inadequate weight loss or unacceptable complication rates. As a result, the JIB is only discussed today for its historical significance. Armed with the knowledge that surgical manipulation of the gastrointestinal (GI) tract could lead to significant and reproducible weight loss, many surgeons embarked on this journey in pursuit of the perfect operation which could produced the desired weight loss with an acceptable complication profile.[17,18,38]

8. Gastric Bypass

The Gastric Bypass (GB) has emerged as the most common operation performed for weight loss in the United States. In fact, it is often referred to as the "gold standard" of bariatric surgery. Its long history of good weight loss with low complication rates have led to this status. The original GB was performed by Mason and Ito in 1967, after they recognized that patients undergoing partial gastrectomy for indications other than weight loss, like peptic ulcer disease, had difficulty gaining weight in the postoperative period.[39] The original version of gastric bypass consisted of a 150-mL gastric pouch and a loop gastrojejunostomy. It has subsequently undergone a number of modifications until it was recognized that a smaller gastric pouch of 20 - 30 mL in conjunction with a Roux-en-Y reconstruction is the most effective combination to achieve maximum weight loss with the lowest rates of amount of complications. The laparoscopic Roux-en-Y gastric bypass (LRYGB) was introduced in 1994 by Wittgrove and Clark.

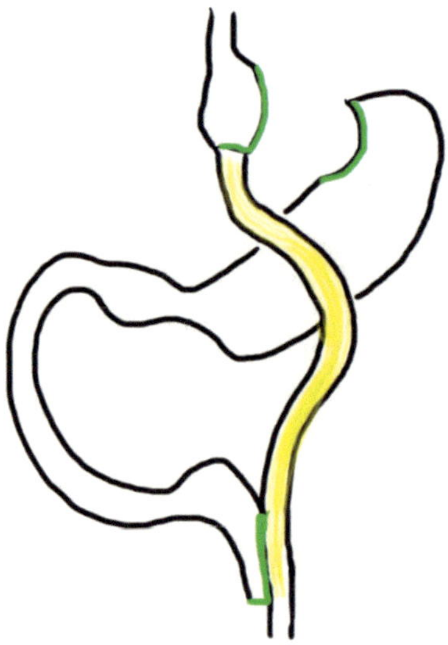

Fig. 5. Gastric Bypass

The operation uses two methods to achieve weight loss. First, the restrictive component of the procedure is created by dividing the stomach to create a smaller gastric pouch. The larger remnant is left in situ. Second, the malabsorptive component is created when the remnant stomach, duodenum, and a short segment of the proximal jejunum is bypassed. Initially the jejunum is divided 30-50 cm distal to the ligament of Treitz. The length of the Roux limb, which consists of the distal transected jejunum, is selected based on the patient's BMI. A 75-100 cm long Roux limb is chosen for a BMI < 50 kg/m^2 and a 150 cm long Roux limb is used for a BMI ≥ 50 kg/m^2. A jejunojejunostomy between the Roux limb and biliopancreatic limb is created in a side-to-side fashion. The Roux limb is brought up to the transected stomach and a gastrojejunostomy is created (see Figure 5).

Several techniques for the creation of the gastrojejunostomy exist. It can be hand sewn or stapled with either a linear stapler or circular stapler. The gastrojejunostomy can be created in a retrogastric or antegastric fashion, while the Roux limb can be passed in an antecolic or retrocolic fashion. The decision for which approach is used ultimately depends on a few factors, but is largely surgeon preference.[17,40,41] There are advantages and disadvantages to each approach and the surgeon should be familiar with these so as to be able to address post-operative complications.

8.1 Weight loss

The overall expectation of the operation is a 60-70% EWL over the course of 12-18 months. During this period of time, close follow-up is essential in order to identify any potential problems which the patient may experience and prevent micronutrient and protein deficiencies.[40]

8.2 Complications

Complications associated with LRYGB are often divided into early and late complications. The most notable early complications after the gastric bypass operation are: bleeding, pulmonary embolism, and anastomotic dehiscence. Pulmonary embolism and anastomotic dehiscence are the two most common reasons for mortality associated with the gastric bypass. The mortality rate varies between reports but generally ranges between 0.5 to 1%.

Bleeding can occur from a number of sites including:

1. Incision/port sites
2. Anastomotic sites (gastrojejunostomy is more common)
3. Gastric pouch or remnant staple line
4. Divided mesentery

The bleeding can be either intra-luminal or extra-luminal. Intraluminal bleeding may present with signs and symptoms of upper or lower GI bleeding such as hematemesis, bright red blood per rectum or melena. Extra-luminal bleeding may only be suspected by clinical findings such as hypotension and tachycardia with a falling hematocrit and decreased urine output. Abdominal distention and abdominal pain are often not reliable physical findings in the morbidly obese patient.

Leakage, likewise, can occur at a number of sites:

1. Gastrojejunostomy
2. Gastric pouch staple line
3. Gastric remnant staple line
4. Jejunojejunostomy

Persistent tachycardia is the hallmark sign for a leak and requires immediate investigation, with a low threshold to return to the operating room. Late complications of the gastric bypass include anastomotic stricture (2-16%). The etiology is unclear, however tissue ischemia or increased tension on the gastrojejunostomy are the most likely reasons. The rate of stenosis is higher when a circular stapler is used for creation of the gastrojejunostomy or when the Roux limb is in an ante-colic position. Marginal ulceration (1-5%), another late complication of RYGB, can develop due to different reasons including re-exposure of the gastrojejunostomy to gastric acid via a gastro-gastric fistula, ischemic changes to the anastomosis most often due to nicotine use, the presence of foreign material (sutures and staples), chronic NSAID use and H. pylori infection.

Iron deficiency (6-52%), vitamin B12 deficiency (3-37%), calcium, thiamine and folate deficiency are the most common micronutrient deficiencies observed in post-bariatric surgery patients. If dietary changes are not maintained, protein malnutrition can result which presents as hair loss. This is reversible if adjustments are made to increase protein intake.

Along with vitamin deficiencies gastric bypass, due to the lack of a pylorus, can result in dumping syndrome. Dumping syndrome occurs in early and late forms. Early dumping syndrome (10 to 30 minutes after ingestion of a meal) is the more common form and occurs in about 25% of patients after gastric surgery. It is characterized by the rapid gastric emptying of hyperosmolar contents into the small bowel. Patients can suffer from abdominal cramps, nausea, explosive diarrhea, tachycardia, lightheadedness and syncope. This is often a self-limited phenomenon and can be treated by dietary modification or manipulation. Late dumping syndrome is usually associated with meals that have high carbohydrate contents. The symptom onset begins from 1 to 4 hours after ingestion of such meals and invariably includes reactive hypoglycemia in addition to some of the vasomotor symptoms seen with early dumping syndrome.

Endoscopic access to the gastric remnant and proximal small bowel becomes challenging and poses potential difficulties in the future, specifically when evaluating for remnant gastric lesions or attempting endoscopic retrograde cholangiopancreatography.[4]

Small bowel obstructions are a standard postoperative risk after any abdominal surgery. They can occur in 1-10% of patients and can be specifically related to trocar sites in laparoscopic surgery. Internal hernias are a special cause of bowel obstructions and have occurred most frequently in the setting of marked weight loss and the creation of inter-mesenteric defects or by failure to close mesenteric defects at the primary operation.

Three potential areas of internal herniation are:

- The mesenteric defect at the jejunojejunostomy
- The space between the transverse mesocolon and Roux-limb mesentery (Peterson's space)
- The defect in the transverse mesocolon if the Roux-limb is passed in a retrocolic fashion

Internal hernias can be intermittent and, therefore, difficult to detect radiographically. Several studies have shown that the "mesenteric swirl" sign on computed tomography (CT) scan is the best indicator of an internal hernia following gastric bypass.[42] Although often debated, closure of all potential sites for internal hernias is highly recommended at the original operation. Long-term follow-up is essential with these patients as complications, such as internal hernias and nutritional deficiencies, can occur at any time. Intimate knowledge of the new anatomy is essential in order to optimally diagnose and treat these potential complications.[43]

9. Biliopancreatic Diversion with Duodenal Switch

The Biliopancreatic Diversion (BPD) was described and championed by Dr. Nicola Scopinaro of Italy in 1979. To date it still remains the most effective surgical intervention for morbid obesity. It is particularly suited for patients who fall in the super-obese category with a BMI greater than $50kg/m^2$. The main limitation has been that which is common to intense malabsorptive procedures: potential significant long-term nutritional deficiencies.

The BPD involves a horizontal gastrectomy that leaves a gastric pouch of about 250 mL that is anastomosed to a 200- to 250-cm Roux limb. The long biliopancreatic limb is anastomosed to this Roux limb at 50 cm from the ileocecal valve to create the common channel (see Figure 6). This results in malabsorptive anatomy with modest restriction and without many of the side effects of the JIB. In 1993 Marceau described modifications to the BPD which have come to be known as the biliopancreatic diversion with duodenal switch (BPD-DS).[10,44-46] In this modification the horizontal gastrectomy was substituted by SG, which allowed for preservation of the pylorus and a decreased incidence of dumping syndrome.

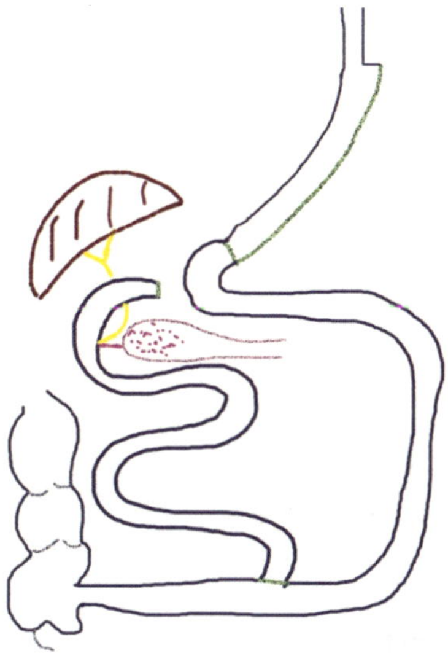

Fig. 6. Biliopancreatic Diversion with Duodenal Switch

Even with the combined restrictive and malabsorptive properties of the gastric bypass, many super-obese patients fail to obtain the desired weight loss. The BPD-DS takes the surgical intensity to another level. It combines a moderate food restriction in the form of a vertical sleeve gastrectomy with the malabsorption of a long intestinal bypass. The sleeve gastrectomy capacity is approximately 100-150 mL. After completion of the sleeve gastrectomy, the pylorus is preserved and the duodenum is transected. The small bowel is then measured and marked 100 cm proximal from the ileocecal valve. This ultimately serves as the site for the anastomosis of a 100 cm common channel. An additional 150 cm of small bowel is measured from the future common channel towards the stomach. The small bowel is then transected at this site. The proximal site of transection is brought up and a duodenoilieal anastomosis is created. The distal small bowel transection site is brought to the 100 cm site and an ileoileal anastomosis performed. Ultimately the alimentary channel is 150 cm and the common channel is 100cm. The remaining small bowel is bypassed.[10,17] Modifications to these measurements are common in clinical practice. The first laparoscopic duodenal switch was performed by Gagner in 2000.

9.1 Weight loss

At 24 months postoperatively the patients can achieve up to 80% EWL with the BPD-DS, and an average of 76% at 10 years. Weight loss certainly exceeds that of the other bariatric procedures but it comes with a greater risk of nutritional complications.

9.2 Complications

Dedicated, long term follow up with nutritional counseling is essential. Patients are educated on the importance of a protein rich, low-carbohydrate diet and the necessity of life-time daily vitamin supplementation which includes iron, calcium, vitamin B12, folate, and a multivitamin. Separate fat soluble vitamin supplementation is also necessary.[44-46]

As with the gastric bypass, other significant complications include bleeding and leaks. Leaks can occur at a number of locations including the gastrectomy site, the anastomosis of the ileum to the duodenum or at the distal Roux-en-Y. These complications require the attention of the knowledgeable and astute physician for diagnosis and management. Internal hernias can also occur if mesenteric defects are not closed or if they reopen after significant weight loss.[47]

10. Laparoscopic Sleeve Gastrectomy with Duodenojejunal Bypass

Laparoscopic Sleeve Gastrectomy with Duodenojejunal Bypass (LSG-DJB) was introduced as a valuable bariatric procedure. The advantage of not having an excluded stomach after SG eliminates the need for technically complicated double-balloon enteroscopy used for surveillance of the excluded stomach after a RYGB. This advantage and the potential significant durable weight loss has made LSG-DJB a very popular surgical intervention in Asia, where the incidence of gastric cancer has been high and obesity is now on the rise.[48] The sleeve gastrectomy is performed, then the first portion of the duodenum is mobilized and subsequently divided with a linear cutting stapler. The biliopancreatic limb is measured to a distance of 150-200 cm and, at this location the small intestine is divided with a linear cutting stapler. A jejunojejunostomy is created, after which the mesenteric defect is closed. A gastrojejunostomy is created in an end-to-side fashion with the distal limb to restore intestinal continuity (see Figure 7). This procedure combines both restrictive and malabsorptive components to achieve weight loss.

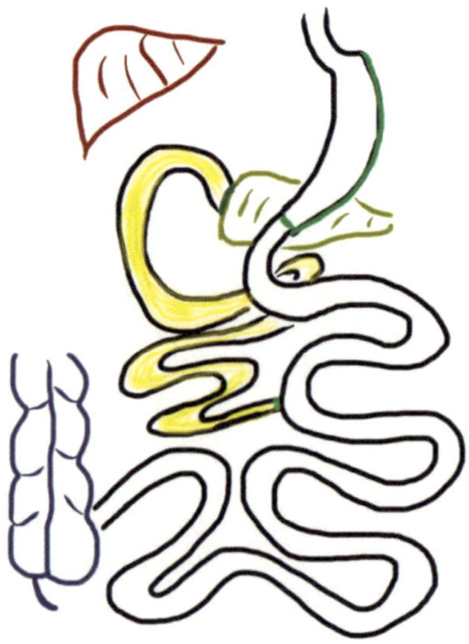

Fig. 7. Laparoscopic Sleeve Gastrectomy with Duodenojejunal Bypass

10.1 Weight loss & complications

Short term EWL after LSG-DJB is comparable to EWL after LRYGB.49 However, long-term data is lacking as this procedure is relatively new. Complications specific for LSG-DJB include bleeding, leak, stenosis at any of the anastomotic sites, marginal ulceration, duodenal stump blowout and dumping syndrome.48

11. Ileal Interposition with Sleeve Gastrectomy

Ileal Interposition with Sleeve Gastrectomy (II-SG) is another operation that has been performed outside of the United States. It was one of many bariatric operations to treat morbid obesity, but also is used in non-obese patients with BMI 21-29 kg/m^2 to treat poorly controlled diabetes. In this case, II-SG is also called the neuroendocrine brake.[50] The sleeve gastrectomy is performed and then the jejunum is divided with a linear stapler 50 cm distal to the ligament of Treitz. The distal ileum is divided 30 cm proximal to the ileocecal valve. Subsequently, the ileum is divided a further 170-200 cm proximally. This segment of ileum is interposed with the proximal jejunum and anastomosed in an isoperistaltic fashion. Then three enteroanastomoses are performed to complete the operation: ileoileostomy, jejunoileostomy, ileojejunostomy (see Figure 8).

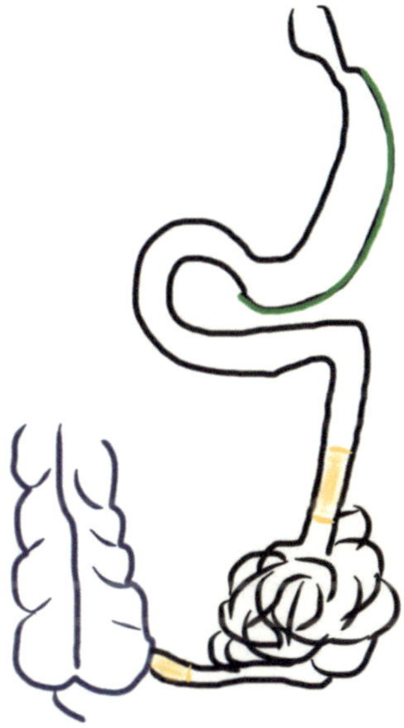

Fig. 8. Ileal Interposition with Sleeve Gastrectomy

11.1 Weight loss & complications

After 5-year follow up, the EWL associated with II-SG is 60%. It is still unclear what percentage of the total weight loss that each part of the operation is responsible for and this requires further investigation. The rate of diabetes remission is reported at 84%.[51] The potential complications of II-SG combine complications of small bowel bypass and SG. The incidence of complications after II-SG is approximately 0.8-2.0% and they include gastric and anastomotic leak, intestinal obstruction, internal hernia, gastric sleeve stricture, GI bleed and nutritional deficiencies.[52]

11.2 Conclusion

Weight loss surgery has been in evolution since the very beginning with the introduction of the JIB. The GB was introduced in the 1960's. Various gastroplasties were in common practice in the 1970s. We returned to the GB in the 1980's given the failure of the gastroplasties. The Scopinaro procedure (BPD) was introduced in the 1979. Modifications of the BPD were introduced in the 1980's. The 1990's brought us the AGBs. The SG became a distinct entity unto itself in the early 21st century and is the newest contender on the field. Finally, we have briefly described two other operations that are not widely used in the U.S. but may become much more common in the future. Not one operation has met all the needs of every patient and as such the search continues for the ultimate operation which will be performed using minimally invasive techniques and produce outstanding and sustainable weight loss with a limited complication profile.

12. References

[1] Ogden CL, Flegal KM, Carroll MD, et al. Prevalence and trends in overweight among US children and adolescents, 1999–2000. JAMA 2002; 288:1728–1732).
[2] Guss SS, Chumlea WC. Tracking of body mass index in children in relation to overweight in adulthood. Am J Clin Nutr. 1999;70(suppl):145S-145S.
[3] National Heart, Lung, and Blood Institute (NHLBI) and National Institute for Diabetes and Digestive and Kidney Diseases (NIDDKD). Clinical guidelines on the identification, evaluation, and treatment of overweight and obesity in adults. The evidence report. Obes Res. 1998;6(suppl 2):51S–210S. Available at: www.nhlbi.nih.gov/guidelines/obesity/ob_gdlns.htm).
[4] Lifestyle, diabetes, and cardiovascular risk factors 10 years after bariatric surgery. Sjöström L, Lindroos AK, Peltonen M, Torgerson J, Bouchard C, Carlsson B, Dahlgren S, Larsson B, Narbro K, Sjöström CD, Sullivan M, Wedel H, Swedish Obese Subjects Study Scientific Group, N Engl J Med. 2004;351(26):2683.
[5] Ten-year trends in health-related quality of life after surgical and conventional treatment for severe obesity: the SOS intervention study. Karlsson J, Taft C, Rydén A, Sjöström L, Sullivan M, Int J Obes (Lond). 2007;31(8):1248.
[6] Swedish obese subjects (SOS)--an intervention study of obesity. Two-year follow-up of health-related quality of life (HRQL) and eating behavior after gastric surgery for severe obesity. Karlsson J, Sjöström L, Sullivan M, Int J Obes Relat Metab Disord. 1998;22(2):113.
[7] Wang Y, Beydoun MA. The obesity epidemic in the United States—gender, age, socioecomomic, racial/ethinic and geographic characteristics: a systematic review and meta-regression analysis. Epidemiol Rev. 2007; 29:6-28
[8] Baskin ML, Ard J, Franklin F, Allison DB. Prevalence of obesity in the United States. Obes Rev.2005 Feb; 6(1):5-6
[9] Korenkov M. Bariatric surgery. Contrib Nephrol. 2006; 151:243-53
[10] NIH Conference: Gastrointestinal surgery for severe obesity: Consensus Development Conference Statement 1991: March 25-27; 9(1)
[11] Bult MJ, van Dalen T, Muller AF. Surgical treatment of obesity. Eur J Endocrinol. 2008Feb; 158(2):135-45
[12] Dixon JB, McPhail T, O'Brien PE. Minimal reporting requirements for weight loss: current methods not ideal. Obese Surg. 2005 Aug; 15(7):1034-9

[13] Oria HE. Reporting Results in Obesity Surgery: Evaluation of a Limited Survey. Obes Surg. 1996 Aug; 6 (4):361-368
[14] Nguyen NT, Ho HS, Palmer LS, Wolfe BM: A comparison study of laparoscopic verses open gastric bypass for morbid obesity. J Am Coll Surg 2000; 191:149-155; discussion 155-157
[15] Nguyen NT, Goldman C, Rosenquist CJ, et al: Laparoscopic versus open gastric bypass: a randomized study of outcomes, quality of life and costs. Ann Surg 2001; 234:279-289; discussion 289-291
[16] Gentileschi P, Kini S, Catarci M, Gagner M: Evidence-based medicine: open and laparoscopic bariatric surgery. Surg Endosc 2002; 16(5):736-744
[17] Buchwald H, Buchwald JN. Evolution of operative procedures for the management of morbid obesity 1950-2000. Obes Surg 2002; 12:705-717
[18] Buchwald H. Overview of bariatric surgery. J Am Coll Surg 2002; 194:367-375
[19] Mason EE. Vertical banded gastroplasty for morbid obesity. Arch Surg 1982; 117:701-706
[20] Sugarman HJ, Starkey JV, Birkenhauer R. A randomized prospective trial of gastric bypass versus vertical banded gastroplasty for morbid obesity and their effects on sweet versus non-sweet eaters. Ann Surg 1987;205:613-624
[21] Van Hout GC, Jakimowicz JJ, Fortuin FA, et al. Weight loss and eating behavior following vertical banded gastroplasty. Obes Surg. 2007 Sep; 17(9):1226-34
[22] Kalfarentzos F, Kechagias I, Soulikia K, et al. Weight loss following vertical banded gastroplasty: intermediate results of a prospective study. Obes Surg. 2001 Jun; 11(3):265-70
[23] Blackburn GL, Hu FB, Harvey AM, Evidence-based recommendations for best practices in weight loss surgery. 2005;13:203.Obes Res
[24] Buchwald H, Avidor Y, Braunwald E, et al. Bariatric surgery: a systematic review and meta-analysis. 2004;292(14):1724.JAMA
[25] Balsiger BM, Poggio, JL, Mai J, et al. Ten and more years after vertical banded gastroplasty as primary operation for morbid obesity. J Gastrointest Surg. 2000 Nov-Dec; 4(6):598-605
[26] Del Amo DA, Diez MM, Guedea ME, et al. Vertical banded gastroplasty: is it a durable operation for morbid obesity? Obes Surg. 2004 Apr; 14(4):536-8
[27] Regan JP, Inabnet WB, Gagner M, et al. Early experience with two-stage laparoscopic Roux-en-Y gastric bypass as an alternative in the super-super obese patient. Obes Surg 2003 Dec; 13(6)861-4
[28] Weight loss, appetite suppression, and changes in fasting and postprandial ghrelin and peptide-YY levels after Roux-en-Y gastric bypass and sleeve gastrectomy: a prospective, double blind study. Karamanakos SN, Vagenas K, Kalfarentzos F, Alexandrides TK Ann Surg. 2008;247(3):401.
[29] Sleeve gastrectomy and gastric banding: effects on plasma ghrelin levels. Langer FB, Reza Hoda MA, Bohdjalian A, Felberbauer FX, Zacherl J, Wenzl E, Schindler K, Luger A, Ludvik B, Prager G. Obes Surg. 2005;15(7):1024).
[30] Arias E, Martinez PR, Ka Ming Li V, Szomstein S, Rosenthal RJ. Mid-term Follow-up after Sleeve Gastrectomy as a Final Approach for Morbid Obesity. Obes Surg. 2009 May; 19(5):544-8
[31] Laparoscopic sleeve gastrectomy as a single-stage procedure for the treatment of morbid obesity and the resulting quality of life, resolution of comorbidities, food tolerance, and 6-year weight loss. Mathieu D`Hondt et al, Surgical Endoscopy (2011) 25:2498-2504, DOI 10.1007/s00464-011-1572-x

[32] Laparoscopic sleeve gastrectomy: surgical technique, indications and clinical results. Braghetto I, Korn O, Valladares H, Gutiérrez L, Csendes A, Debandi A, Castillo J, Rodríguez A, Burgos AM, Brunet L, Obes Surg.,2007;17(11):1442

[33] Laparoscopic sleeve gastrectomy: a multi-purpose bariatric operation. Baltasar A, Serra C, Pérez N, Bou R, Bengochea M, Ferri L, Obes Surg. 2005;15(8):1124

[34] Dixon JB, O'Brien PE. Selecting the optimal patient for the Lap-Band placement. Am J Surg 2002; 184:17S-20S

[35] O'Brien PE, Dixon JB. Weight loss and early and late complications-the international experience. Am J Surg 2002; 184:42S-45S

[36] Kuzmak LI. A review of seven years' experience with silicon gastric banding. Obes Surg 1991; 1:403-408

[37] Belachew M, Legrand MJ, Defechereux TH, et al. Laparoscopic adjustable silicone gastric banding in the treatment of morbid obesity: a preliminary report. Surg Endosc 1994; 8:1354-1356

[38] Buchwald H, Rucker RD. The rise and fall of jejunoileal bypass. In: Nelson RL, Nyhus LM, eds. Surgery of the small intestine. Norwalk, CT: Appleton Century Crofts; 1987; 529-541

[39] Gastric bypass. Mason EE, Ito C, Ann Surg. 1969;170(3):329

[40] Brolin RE, Kenler HA, Gorman JH, et al. Long-limb gastric bypass in the superobese; apropective randomized study. Ann Surg 1992; 215:387-395

[41] Wittgrove AC, Clark GW, Tremblay LJ. Laparoscopic gastric bypass, Roux-en-Y: preliminary report of five cases. Obes Surg 1994; 4:353-357

[42] Sensitivity and specificity of eight CT signs in the preoperative diagnosis of internal mesenteric hernia following Roux-en-Y gastric bypass surgery. Iannuccilli JD, Grand D, Murphy BL, Evangelista P, Roye GD, Mayo-Smith W. Clin Radiol. 2009;64(4):373)

[43] Rogula T, Yenumula PR, Schauer PR. A complication of Roux-en-Y bypass: intestinal obstruction. Surg Endosc 2007 Nov; 21(11):1914-8

[44] Scopinaro N, Gianetta E, Civalleri D, et al. Bilio-pancreatic bypass for obesity: II. Initial experience in man. Br J Surg 1979; 66:618-620

[45] Hess DW, Hess DS. Biliopancreatic diversion with a duodenal switch. Obes Surg, 1998; 8:267-282

[46] Marceau P, Hould FS, Simard S, et al: (1998) Biliopancreatic diversion with duodenal switch. Word J Surg 1998; 947-954

[47] Gagner M. Laparoscopic Bilipancreatic Diversion with Duodenal Switch. In: Inabnet WB, Demaria EJ, Ikrammuddin S, eds. Laparoscopic Bariatric Surgery. Philadelphia, PA: Lippincott Williams & Wilkins; 2005; 133-142

[48] Laparoscopic Sleeve Gastrectomy with Duodenojejunal Bypass: Technique and Preliminary Results. Kazunori Kasama et al, Obes. Surg. 2009. 19:1341-1345

[49] Laparoscopic Sleeve Gastrectomy with Duodenojejunal Bypass: Technique and Preliminary Results. Kazunori Kasama et al, Obes. Surg. 2009. 19:1341-1345.

[50] DePaula AL, Macedo ALV, Rassi N, Machado CA, Schraibman, V, Silva LQ, Halpern H (2008) Laparoscopic treatment of type 2 diabetes mellitus for patients with a body mass index less than 35. Surg Endosc 22:706–16

[51] Systematic review of sleeve gastrectomy as staging and primary bariatric procedure. Brethhauer SA, Hammel JP, Schauer PR, Surg Obes Relat Diseas. 2009;5:469-75

[52] Surgical Treatment of Morbid Obesity: Mid term outcomes of the Laparoscopic Ileal Interposition Associated to a Sleeve Gastrectomy in 120 Patients. Aureo L DePaula et al, Obesity surgery (2011), 21:668-675

2

Effect of Obesity on Circulating Adipokines and Their Expression in Omental Adipose Tissue of Female Bariatric Surgery Patients

John N. Fain
Department of Molecular Sciences,
University of Tennessee Health Science Center, Memphis,
USA

1. Introduction

This chapter is a review of the effects of excessive, formerly known as morbid, obesity on circulating levels and gene expression of adipokines and related factors in the visceral omental adipose tissue of women undergoing bariatric surgery. The current paradigm is that most of the deleterious metabolic effects of excessive obesity are due to Type 2 diabetes and/or hypertension secondary to the mild inflammatory process resulting from visceral adiposity. The visceral adipose tissue, which is primarily omental fat, acts as an endocrine tumor secreting adipokines that result in hypertension and diabetes. These deleterious effects are reversible after bariatric surgery due to a massive reduction in adipose tissue mass.

The circulating levels and gene expression in fat of many adipokines are affected by excessive obesity. However, a major problem is determining which adipokine alterations are causally related and which are secondary effects of the inflammatory state seen in obesity. Many reports have focused on only one adipokine and suggested that it has a causal relationship but at least 40 adipokines have been linked to excessive obesity by one or more investigators. The relative role of each of these adipokines in human obesity is discussed in this review. It should be noted that the term adipokine refers to any factor, including cytokines, whose circulating levels are affected by release from either the fat or nonfat cells of human adipose tissue.

2. The deleterious effects of human obesity are secondary to enhanced accumulation of visceral adipose tissue

The visceral omental fat of women is important because

i. it plays a key role in the pathogenesis of the deleterious metabolic consequences of obesity and
ii. women comprise 80 to 90% of bariatric surgery patients and
iii. most intra-abdominal fat is omental fat. The omentum also has a central role in an inflammatory response that involves macrophages in defending against peritonitis

(Platell et al., 2000). In obesity per se, this macrophage infiltration into the omentum may result in an enhanced inflammatory response that promotes insulin resistance and ultimately diabetes/hypertension and it has been reported that omentectomy in connection with open bariatric surgery resulted in an enhanced insulin sensitivity as compared to patients undergoing open bariatric surgery without omentectomy (Thorne et al., 2002).

Extreme obesity results in increased risk for hypertension and/or diabetes (Cottam et al., 2004, Pories, 2008, Sugerman et al., 2003). The type 2 diabetes is reversible since, after weight loss of approximately 40 kg or more due to bariatric surgery, the diabetes disappears in over 80% of humans (Pories, 2008; Sugerman et al., 2003). Not all extremely obese individuals develop diabetes or hypertension and for these individuals there is no increased risk of morbidity (Livingston & Ko, 2005). However, there is increasing evidence that the accumulation of visceral omental fat is associated with the development of diabetes/hypertension (Despres & Lemieux, 2006). It is recognized that waist circumference is an effective and inexpensive measure of visceral fat accumulation (Scherzer et al., 2008; Shen et al., 2006) and is a better predictor of coronary heart disease than is BMI (Canoy et al., 2007; Despres et al., 2008; Pischon et al, 2008). Waist circumference correlates with visceral fat accumulation as measured by MRI (Scherzer et al., 2008), DEXA (Shen et al., 2006) or fat mass as measured by bioelectrical impedance (Madan et al., 2006).

3. Most release of adipokines is by the nonfat cells in human adipose tissue except for leptin

Originally it was postulated that most of the adipokine release by adipose tissue was due to the fat cells but it is now clear that leptin is the only adipokine released exclusively by the fat cells. In fact, over a 48h incubation, the release of leptin was 1800% of that by the nonfat cells derived from the same amount of human adipose tissue, while that of adiponectin, amyloid proteins 1&2, haptoglobin and NGF was only 64, 144, 75 and 72% respectively of that by nonfat cells (Fain, 2006). Release of MIF and PAI-1 by fat cells was 37 and 23% of that by nonfat cells while that of cathepsin S, HGF, IL-1β, IL-1Ra, IL-6, IL-8, IL-10 MCP-1, TGF-β1, VCAM-1 and VEGF was 12% or less of that by nonfat cells (Fain, 2006). Clearly, the majority of the inflammatory adipokines are released by the nonfat cells of human adipose tissue, which is hardly surprising since per g of fat in obese women two-thirds of the cells are nonfat cells (Fain, et al., 2006) and it is established that obesity is accompanied by macrophage infiltration into human adipose tissue (Weisberg et al., 2003; Xu et al., 2003).

4. Relationship between circulating levels of adipokines and obesity

There is evidence that the circulating levels of many adipokines are elevated in obesity (Fain, 2010). Since the deleterious effects of obesity on diabetes is reversed in over 80% of the patients after bariatric surgery which reduced the BMI from above 45 to 35 or less (Pories, 2008), it is clear that the appropriate criteria for correlating decreases or increases in circulating adipokines is what happens over the range of BMI values from 30 to 70. Another way of assessing effects of obesity is to examine which adipokines show decreases in their circulating levels after bariatric surgery. An additional problem with regard to circulating adipokines is that the circulating levels of some are either at or below the limits of sensitivity for their assay and this is a special problem with regard to TNFα and IL-1β. These adipokines may be very important in the inflammatory response seen in obesity but they primarily act as local autocrine or paracrine mediators of inflammation rather than as circulating hormones.

The effects of obesity and coronary artery disease on circulating levels of 16 adipokines are summarized in Table 1. The coronary artery disease patients were 16 individuals undergoing coronary artery bypass surgery. They had an average BMI of 30.1 and were compared with 12 controls undergoing open heart surgery for other reasons. The controls had a BMI of 27.3 and were younger than the coronary artery disease patients. The data were adjusted for age which eliminated effect of CAD on circulating levels of IL-8 and osteoprotegerin leaving only CD14 and adipsin as adipokines affected by coronary artery disease (Sacks et al., 2011). In contrast, obesity over the BMI range of 38 to 66 [mean was 50], in women undergoing bariatric surgery increased the circulating levels of adipsin, FABP4, and secretory phospholipase A_2 [PLA_2] (Table 1).

Circulating levels are elevated in obesity	**Circulating levels are elevated in CAD**	**Circulating levels are not elevated by excessive obesity or CAD**		
Adipsin	Adipsin	CD-163	IL-8	βNGF
FABP4	CD14	sFLT1	Lipocalin-2	RANTES
IL-1Ra		GPX-3	MCP-1	IL-10
$sPLA_2$		ZAG	Osteoprotegerin	

Table 1. Comparison of effects of obesity versus CAD on circulating levels of 17 adipokines. The effects of severe coronary artery disease (CAD) are taken from the report by (Sacks et al., 2011) while the data for obese women is for the same circulating adipokines with significant positive correlation coefficients [Pearson r of ≥ 0.51] between waist circumference and circulating levels in 12-23 bariatric surgery patients not taking drugs for hypertension with BMI values ranging from 38 to 66 and waist circumference from 107 to 168 cm (Fain, 2011).

Only with IL-1Ra was a significant positive correlation seen between waist circumference and circulating levels as well as mRNA expression in omental fat of severely obese female bariatric patients (Fain, 2011). There was no significant correlation between waist circumference and mRNA level for FABP4, adipsin, & PLA_2 in omental fat (Fain, 2011). Circulating levels of adipsin, FABP4 & PLA2 correlated with waist circumference but not with mRNA levels in omental fat. These data suggest that if mRNA levels in omental fat are equivalent to protein expression, then the circulating levels are not regulated solely by omental fat mRNA expression. It may well be that the source of these adipokines is other fat depots. Alternatively the data could be interpreted as compatible with the hypothesis that protein expression is not equivalent to gene expression.

I have examined the effects of obesity in women on gene expression of almost all the putative adipokines discussed in the next section, except for CRP, which is not released by human fat (Fain, 2006). I found significant positive correlations between waist circumference and mRNA levels in human omental fat for 4 of the 40 proteins: amyloid A [r = 0.57], PAI-1 [r = 0.53], IL-1Ra [r = 0.45] and leptin [r = 0.48] (Fain, 2011). Of these proteins only amyloid A and leptin are preferentially expressed in the fat cells of human omental fat (Fain, 2010).

5. Individual adipokines

The following sections discuss 40 putative adipokines listed in alphabetical order that have been linked to obesity and inflammation. It should be noted that correlations between waist circumference or BMI and circulating levels of any protein indicate only that the protein is a marker molecule rather than the maker of obesity. In view of the many known circulating marker molecules for obesity, caution should be exercised and direct proof demanded before any causal relationship is established. Furthermore, most reports are linked to a particular molecule and the professional careers of the authors are directly linked to their ability to persuade others that the particular marker of interest to them is causally linked to obesity.

5.1 Adiponectin

Adiponectin is a protein that circulates at relatively high levels in humans and is related to the C1q complement factor. Adiponectin, unlike leptin, is not produced solely by fat cells in humans (Fain et al., 2008c). Within 10 years of its discovery adiponectin was accepted as an anti-diabetic, anti-atherosclerotic and anti-inflammatory agent secreted by adipocytes whose low levels in obesity were related to the insulin-resistance in obesity (Trujillo & Scherer, 2005). While the circulating levels of most adipokines are elevated in obesity, this is not the case for adiponectin whose circulating levels negatively correlate with BMI values between 18 and 30, but in males there was no further drop in circulating adiponectin at BMI values above 32 (Arita et al., 1999). Negative effects of obesity on circulating adiponectin have been reported comparing individuals with mean BMI values of 27 versus 35 by Engeli et al., (2003) and by Hoffstedt et al., (2004) comparing humans with BMI values of 24 versus 37. One complexity with regard to circulating levels of adiponectin (Hung et al., 2008) and leptin (Thomas et al., 2000) is that they are both higher in women than in men but the significance of this is not yet understood.

Elevated concentrations of circulating adiponectin have been associated with a lower incidence of type 2 diabetes (Li et al., 2009; Zhu et al., 2010). However, circulating adiponectin is actually positively correlated with all cause mortality as well as cardiovascular mortality in type 2 diabetics (Forsblom et al., 2011). In another study Luc et al., (2010) found no correlation between total circulating adiponectin and cardiovascular disease in men enrolled in the PRIME study. Elevated levels of adiponectin have also been associated with stroke mortality (Nagasawa et al, 2011). Clearly low adiponectin levels in plasma of obese individuals may not necessarily be linked to increased mortality or development of type 2 diabetes and are not consistently seen. I conclude that adiponectin is not produced solely by fat cells and the function of adiponectin remains to be elucidated as well as whether it is causally linked to the development of type 2 diabetes in obesity. It may just be a unique marker of obesity whose levels are sometimes, but not always, lower in obesity.

5.2 Adipsin/complement D

Adipsin is another name for complement factor D that is a novel serine protease whose only known substrate is another complement serine protease known as factor B (Volanakis and Narayan, 1996). Complement factor D was re-discovered and named adipsin since it was found in murine adipocytes and circulating levels were lower in several animal models of obesity (Rosen et al., 1989). However, Napolitano et al., (1994) found that in humans just the opposite was seen in that circulating levels of adipsin positively correlated with the extent of obesity. I found a similar correlation between circulating adipsin and BMI but there was no effect of obesity on the gene expression of adipsin in omental adipose tissue of obese women (Fain, 2011). The complement system is an essential element in our innate defense system and it is possible that the increase in adipsin/complement D seen in human obesity is a reflection of an enhanced inflammatory response to obesity. What accounts for the elevations in circulating adipsin/complement D in obesity is unclear, but it is an obesity marker.

5.3 Amyloid A

The serum amyloid A proteins are major acute-phase reactants released by the liver whose circulating levels increase dramatically in inflammation and obesity (Poitou et al., 2005; 2006; Yang et al., 2006a). Circulating levels of amyloid A (Yang et al., 2006a) as well as gene expression in adipose tissue (Yang et al., 2006a; Fain, 2011) correlated with BMI. In fact of over 100 genes whose expression was correlated in omental adipose tissue with BMI, the highest positive correlation was seen for amyloid A (Fain 2011). A major expression site of Amyloid A is adipose tissue, which is postulated to contribute to circulating levels (Poitou et al., 2005; Sjoholm et al., 2005) and Yang et al (2006a) have suggested that amyloid A is both a proinflammatory and lipolytic adipokine in humans. Whether this is the case remains to be demonstrated but these are intriguing possibilities.

5.4 Angiotensin converting enzyme (ACE)

ACE is a zinc metallopeptidase that cleaves the C-terminal dipeptide from angiotensin I to form Angiotensin II. The presence of the major components of the renin-angiotensin system in human adipose tissue has led to the suggestion that its regulation and function are involved in the hypertension linked to visceral adiposity (Giacchetti et al., 2002). The circulating levels of ACE are unchanged in obesity as is its gene expression in adipose tissue of humans but there is a positive correlation with blood pressure (Gorzelniak et al, 2002). It has been difficult to get evidence for a key role of ACE but recently it was reported that ACE inhibition using captopril treatment of mice on a high fat diet reduced the extent of obesity and the expression of markers of inflammation in murine adipose tissue (Premaratna et al. 2011). Lee at al (2008a) reported that in obese rats, angiotensin receptor blockade reduced insulin resistance by modification of adipose tissue metabolism. Abuissa et al (2005) demonstrated that anti-hypertensive agents such as ACE inhibitors or angiotensin receptor blockers can reduce the onset of diabetes in humans by approximately 25%. However, there is no evidence that circulating levels of ACE are altered in obesity.

5.5 Angiotensinogen

This protein is made in large quantities by the liver and secreted into the circulation where it can be cleaved by renin and/or cathepsin D to form angiotensin I. Karlsson et al (1998) demonstrated that angiotensinogen is also made in adipose tissue and is enriched in adipocytes, which was confirmed by Fain et al., (2008a). The reason for this is still not well understood but it could be a link between obesity and hypertension. Gorzelniak et al (2002) reported that angiotensinogen gene expression in human subcutaneous adipocytes was negatively correlated with the BMI of the adipocyte donors and this may be an adaptive response to reduce angiotensin II formation in obesity. Angiotensinogen gene expression has consistently been reported to be lower in subcutaneous than in omental adipose tissue of humans (Giacchetti et al., 2002, van Harmelen et al., 2000; Fain, 2010) but the significance of this is also unknown. However, this might be linked to the deleterious effects of visceral obesity on the development of hypertension and diabetes in obese humans but the role of angiotensinogen made in fat is unclear.

5.6 Apelin

Apelin is a novel bioactive peptide that is the endogenous ligand of the orphan G protein-coupled receptor AJP (Masri et al., 2005; Castan-Laurell et al., 2011). The circulating levels of apelin and leptin are elevated in obesity but unlike leptin, the gene expression of apelin is found to the same extent in both nonfat and fat cells of human adipose tissue (Boucher et al., 2005; Heinonen et al., 2005). The apelin receptor is expressed on the surface of T lymphocytes and endothelial cells (Masri et al., 2005) and the enhanced levels seen in obesity may reflect release by nonfat cells of fat. A null mutation of the apelin receptor in mice had little effect except for an enhanced vasopressor response to apelin (Ishida et al., 2004). Hung et al (2011) found that inhibitors of the renin-angiotensin system enhanced the secretion of apelin by adipocytes. Fain (2011) found that extremely obese women taking anti-hypertensive agents had decreased expression of apelin in their omental adipose tissue that was accompanied by an enhanced expression of the renin receptor and CD150/SLAMF-1. These data suggest a counter regulatory role of apelin signaling to that of the angiotensin with regard to blood pressure regulation in humans.

5.7 Cathepsin S

Cathepsins are endopeptidase cysteine proteases that are secreted by inflammatory cells. Lafarge et al., (2010) suggested that cathepsin S is one of the most dysregulated genes in adipose tissue of obese subjects since its expression and circulating levels positively correlated with BMI. While in humans there are other cathepsins, it is cathepsin S that is more influenced by obesity (Naour et al., Lafarge et al., 2010). It has been suggested that cathepsin S is the link between obesity and inflammation in obesity (Taleb and Clement, 2007) but all the studies to date are correlative. For example Jobs et al., (2010) found a high correlation between circulating cathepsin S and c-reactive protein [CRP] but what this means is unclear since both are inflammatory response proteins made by the liver. It is perhaps better to describe the elevations in cathepsin S seen in obesity as a response to the inflammation with no proof yet for any type of causal relationship.

5.8 CD14

CD14 is a glycolipid-anchored membrane protein that functions as a receptor for the complex of lipopolysaccharide binding protein plus lipopolysaccharide and is also released into the circulation. In knockout mice lacking CD14 there is less diet-induced obesity and macrophage accumulation in adipose tissue (Cani et al., 2007; Roncon-Albuquerque et al., 2008). CD 14 is a co-receptor with toll-like receptor 4 [TLR4] for activation of macrophages by lipopolysaccharide and by free fatty acids, which Fessler et al (2009) have postulated to be the link between obesity and inflammation. However, there is no evidence that obesity affects the circulating levels of CD 14 (Fain, 2011; Manco et al., 2007) despite the fact that release of CD14 by explants of human omental adipose tissue was enhanced in fat from obese individuals (Fain et al., 2010). I conclude that circulating CD 14 is not an obesity marker.

5.9 C reactive protein [CRP]

CRP is a prototypical acute phase protein released by the liver and its circulating levels can increase by 10,000-fold within hours of infection or injury. Recently CRP has been proposed as a predictive biomarker for cardiovascular disease risk although it has poor predictive value in humans (Levinson et al., 2004). Yudkin et al., (1999) originally reported that obesity is associated with elevated release of IL-6 by human adipose tissue and enhanced circulating levels of IL-6 and CRP. These results have been confirmed by Festa et al., (2001), Hanusch-Enserer et al., (2003) and Maachi et al., (2004). There is virtually no synthesis of CRP by adipose tissue and the small amount of release seen in vitro could be due to release of CRP taken up from the circulation (Fain, 2006). CRP levels in humans correlate with those of serum amyloid (Larsson and Hansson, 2003) suggesting that both are inflammatory markers released by the liver in response to the low-grade inflammation induced by obesity. At least for CRP in mice there is direct evidence that it is not involved in the development of atherosclerosis, clearly indicating that it is a marker not a maker of atherosclerosis (Nilsson, 2005).

5.10 Endothelin-1

Endothelin is a potent vasoconstrictor peptide that is released by endothelial cells. Yudkin (2007) pointed out that obese humans show endothelial dysfunction that may be due to vascular insulin resistance. Takahashi et al., (1990) had earlier reported that circulating levels of endothelin-1 are 3-fold higher in diabetics than in non-diabetic humans. Van Harmelen et al., (2008) reported that the release of endothelin-1 by subcutaneous adipose tissue in vivo was greater in obese individuals and that endothelin blocked the anti-lipolytic action of insulin in omental but not subcutaneous adipocytes. Gogg et al., (2009) subsequently reported that in microvascular endothelial cells isolated from subcutaneous adipose tissue of type 2 diabetics, insulin action was impaired at the level of IRS-1 and the PI 3-kinase pathways. They suggested that enhanced endothelin-1 was responsible for this impairment. These results suggest that studies should be designed to test the hypothesis that impaired insulin action in obesity is secondary to enhanced endothelin-1 release by endothelial cells.

5.11 Fatty acid binding protein 4 [FABP-4]

FABP4 is a member of a family of lipid chaperone proteins that bind with high affinity hydrophobic ligands such as long chain fatty acids (Furuhashi et al., 2008). FABP4 is also known as aP2 and appears to be involved in the movement of fatty acid out of the fat cell during lipolysis (Coe et al., 1999). In the absence of FABP4 there is enhanced accumulation of fatty acids in fat cells (Coe et al., 1999) and reduced expression of inflammatory cytokines in macrophages (Furahashi et al, 2008). Hotamisligil et al., (1996) reported that in FABP4-knockout mice, obesity still developed on a high-fat diet but insulin resistance or diabetes was not seen. These data support the hypothesis that the link between obesity and inflammation in adipose tissue is enhanced lipolysis and free fatty acid release seen in the enlarged fat cells that accumulate in obese animals. In the absence of FABP4 the release of fatty acids by fat cells is impaired which results in reduced lipolysis. In obesity the circulating levels of FABP4 show a positive correlation with BMI (Xu et al., 2007; Terra et al., 2011; Fain, 2011). This suggests that the levels of FABP4 are elevated in obesity ensuring that fatty acid release is enhanced and the TLR4 receptors are activated in the monocytes and neutrophils surrounding the fat cells. This results in inflammatory adipokine release and recruitment of macrophages (Fessler et al., 2009). An alternative hypothesis is that the TLR4 receptors are less important in transmitting free fatty acid effects and that the role of FABP4 in macrophages is to move toxic free fatty acids into the macrophages. Furuhashi et al., (2007) have pointed out that inhibition of this protein with small molecules might be an effective way to prevent the development of diabetes in obesity. However, Lan et al., (2011) reported that such a drug ameliorated dyslipidemia but not the insulin resistance due to diet-induced obesity in mice.

5.12 Glutathione peroxidase 3 [GPX-3]

GPX-3 along with glutathione reductase are enzymes involved in the removal of hydrogen peroxide formed in mitochondria and are thus able to reduce the level of reactive oxygen species in cells (Haddad and Harb, 2005). Circulating levels of GPX-3 are down in patients with coronary atherosclerosis but by only 14% (Dogru-Abbasoglu et al., 1999) and slightly lower in obese humans as well (Lee et al, 2008b). However, negative effects of GPX-3 knockout studies in mice on the development of obesity (Yang et al, 2009) and of obesity in women on circulating levels of GPX-3 (Fain, 2011) suggest that the role of this enzyme in obesity is unclear. In conclusion, the general consensus is that obesity does not result in enhanced circulating levels of GPX-3.

5.13 Haptoglobin

Haptoglobin is an acute phase protein primarily synthesized in the liver of humans that binds hemoglobin (Quaye, 2008). Obesity is associated with elevated circulating levels of haptoglobin (Scriba et al., 1979; Chiellini et al., 2004). In murine in vitro differentiated adipocytes a proteomic approach identified haptoglobin as the most abundant protein secreted by these cells (Kratchmarova et al., 2002). However, in human adipose tissue haptoglobin release in vitro by both the nonfat and the fat cells was 1 to 5% of that for IL-8, IL-6 or adiponectin (Fain et al., 2004b). They concluded that adipose tissue release of haptoglobin probably contributed very little to circulating levels as did Taes et al., (2005). In contrast, Chiellini et al., (2004) concluded that haptoglobin was a novel marker of adiposity and that adipose tissue contributes to circulating levels in humans was important. Unfortunately haptoglobin does not appear to be a novel or unique marker for adiposity but a member of the acute phase response family released by liver whose circulating levels are elevated in mild inflammatory states such as those seen in obesity.

5.14 Interleukin-1β [IL-1β] and IL-1 receptor antagonist [IL-1 Ra]

IL-1β and TNFα are generally thought of as prototypical pro-inflammatory cytokines. Blockade of both pathways, but neither one alone, inhibited the inflammatory response based on IL-8 and IL-6 release by 40 to 50% when explants of human visceral omental adipose tissue are incubated for 48 h (Fain et al., 2005a). In interleukin-1 receptor knockout mice the insulin resistance and adipose tissue inflammation induced by a high fat diet is abolished suggesting a key role for IL-1β in the inflammatory response due to obesity (McGillicuddy et al., 2011). IL-1β is primarily paracrine factor acting locally since circulating levels are below the sensitivity of available assays (Jung et al., 2010). However, IL-1β gene expression in both adipose tissue and liver decreases 6 months after bariatric surgery indicating a reduction in the chronic inflammatory state (Moschen et al., 2011).

In contrast, the circulating levels of IL-1 Ra are elevated in obesity (Fain, 2011; Juge-Aubry et al., 2003: Jung et al., 2010; Meier et al., 2002). Furthermore the gene expression of this protein, unlike that of IL-1β, in omental adipose tissue of humans correlates with waist circumference or BMI of obese women (Fain, 2011). IL-1Ra is a physiological antagonist of IL-1β since it competes with the IL-1 receptors for the available IL-1β and is sold as an injectable drug [anakinra] for the reduction of immune-mediated inflammatory conditions (Goldbach-Mansky, 2009). The elevated circulating levels of IL-1Ra that are seen in obesity as well as enhanced formation in adipose tissue in obesity are perhaps the best evidence that IL-1β formation is enhanced in obesity. Fain (2011) found that the mRNA expression in omental fat of IL-1Ra was the only one showing a positive correlation between waist circumference and mRNA levels in massively obese women taking anti-hypertensive drugs. In contrast, a positive correlation was seen for p67 phox, PAI-1 and 11β HSD1 mRNA expressions only in women not taking anti-hypertensive drugs. What this means is unclear but suggests that unexpected interactions exist between obesity and hypertension with regard to mRNA expression in omental fat.

5.15 Interleukin-6 [IL-6]

IL-6 is a well-established stimulator of acute-phase protein secretion by liver that can produce dramatic increases in circulating CRP, amyloid protein and haptoglobin (Heinrich et al., 1990). Yudkin et al., (2000) postulated that enhanced formation of IL-6 is important in the development of coronary heart disease based on the assumption that IL-6 is the most important mediator of an inflammatory response. It is established that obesity results in elevations in circulating IL-6 (Khaodhiar et al., 2004; Vozarova et al., 2001). While in adipose tissue the IL-6 content positively relates to an enhanced insulin resistance (Bastard et al., 2002) there is evidence that IL-6 is beneficial for insulin action on muscle (Carey and Febbraio, 2004; Kim et al., 2009). Furthermore IL-6 knockout mice develop obesity indicating complexities in IL-6 action in rodents (Wallenius, et al., 2002). Whatever its function, the circulating levels of IL-6 are clearly elevated in obesity.

5.16 Interleukin-8 [IL-8]

IL-8 is the prototypical human chemokine that is involved in the recruitment of circulating neutrophils to its site of release (Reape and Groot, 1999). Circulating levels of IL-8 are elevated in obesity (Bruun et al., 2003; Straczkowski et al., 2002). Release by adipose tissue explants, but not by adipocytes, of women with an average BMI of 42, was elevated as compared to those with a BMI of 32 (Fain et al., 2004a). IL-8 release was primarily by the nonfat cells of adipose tissue and release by omental was greater than that by subcutaneous adipose tissue explants incubated in vitro for 48 h (Bruun et al., 2004). It is possible that IL-8 is more important than any other adipokine in the inflammatory response to obesity especially with regard to recruitment of neutrophils and conversion to macrophages in adipose tissue.

5.17 Interleukin-10 [IL-10]

IL-10 is a cytokine commonly thought to have anti-inflammatory properties whose secretion by macrophages is coordinated with that of pro-inflammatory cytokines in that lipopolysaccharide will increase the release of IL-10 as well as inflammatory cytokines (Mocellin et al., 2003). In vitro studies with human adipose tissue indicated that IL-10 release is predominantly by the nonfat cells such as macrophages and is enhanced in adipose tissue from obese women (Fain, 2010). While adipose tissue macrophages are predominately of the classic-anti-inflammatory M2 phenotype, based on surface markers expression, they secrete higher amounts of pro-inflammatory adipokines such as TNF-α, IL-6, Il-1β and MCP-1 than the M1 macrophages (Zeyda et al., 2007). Esposito et al., (2003) reported that circulating levels of IL-10 were elevated in obesity in women and reduced, along with those of IL-6 and CRP, in obese women without the metabolic syndrome after a significant [11 kg] loss of weight. However, Fain (2011) reported no effect of BMI on circulating levels of IL-10 and Manigrasso et al., (2005) reported that after body weight reduction of 8 kg in android obese women there was no significant change in circulating levels of adiponectin or IL-10 while low adiponectin correlated with low IL-10 levels. Apparently, there is no large or reproducible effect of obesity on circulating levels of IL-10 and whether it is always an anti-inflammatory adipokine is unclear (Mocellin et al., 2003).

5.18 Leptin

Leptin was discovered in 1994 through positional cloning of the mouse *ob* gene (Zhang et al., 1994) and its absence leads to massive obesity in mice and men as well as delayed sexual maturation and immune defects (Dagogo-Jack, 2001; Gautron and Elmquist, 2011). However, few cases of human obesity are due to an absence of leptin since the vast majority of obese humans have elevated levels of leptin that correlate with BMI (Considine et al., 1996). There are sex differences as well since the circulating levels of leptin are higher in women than in men at all BMI values (Smirnoff et al., 2001). Furthermore, similar correlations of circulating values with BMI were soon reported for acute phase proteins such as amyloid and CRP as well as with soluble TNF receptors and PAI (van Dielen et al., 2001). Their report and many others have amply demonstrated that elevated body fat content is associated with a pro-inflammatory state and enhanced circulating levels of leptin. Furthermore, Kshatriya, et al., (2011) recently suggested that leptin might have a pathophysiological role in the development of hypertension and vascular heart disease in obesity.

Whether leptin is a pro-inflammatory hormone in obese humans is unclear but unlike all the known inflammatory factors it is released only by fat cells. The in vitro release of leptin is almost exclusively by fat cells as compared to the nonfat cells derived from human visceral omental adipose tissue while release of LPL is about 80%, amyloid about 60 % and adiponectin about 40% of total release by fat cells plus nonfat cells (Fain, 2010). To date, leptin appears to be the only protein made exclusively by fat cells and its formation apparently reflects fat cell size as reviewed by Fain and Bahouth (2000). In incubated fat cells or adipose tissue explants the greatest stimulation of leptin release is due to glucocorticoids which may be secondary to their anti-inflammatory effect (Fain et al., 2008d) and in vivo administration of glucocorticoids elevated circulating levels of leptin (Dagogo-jack, 2001). However, the link between fat cell size and enhanced leptin release remains to be demonstrated but one theoretical possibility is stretch receptors within fat cells.

5.19 Lipocalin-2

This protein was originally found as a protein secreted by human neutrophils. All lipocalins have an eight-stranded continuously hydrogen-bonded antiparallel β-barrel that can bind and transport a wide variety of small hydrophobic molecules such as fatty acids (Zhang et al., 2008). Based on studies in rodents, Yan et al., (2007) and Wang et al., (2007) concluded that lipocalin-2 was an inflammatory marker released by adipocytes whose release was enhanced by obesity. However, Jun et al., (2011) found no effect of global ablation of lipocalin-2 on obesity-mediated insulin resistance in vivo. In obese humans no statistically significant effect of BMI was found on circulating levels of lipocalin-2 (Stejskal et al., 2008) and this was confirmed by Fain (2011). Furthermore lipocalin-2 was found in and released almost exclusively by the nonfat cells rather than the fat cells isolated from human omental adipose tissue (Fain, 2010). Total lipocalin-2 release by explants of incubated human omental adipose tissue in vitro positively correlated with BMI of the humans from whom fat was obtained as was the case for release of pro-inflammatory adipokines such as IL-8, IL-10, CD14, and RANTES (Fain, 2010). However, the circulating levels of IL-8, IL-10, CD14, and RANTES did not correlate with BMI (Fain, 2011). Lipocalin-2 thus appears to be an inflammatory marker whose circulating levels are not invariably elevated in obesity.

5.20 Lipoprotein lipase [LPL]

This multi-functional enzyme is the rate-limiting enzyme for the hydrolysis of circulating lipids containing triglycerides (Wang and Eckel, 2009). LPL was shown by Rodbell (1964) to be preferentially released by fat cells rather than the non-fat cells of rat adipose tissue. Similar results are seen in human omental adipose tissue and the total release of LPL by adipose tissue correlated with BMI (Fain, 2010). The circulating levels of LPL have been reported to be unrelated to BMI (Kobayashi et al, 2007; Magkos et al., 2009). However, the elevated subcutaneous adipose tissue expression of LPL was reduced to control values in individuals 12 months after bariatric surgery (Pardina et al., 2009). Fain (2010) also found a positive correlation between BMI and the release of LPL by explants of human omental fat incubated in vitro. The available data indicate that LPL protein expression in adipose tissue, but not the circulating levels, correlate positively with obesity.

5.21 Macrophage migration inhibitory factor [MIF]

MIF is a pro-inflammatory cytokine that is involved in many inflammatory disorders (Donn and Ray, 2004; Kleemann and Bucala, 2010). Both MIF and MCP-1 seem to be especially important in macrophage recruitment into adipose tissue. Verschuren et al., (2009) found that in MIF knockout mice the development of obesity with age was not affected but the development of the inflammatory cascade and insulin resistance were markedly reduced. MIF release in vitro by incubated explants of human adipose tissue or adipocytes (Skurk et al., 2005) had a positive correlation coefficient of approximately 0.5 with BMI of the fat donors. Dandona et al., (2004) reported a similar correlation between circulating levels of MIF and BMI. Church et al., (2005) reported that a weight loss of approximately 14 kg over 8.5 months resulted in a 40% decrease in circulating levels of MIF. MIF appears to be an obesity-linked inflammatory factor whose circulating levels are elevated in obesity.

5.22 Monocyte chemoattractant protein 1 [MCP-1]

MCP-1 is also known as chemokine CCL2 and is a mononuclear cell chemoattractant protein that is a pro-inflammatory adipokine (Frangogiannis, 2004). Circulating levels of MCP-1 have been reported to be elevated in obese humans (Malavazos et al., 2005) and to have a positive correlation with BMI (Christiansen et al., 2005). However, neither Miller et al., (2002) or Fain (2011) found any effect of obesity on circulating levels of MCP-1. Madani et al., (2009) reported that MCP-1 and IL-6, but not RANTES, were released in vivo by human abdominal subcutaneous adipose tissue to a far greater extent in individuals with a BMI of 43 as compared to controls with a BMI of 25. Dahlman et al (2005) found that obesity increased the mRNA level of MCP-1 in human subcutaneous adipose tissue by 2.6-fold. The in vitro release of MCP-1 by adipose tissue explants was also increased by 6 to 10-fold without any change in the in vivo release. These data indicate that while obesity enhances MCP-1 release by adipose tissue there appears to be little contribution of adipose tissue to its circulating levels.

5.23 Nesfatin-1

This novel anorexigenic peptide is processed from nucleobindin-2 and released by adipose tissue (Ramanjaneya et al., 2010). While they reported a positive correlation of 0.63 between circulating levels of nesfatin-1 and BMI, the opposite was reported by Tsuchiya et al., (2010). However, Tan et al., (2011) found a positive correlation of 0.83 between the circulating nesfatin-1 and BMI, in 38 subjects [20 were women] with BMI values ranging from 16 to 38. It is unlikely that nesfatin-1 is derived from nucleobindin-2 gene expression solely in fat cells as is the case with leptin. I [unpublished studies] have found that the ratio of nucleobindin-2 gene expression in fat as compared to nonfat cells derived from human omental adipose tissue was 0.44 while that for leptin was 28. Furthermore, nucleobindin-2 is a ubiquitous Ca^{2+} binding protein that may participate in Ca^{2+} storage in the Golgi as well as in other biological processes involving DNA-binding and protein-protein interactions (de Alba and Tjandra, 2004). There is also evidence that it associates with cyclooxygenase-2 in human neutrophils (Leclerc et al., 2008). It is strange that nesfatin-1 is derived from a precursor protein with so many functions. However, it is possible that nesfatin-1 is formed in fat cells from nucleobindin-2. This hypothesis remains to be tested and at the moment the relationship of nesfatin-1 to fat cell metabolism is unclear and it also remains to be proven that nesfatin-1 is formed and released by fat cells much less that it functions physiologically as an anorexigenic peptide.

5.24 Omentin/intelectin

Omentin has been described as a novel adipokine secreted by omental adipose tissue (Schaffler et al., 2005; Yang et al., 2006b; Tan et al., 2008) but it is actually a lectin that binds to the galactofuranose moiety in the carbohydrate chains of bacterial cell walls (Tsuji et al., 2001). Omentin/intelectin is involved in mucosal defense mechanisms in the small intestinal brush border (Wrackmeyer et al., 2006). Fain et al., (2008b) found that omentin/intelectin gene expression was almost exclusively in the nonfat cells of omental fat and its expression in epicardial fat was 100-fold higher than that in subcutaneous fat. This is what is expected if omentin is made in endothelial cells of blood vessels derived from mesothelial cells of the sphlanchopleuric mesoderm of the gut. Thus it is hardly surprising that circulating levels of omentin/intelectin are negatively correlated with the extent of carotid intima-media thickness (Shibata et al., 2011) since they are probably derived from the endothelial cells of the blood vessels. Female subjects have higher circulating levels of omentin than male subjects and those levels correlate with the circulating levels of adiponectin, both being negatively associated with insulin resistance (Yan et al., 2011). These findings confirm the original report by de Souza Batista et al., (2007) that circulating levels of omentin/intelectin are negatively correlated with BMI and insulin resistance. I conclude that omentin/intelectin is not really an adipokine but a circulating factor derived from the endothelial cells of all the blood vessels in the abdominal cavity. It appears to be a marker of endothelial cells rather than of fat cells.

5.25 Orsomucoid/α1 acid glycoprotein

Orsomucoid is also known as α1 acid glycoprotein and is one of the most abundant plasma proteins (Lee et al., 2010). It is an acute phase protein secreted by the liver in response to stress and inflammation. In mice, it is also induced in the adipose tissue in obesity and its formation is not further enhanced by inflammatory stimuli or reduced in the diabetic state (Lin et al., 2001; Lee et al., 2010). It is clearly not an inflammatory adipokine since in human omental adipose tissue incubated in primary culture, its gene expression is markedly enhanced by dexamethasone which inhibited expression of inflammatory adipokines (Fain et al., 2010b). In humans, circulating levels of orsomucoid are not lower in diabetic subjects and show a weak positive correlation with BMI as expected of an inflammatory response protein (Akbay et al., 2004; Maachi et al., 2004). Orsomucoid appears to be a unique inflammatory response protein whose circulating levels poorly respond to the degree of obesity or diabetes in humans.

5.26 Osteoprotegerin [OPG]

OPG is a secreted glycoprotein of the TNF receptor family that is released by many cells including those in atherosclerotic plaque lesions in response to inflammatory stimuli (Venuraju et al., 2010). There is evidence in humans for a positive relationship between circulating levels of OPG and the severity of atherosclerosis (Venuraju et al., 2010). However, circulating levels of OPG increase with age (Gannage-Yared et al., 2008; Sacks et al., 2011) and after correcting for age there was no effect of severe coronary artery disease on circulating levels of OPG (Sacks et al., 2011). Obesity effects on circulating OPG have been contradictory to say the least. Gannage-Yared et al., (2008) and Fain (2011) reported no change while Holecki et al., (2007) and Ashley et al., (2011) reported decreases in obesity. Venuraju et al., (2010) concluded that there is no consensus on the relationship between BMI or other cardiovascular risk factors and the circulating levels of OPG much less the function of this protein in humans.

5.27 Plasminogen activator inhibitor protein-1 [PAI-1]

PAI-1 is also known as serpin E1 and is a member of the serpin family of serine protease inhibitors. PAI-1 is the predominant inhibitor of the fibrinolytic system (Alessi et al., 2007). The release of PAI-1 by visceral adipose tissue is primarily by nonfat cells such as macrophages and greater than that by subcutaneous human fat (Bastelica et al., 2002; Fain et al., 2004a). Total release by human fat in vitro correlates with BMI (Fain, 2010) and the gene expression of PAI-1 in visceral omental fat of obese women correlated to a greater extent with BMI than that of inflammatory adipokines such as TNFα, MCP-1, IL-1β, IL-6, IL-8 or MIF (Fain, 2011). Alessi et al., (2007) have reviewed the evidence that circulating PAI-1 levels are enhanced in obesity and are primarily produced by macrophages in adipose tissue. While Lindeman et al., (2004) confirmed the high correlation between visceral fat and circulating PAI-1, their in vivo measurements of release from visceral fat were negative. They concluded that the relationship between PAI-levels and visceral fat is as co-correlates rather than a causal relationship.

5.28 Secretory type II phospholipase A_2 [PLA_2]

PLA_2 is an acute phase protein that is able to degrade phospholipids present in lipoproteins and cell membranes thus releasing inflammatory molecules (Rosenson and Gelb, 2009). It is reported to be, like CRP, an independent risk factor for coronary heart disease (Kugiyama et al., 1999). Circulating levels of PLA_2 are higher in women than in men and reported to be positively correlated with waist circumference in obese women (Rana et al., 2011; Weyer et al., 2002; Fain, 2011). It has been claimed that PLA_2 is secreted by epicardial adipose tissue and over expressed in humans with coronary artery disease (Dutour et al., 2010) but Sacks et al., (2011) failed to see elevations in circulating PLA_2 in humans with severe coronary artery disease or any difference in its gene expression in epicardial, sternal or substernal fat of controls as compared to those with coronary artery disease. I conclude that PLA_2 is primarily an obesity marker.

5.29 Regulated on activation, normal T cell expressed and secreted [RANTES]

In obese mice, both the levels of mRNA in fat and protein secretion of RANTES are enhanced by obesity that is accompanied by increased accumulation in adipose tissue of T cells as well as macrophages (Wu et al., 2007). Maury et al., (2007) reported that RANTES was released in greater amounts by fat cells isolated from the omental adipose tissue of obese humans but Fain et al., (2010a) found no effects of obesity on the total release of RANTES by explants of human adipose tissue in primary culture. Furthermore, Madani et al., (2009) found no effect of obesity on in vivo release of RANTES by human subcutaneous adipose tissue under conditions where increases in IL-6 and MCP-1 could be readily detected. Madani et al., (2009) also observed that circulating levels of RANTES were far higher than could be accounted for release by adipose tissue. They concluded that it is more likely that RANTES acts on adipose tissue.

5.30 Renin receptor protein

This is an intracellular protein that is expressed in the nonfat cells of human adipose tissue. It may increase angiotensin I generation from angiotensinogen by enhancing the uptake of circulating renin thus enhancing the activity of the renin-angiotensin system in visceral adipose tissue (Engeli et al., 1999; Achard et al., 2007). In severely obese (BMI of 49) non-diabetic women taking anti-hypertensive agents the gene expression in omental adipose tissue of the renin receptor was increased by 60% while that of ACE and angiotensinogen was unaffected (Fain, 2011). Fowler et al., (2009) have shown in rodents that adipose tissue may control its own local renin concentration independent of plasma renin. These data suggest that the renin receptor protein is important in local regulation of angiotensin II formation in adipose tissue. This is a promising area for future studies and suggests that the regulation of the renin-angiotensin system in adipose tissue is both more important and more complex than originally envisioned.

5.31 Resistin

Steppan et al., (2001) based on studies in rodents, postulated that resistin was secreted by fat cells and was the missing link between obesity and diabetes. However, studies in human adipose tissue have shown that resistin is neither released by fat cells (Fain et al., 2003) nor are detectable amounts of resistin mRNA expressed in human fat cells (Nagaev and Smith, 2001; Savage et al., 2001; Janke et al., 2002; Fain, 2010). It is now accepted that resistin is produced largely by macrophages (Lehrke et al., 2004) and not linked to markers for insulin resistance or adiposity (Hasegawa et al., 2005). The consensus is that circulating resistin is not derived from adipose tissue but is involved in inflammation under some conditions. Clearly in humans, resistin is not an important factor released by fat cells that links insulin resistance and obesity.

5.32 Retinol binding protein 4 [RBP-4]

This protein is a member of the lipocalin family of molecules that bind small hydrophobic molecules such as retinol and is expressed at high levels in liver as well as adipose tissue (Kotnik et al., 2011). Like leptin, but unlike most putative adipokines, it is expressed exclusively in the fat cells of human adipose tissue (Fain, 2010). The laboratory of Barbara Kahn suggested that RBP-4 is causally related to insulin resistance in obesity and type 2 diabetes (Yang et al., 2005; Graham et al., 2006). However, Kotnik et al., (2011) suggested that the evidence for an association between obesity and circulating as well as adipose tissue levels of RBP4 is not a consistent finding in clinical studies. Some of these differences could be due to confounding factors such as procedures for collection of blood and the antibodies used for the assays as well as sex differences, age, retinol status, iron status and kidney function which have all been shown to affect circulating levels of RBP4. Most probably, as suggested by Yao-Borengasser et al., (2007), RBP-4 gene expression in human fat correlates with inflammation rather than insulin resistance and the great hope that this would be a link between obesity and insulin resistance is still just a great hope.

5.33 Thrombospondin-1 [TSP1]

TSP1 is an inhibitor of angiogenesis that is able to activate the latent TGFβ1 complex and interact with CD36 on endothelial cells leading to apoptosis (Bornstein, 2009). Varma et al., (2008) postulated that TSP-1 is an adipokine associated with obesity, inflammation and insulin resistance. While they workers reported that its gene expression in fat cells was 4-fold that of nonfat cells, Fain (2010) found only a non-significant 1.8-fold increase in fat cells over that in nonfat cells of omental adipose tissue. Bornstein (2009) pointed out that TSP-1 is synthesized and secreted by a wide variety of cells in culture including endothelial cells, fibroblasts and smooth muscle cells. Clearly TSP-1 is not an adipokine in the sense of being a protein preferentially expressed in fat cells but is rather found in all cells examined to date. The major function of TSP-1 is to regulate angiogenesis and knockout mice have an increased density of capillaries in cardiac and skeletal muscle. Endothelial-derived TSP-1 has also been claimed to promote macrophage recruitment (Kirsch et al., 2010). Varma et al., (2008) reported a small but positive correlation between gene expression of TSP-1 in adipose tissue and BMI with no effect of prior metformin administration. However, Tan et al., (2009) found that 6-months treatment with metformin of women with PCOS elevated the low circulating levels of TSP-1. The available evidence does not support the claim that TSP-1 is an adipokine released by fat cells that has any causal relationship to obesity and insulin resistance.

5.34 TGF-β1

TGF-β1 is now accepted to be multifunctional regulator of the immune and inflammatory processes and works through regulating the activity of Smad proteins (Shi and Massague, 2003). Smad-3 deficient mice are protected from diet-induced obesity and diabetes and the adipocytes had marked increases in mitochondrial biogenesis and respiration accompanied by increased PGC-1α mRNA (Yadav et al., (2011). There is other evidence for perturbation of mitochondrial function, specifically reactive oxygen species formation, due to TGF-β1 since it enhanced mitochondrial reactive oxygen species formation in rodent hepatocytes (Albright et al., 2003) while preventing cell death due to caspase activation in synovial cells (Kawakami et al., 2004).

In obese hypertensive humans, circulating levels of TGF-β1 correlated with BMI (Scaglione et al., 2003) but not in a study where only 10% of the humans were hypertensive (Bastelica et al., 2002). In another study comparing circulating TGF-β1 in women with an average BMI of 32 against lean controls with a BMI of 21, the values were actually higher in the lean controls (Corica et al., 1997). However, both protein and gene expression (Alessi et al., 2000) of TGF-β1 in human adipose tissue positively correlates with BMI as does release of TGFβ1 by human adipose tissue in primary culture (Fain et al., 2005b). The formation and release of TGFβ1 by human adipose tissue is almost exclusively by the nonfat cells and is not inhibited by dexamethasone, as is the case for release of inflammatory adipokines such as the interleukins and IL-1Ra (Fain et al., 2005b; Fain et al., 2010b). While circulating levels of TGFβ1 do not appear to be elevated in obesity, one caveat is that what is measured is actually the latent form of TGFβ1. This accounts for most of the circulating TGFβ1 and obesity could affect conversion to the active form with a much shorter half-life (Flaumenhaft et al., 1993). I conclude that TGFβ1 is formed by the nonfat cells in human adipose tissue and acts as a local paracrine/autocrine factor that is required for the development of obesity and insulin resistance. However, this does not necessarily mean that it plays a causal role since it is a multifunctional regulator of cellular metabolism. The recent findings of Yadav et al., (2011) suggest that the inhibition of TGFβ1 release and/or action might have favorable effects on the development of insulin resistance in obesity by uncoupling respiration in white fat thus preventing fatty acid accumulation.

5.35 Tumor necrosis factor α [TNFα]

Hotamisligil et al., (1993) found elevated levels of TNFα and its gene expression in several rodent models of obesity and diabetes and neutralization of TNFα significantly reduced insulin resistance. In humans, Hotamisligil et al., (1995) found that obesity greatly enhanced TNFα release by adipose tissue explants and its gene expression in adipose tissue correlated with both BMI and circulating levels of insulin, which is a marker for insulin resistance. Fain et al., (2004c) confirmed that the release of TNFα by both explants of human adipose tissue and adipocytes positively correlates with the BMI of the fat donors but the release of TNFα is primarily by the non-fat cells. In obesity there is increased accumulation of macrophages in adipose tissue and these cells release massive amounts of cytokines such as TNFα (Xu et al., 2003; Weisberg et al., 2003). However, Kern et al., (1995) and Fain et al., (2004c) found that TNFα is also released by nonfat cells other than macrophages in human adipose tissue. There is a reproducible correlation between BMI and TNFα release by human adipose tissue explants (Fain et al., 2004c; Arner et al., 2010) or adipocytes (Fain et al., 2004c). However, this has not been seen in all studies with respect to TNFα gene expression in adipose tissue and BMI (Kern et al., 1995; Koistinen et al., 2000).

It has been difficult to obtain evidence in humans by blocking TNFα action in vivo with etanercept that this improves insulin sensitivity (Lo et al., 2007). However, Fain et al., (2005a) found that blocking endogenous TNFα action on incubated human fat explants using etanercept had little effect on the release of IL-6 or IL-8. However, in combination with an antibody that blocked the action of endogenous IL-1β there was a 55 to 60% decrease in the release of IL-6 and IL-8. There is little evidence that TNFα circulates as an adipokine. Rather it acts as an autocrine/paracrine factor since circulating levels are generally below the sensitivity of available assays. There is no evidence for its release in vivo into the circulation under conditions where release of IL-6 could be detected (Mohamed-Ali et al., 1997). I conclude that TNFα is an important component of the inflammatory response acting as an autocrine/paracrine adipokine along with IL-1β to activate the inflammatory cascade in adipose tissue in all cells resulting in enhanced release of pro-inflammatory adipokines such as IL-6 and IL-8. It will be important to understand how human adipocytes even after isolation from the adipose tissue environment and washed several times still show rates of TNFα release that reflect the BMI of the person from whom the adipocytes were obtained. The simplest explanation is that this reflects the average fat cell size as shown by Arner et al., (2010) and that 'stretch receptors' are involved that stimulate TNFα and leptin release.

5.36 Tumor necrosis factor receptor 2 [TNFR2]

The actual receptor for TNFα is TNFR1 but there is also a second soluble form of the receptor known as TNFR2 that can be cleaved from the TNFR1 or expressed directly and its expression in adipose tissue is markedly enhanced in obesity (Hotamisligil et al., 1997). Similar increases in circulating TNFR2 but not TNFR1 have been seen in obese humans (Fernandez-Real et al., 1998). These data suggest that increased formation of the TNFR2 is part of a feedback system designed to reduce the effects of TNFα since the soluble TNFR2 protein binds to and thus reduces the level of active TNFα.

5.37 Vascular endothelial growth factor A [VEGF] and VEGFR1 & 2

There is evidence that VEGF is involved in angiogenesis in adipose tissue which is a highly vascularized tissue (Cao, 2010) and that adipose tissue mass can be regulated through the vasculature (Rupnick et al., 2002). In overweight/obese humans, there is an inverse correlation between obesity and pO_2, temperature, capillaries per 1000 μm^2 and VEGF gene expression suggesting that the reduced pO_2 did not result in VEGF release and neovascularization (Pasarica et al., 2009). Kabon et al., (2004) had previously reported that obesity decreased adipose tissue oxygenation in humans. Thus the question is why in obesity the reduced pO_2 in the expanding fat mass does not result in release of VEGF and growth of more blood vessels to enhance pO_2. But obesity in humans does enhance the circulating levels of VEGF and the best correlation [Pearson r of 0.49] was seen with visceral fat mass (Miyazawa-Hoshimoto et al., 2003). Cao (2010) has suggested that adipose tissue angiogenesis is a good therapeutic target for the treatment of obesity. However, we know so little about what regulates the growth of adipocytes and the endothelial cells of the blood vessels that we are literally groping in the dark. One way to regulate the activity of VEGF is through the formation and release of the soluble form of the VEGFR-1 receptor, known as sFlt-1, which competes with the VEGFR1 and VEGFR2 receptors for binding of VEGF. Obesity in rodents and man is associated with reduced mRNA content as well as release of sFlt1 while in isolated human adipocytes hypoxia enhances the expression of VEGF but not of sFlt1 (Herse et al., 2011).

5.38 Vaspin

This protein was originally described as a serine protease inhibitor derived from visceral adipose tissue (Hida et al., 2005) but Kloting et al., (2006) reported that it was present to the same extent in visceral as in subcutaneous adipose tissue of humans. It is not found in fat cells of human visceral omental adipose tissue but is found in the nonfat cells (Fain, 2010). Circulating levels of vaspin are not elevated in massively obese women (Auguet et al., 2011). Similarly a 10-month lifestyle intervention program led to a favorable change in metabolic parameters and circulating adiponectin but not vaspin (Kim et al., 2011). I conclude that vaspin is probably not an adipokine but rather a member of the serpin protease family with unknown functions whose circulating levels are not appreciably altered in obesity.

5.39 Visfatin/PBEF/Nampt

This putative adipokine was originally described as a protein selectively expressed in visceral fat with insulin-mimetic properties whose circulating levels are elevated in obesity (Fukuhara et al., 2005). However, this protein turned out to be identical to PBEF [pre-B-colony-enhancing factor] and Nampt [nicotinamide phosphoribosyltransferase]. Furthermore, the claim that visfatin was an insulin-like peptide has been withdrawn (Sommer et al., 2008) and its gene expression in human visceral fat is no higher than in subcutaneous fat (Berndt et al., 2005; Fain, 2010). Circulating concentrations of visfatin as measured by an ELISA specific for full-length visfatin are not elevated in obesity (Retnakaran et al., 2008; Korner et al., 2007). Visfatin gene expression is primarily in the nonfat cells of human adipose tissue (Fain et al., 2010a) and it is unclear at this time whether it is more than an intracellular enzyme involved in NAD biosynthesis in all fat depots not just visceral adipose tissue.

5.40 Zinc $\alpha 2$ glycoprotein [ZAG]

This protein has been postulated to be an adipokine modulator of body fat mass (Bing et al., 2010). However, ZAG is a novel adhesive protein (Takagaki et al., 1994) secreted by epithelial cells, sweat glands and many tumors that is found in high concentrations in seminal plasma

(Bing et al., 2010). ZAG is identical to a lipid mobilizing factor isolated from the urine of humans with cancer cachexia that causes selective loss of fat in rodents but there is no evidence that ZAG either enhances lipid mobilization or lipid utilization in humans (Bing et al., 2010). ZAG has been postulated to be a candidate gene for obesity, but like adiponectin and unlike most adipokines, its gene expression in adipose tissue is lower in obese than in lean humans (Bing et al., 2010). There is also an inverse relationship between circulating levels of ZAG in humans and insulin resistance but no effect of BMI on circulating levels of ZAG (Ceperuelo-Mallafre et al., 2009). However, Selva et al., (2009) reported just the opposite results, with obesity lowering both circulating levels and gene expression of ZAG in adipose tissue but no correlation was observed between ZAG levels and insulin resistance. ZAG, like adiponectin, is preferentially expressed in the fat cells of human omental adipose tissue where it is expressed at higher levels than in subcutaneous adipose tissue (Fain, 2010). While the available data are conflicting with regard to circulating levels of ZAG, there is consensus that gene expression of ZAG in adipose tissue correlates with that of adiponectin (Mracek et al., 2010) and that weight loss reduces insulin resistance in humans while enhancing gene expression of ZAG in adipose tissue. However, what we have are correlations and there is no consistent relationship between circulating levels of ZAG and obesity.

6. Summary of adipokines most likely linked in a causal way to morbid obesity

Of the 40 adipokines mentioned in the previous sections, the circulating levels of only adiponectin and ZAG appear to be reduced under some conditions by obesity. The circulating levels of 14 of the remaining 38 putative adipokines are elevated in obesity, and of these only leptin appears to be released exclusively by the fat cells of human adipose tissue as shown in Table 2.

Circulating adipokines released only by fat cells	Circulating adipokines released by fat cells and non fat cells	Circulating adipokines released primarily by non fat cells	Circulating factors released primarily by liver
Leptin	Amyloid A	Adipsin	Cathepsin S
	FABP4	Apelin	CRP
	VEGF	IL-6 & IL-8	Haptoglobin
		MIF	
		PAI-1	
		IL-1Ra	
		$sPLA_2$	

Table 2. Circulating adipokines whose release is reproducibly elevated in obesity over BMI values from 25 to 70

While amyloid A, FABP4 and VEGF levels are elevated in obesity there is no proof that their circulating levels are derived primarily from adipose tissue release. Furthermore, there is ample evidence that both the fat cells and the nonfat cells of adipose tissue release all three and with amyloid A, the liver makes and releases large amount of this acute phase protein. I refer to amyloid A as an adipokine because it is formed and released by adipose tissue in appreciable amounts in contrast to CRP where the release by adipose tissue is too small to contribute to circulating levels. Except for leptin, there is no evidence that the circulating levels of the other putative adipokines are derived exclusively from adipose tissue or even that release by adipose tissue regulates their circulating levels. Probably the circulating levels of adipsin, apelin and IL-6 are influenced primarily by release by lymphoid tissues but in any case it is unlikely that release by adipose tissue is derived from fat cells. Finally, we have acute phase proteins such as CRP and haptoglobin whose circulating levels are elevated in obesity along with that of cathepsin S and are released primarily by liver in response to circulating inflammatory factors such as IL-6.

Interestingly in female bariatric surgery patients, the mRNA levels in omental adipose tissue positively correlated with visceral obesity as measured by waist circumference for only four of the 12 adipokines whose circulating levels are consistently elevated in obesity as shown in Table 3. Furthermore, except for IL-1Ra, the increased mRNA expression in omental adipose tissue in obese women was abolished in those taking anti-hypertensive drugs (Fain, 2011). It is unclear why only IL-1Ra mRNA expression correlate with waist circumference but not that for MIF, IL-8 and IL-6. This suggests that hypertension in obese women has profound effects upon mRNA levels and abolishes the effect of obesity. The increase in leptin is expected and so far it is the only adipokine released solely by fat cells whose circulating levels are elevated in obesity. The elevated mRNA levels in visceral omental adipose tissue and circulating levels of both PAI-1 and Amyloid A suggest that these proteins may have a special role in visceral obesity.

Positive correlations for these adipokines with severe obesity in women and

mRNA levels in Omental fat	**Circulating levels**		
Amyloid A	Amyloid A	Adipsin	IL-8
IL-1Ra	IL-1Ra	Apelin	MIF
Leptin	Leptin	FABP4	$sPLA_2$
PAI-1	PAI-1	IL-6	VEGF

Table 3. Comparison of effects of severe obesity in women based on gene expression in visceral omental adipose tissue as compared to effects on circulating levels. The data on mRNA levels are from Fain (2011) and on circulating levels the data reviewed in sections 5.1 to 5.40 of this chapter.

The division between primary signals, pro- and anti-inflammatory molecules, secondary response molecules and unlikely adipokines is outlined in Table 4. The levels of secondary response molecules are elevated in obesity but are probably not regulated by release from adipose tissue. In contrast unlikely adipokines are those proteins whose circulating levels are not appreciably altered in obesity and are derived from sources other than adipose tissue in humans. The primary response signal in obesity is probably related to the expansion of the fat cells, which results in enhanced release of both fatty acids and leptin. Either or both of these signals could act as autocrine/paracrine factors to enhance the release of inflammatory mediators by both the fat and nonfat cells of visceral omental adipose tissue. This is accompanied by decreased release of adiponectin and enhanced release of IL-1Ra, IL-10 and TNF-R2 that act as anti-inflammatory mediators to reduce inflammation. The inflammatory response is associated with enhanced formation of the so-called secondary response molecules whose role in promoting insulin resistance is unclear while apelin is linked in some way to the renin-angiotensin system and hypertension.

Primary signals	Pro-inflammatory mediators	Anti-inflammatory mediators	Secondary response molecules	Unlikely adipokines in humans		
Fatty acids	IL-1β	Adiponectin	Adipsin	Cathepsin S	Nesfatin	RBP-4
Leptin	IL-6	IL-1Ra	Amyloid A	CD14	Omentin	TSP-1
	IL-8	IL-10	Apelin	CRP	Orsomucoid	Vaspin
	MCP-1	TNF-R2	FABP4	Endothelin-1	OPG	Visfatin
	MIF		PAI-1	Haptoglobin	RANTES	ZAG
	TNFα		$sPLA_2$	Lipocalin-2	Resistin	

Table 4. Separation of putative adipokines by their role in the inflammatory response seen in obesity

It should be noted that correlations of obesity with regards to mRNA levels in omental adipose tissue and elevations in the circulating levels of any protein do not prove a cause and effect relationship and most likely these are marker not maker molecules of obesity. Furthermore, it is likely that additional proteins other than those listed as unlikely adipokines will be found whose circulating levels are altered in obesity under some circumstances. Of the 12 listed in Table 3 as adipokines whose circulating levels are elevated in obesity, only leptin still remains as a primary response signal by fat cells in obesity.

7. References

Abuissa H, Jones, PG, Marso SP, O'Keefe JH Jr. (2005). Angiotensin-converting enzyme inhibitors or angiotensin receptor blockers for prevention of type 2 diabetes: a meta-analysis of randomized clinical trials. *Journal of the American College of Cardiology*, Vol.46, No.5, (September 2005), pp. 821-826, PMID 16139131

Achard V, Boullu-Ciocca S, Desbriere R, Nguyen G, Grino M (2007). Renin receptor expression in human adipose tissue. *American Journal of Physiology Regulatory, Integrative and Comparative Physiology*, Vol.292, No.1, (January 2007) pp. R274-R282, PMID 17197644

Akbay E, Yetkin I, Ersoy R, Kulaksizoglu S, Toruner F, Arslan M (2004). The relationship between levels of alpha1-acid glycoprotein and metabolic parameters of diabetes mellitus. *Diabetes Nutrition & Metabolism*, Vol.17, No.6, (December 2004) pp. 331-335, PMID 15887626

Albright CD, Salganik RI, Craciunescu CN, Mar MH, Zeisel SH (2003). Mitochondrial and microsomal derived reactive oxygen species mediate apoptosis induced by transforming growth factor-beta1 in immortalized rat hepatocytes. *Journal of Cellular Biochemistry*, Vol.89, No.2, (May 2003) pp. 254-261, PMID 12704789

Alessi MC, Bastelica D, Morange P, Berthet B, Leduc I, Verdier M, Geel O, Juhan-Vague I (2000). Plasminogen activator inhibitor 1, transforming growth factor-beta1, and BMI are closely associated in human adipose tissue during morbid obesity. *Diabetes*, Vol.49, No.8, (August 2000) pp. 1374-1380, PMID 10923640

Alessi MC, Poggi M, Juhan-Vague I (2007). Plasminogen activator inhibitor-1, adipose tissue and insulin resistance. *Current Opinion in Lipidology*, Vol.18, No.3, (June 2007) pp. 240-245, PMID 17495595

Arita Y, Kihara S, Ouchi N, Takahashi M, Maeda K, Miyagawa J, Hotta K, Shimomura I, Nakamura T, Miyaoka K, Kuriyama H, Nishida M, Yamashita S, Okubo K, Matsubara K, Muraguchi M, Ohmoto Y, Funahashi T, Matsuzawa Y (1999). Paradoxical decrease of an adipose-specific protein, adiponectin, in obesity. *Biochemical and Biophysical Research Communications*, Vol.257, No.1, (April 1999) pp. 79-83, PMID 10092513

Arner E , Ryden M, Arner P (2010). Tumor necrosis factor α and regulation of adipose tissue. *New England Journal of Medicine*, Vol.362, No.12, (March 2010) pp. 1151-1153, PMID 20335599

Ashley DT, O'Sullivan EP, Davenport C, Devlin N, Crowley RK, McCaffrey N, Moyna NM, Smith D, O'Gorman DJ (2011). Similar to adiponectin, serum levels of osteoprotegerin are associated with obesity in healthy subjects. *Metabolism*, Vol.60, No.7, (July 2011) pp. 994-1000, PMID 21087777

Auguet T, Quintero Y, Riesco D, Morancho B, Terra X, Crescenti A, Broch M, Aguilar C, Olona M, Porras JA, Hernandez M, Sabench F, del Castillo D, Richart C (2011). New adipokines vaspin and omentin. Circulating levels and gene expression in adipose tissue from morbidly obese women. *BMC Medical Genetics*, Vol.12, No.60, (April 2011), PMID 21526992

Bastard JP, Maachi M, Van Nhieu JT, Jardel C, Bruckert E, Grimaldi A, Robert JJ, Capeau J, Hainque B (2002). Adipose tissue IL-6 content correlates with resistance to insulin activation of glucose uptake both in vivo and in vitro. *The Journal of Clinical Endocrinology & Metabolism*, Vol.87, No.5, (May 2002) pp. 2084-2089, PMID 11994345

Bastelica D, Morange P, Berthet B, Borghi H, Lacroix O, Grino M, Juhan-Vague I, Alessi MC (2002). Stromal cells are the main plasminogen activator inhibitor-1-producing cells in human fat: evidence of differences between visceral and subcutaneous deposits. *Arteriosclerosis, Thrombosis, and Vascular Biology*, Vol.22, No.1, (January 2002) pp. 173-178, PMID 11788479

Berndt J, Kloting N, Kralisch S, Kovacs P, Fasshauer M, Schon MR, Stumvoll M, Bluher M (2005). Plasma visfatin concentrations and fat depot-specific mRNA expression in humans. *Diabetes*, Vol.54, No.10, (October 2005) pp. 2911-2916, PMID 16186392

Bing C, Mracek T, Gao D. Trayhurn P (2010). Zinc-α2-glycoprotein: an adipokine modulator of body fat mass? *International Journal of Obesity (London)*, Vol.34, No.11, (November 2010) pp. 1559-1565, PMID 20514048

Bornstein P (2009). Thrombospondins function as regulators of angiogenesis. *Journal of Cell Communication and Signaling*, Vol.3, No.3-4, (December 2009) pp. 189-200, PMID 19798599

Boucher J, Masri B, Daviaud D, Gesta S, Guigne C, Mazzucotelli A, Castan-Laurell I, Tack I, Knibiehler B, Carpene C, Audigier Y, Saulnier-Blache JS, Valet P (2005). Apelin, a newly identified adipokine up-regulated by insulin and obesity. *Endocrinology*, Vol.146, No.4, (April 2005) pp. 1764-1771, PMID 15677759

Bruun JM, Lihn AS, Madan AK, Pedersen SB, Schiott KM, Fain JN, Richelsen B (2004). Higher production of IL-8 in visceral vs. subcutaneous adipose tissue. Implication of nonadipose cells in adipose tissue. *American Journal of Physiology Endocrinology and Metabolism*, Vol.286, No.1, (January 2004) pp. E8-E13, PMID 13129857

Bruun JM, Verdich C, Toubro S, Astrup A, Richelsen B (2003). Association between measures of insulin sensitivity and circulating levels of interleukin-8, interleukin-6 and tumor necrosis factor-alpha. Effect of weight loss in obese men. *European Journal of Endocrinology*, Vol.148, No.5, (May 2003) pp. 535-542, PMID 1272053

Cani PD, Amar J, Iglesias MA, Poggi M, Knauf c, Bastelica D, Neyrinck AM, Fava F, Tuohy KM, Chabo C, Waget A, Delmee E,

Cousin B, Sulpice T, Chamontin B, Ferrieres J, Tanti JF, Gibson GR, Casteilla L, Delzenne NM, Alessi MC, Burcelin R (2007). Metabolic endotoxemia initiates obesity and insulin resistance. *Diabetes*, Vol.56, No.7, (July 2007) pp. 1761-1772, PMID 17456850

Canoy D, Boekholdt SM, Wareham N, Luben R, Welch A, Bingham S, Buchan I, Day N, Khaw KT (2007). Body fat distribution and risk of coronary heart disease in men and women in the European Prospective Investigation Into Cancer and Nutrition in Norfolk cohort: a population-based prospective study. *Circulation*, Vol.116, No.25, (December 2007) pp. 2933-2943, PMID 18071080

Cao Y (2010). Adipose tissue angiogenesis as a therapeutic target for obesity and metabolic diseases. *Nature Reviews. Drug Discovery*, Vol.9, No.2, (February 2010) pp. 107-115, PMID 20118961

Carey AL, Febbraio MA (2004). Interleukin-6 and insulin sensitivity: friend or foe? *Diabetologia*, Vol.47, No.7, (July 2004) pp. 1135-1142, PMID 15241593

Castan-Laurell I, Dray C, Attane C, Duparc T, Knauf C, Valet P (2011). Apelin, diabetes, and obesity. *Endocrine*, Vol.40, No.1, (August 2011) pp. 1-9, PMID 21725702

Ceperuelo-Mallafré V, Näf S, Escoté X, Caubet E, Gomez JM, Miranda M, Chacon MR, Gonzalez-Clemente JM, Gallart L, Gutierrez C, Vendrell J (2009). Circulating and adipose tissue gene expression of zinc-alpha2-glycoprotein in obesity: its relationship with adipokine and lipolytic gene markers in subcutaneous and visceral fat. *The Journal of Clinical Endocrinology & Metabolism*, Vol.94, No.12, (December 2009) pp. 5062-5069, PMID 19846741

Chiellini C, Santini F,Marsili A, Berti P, Bertacca A, Pelosini C, Scartabelli G, Pardini E, Lopez-Soriano J, Centoni R, Ciccarone AM, Benzi L, Vitti P, Del Prato S, Pinchera A, Maffei M (2004). Serum haptoglobin: a novel marker of adiposity in humans. *The Journal of Clinical Endocrinology & Metabolism*, Vol.89, No.6, (June 2004) pp. 2678-2683, PMID 15181041

Christiansen T, Richelsen B, Bruun JM (2005). Monocyte chemoattractant protein-1 is produced in isolated adipocytes, associated with adiposity and reduced after weight loss in morbid obese subjects. *International Journal of Obesity (London)*, Vol.29, No.1, (January 2005) pp. 146-150, PMID 15520826

Church TS, Willis MS, Priest EL, Lamonte MJ, Earnest CP, Wilkinson WJ, Wilson DA, Giroir BP (2005). Obesity, macrophage migration inhibitory factor, and weight loss.

International Journal of Obesity (London), Vol.29, No.6, (June 2005) pp. 675-681, PMID 15795748

Coe NR, Simpson MA, Bernlohr DA (1999). Targeted disruption of the adipocyte lipid-binding protein (aP2 protein) gene impairs fat cell lipolysis and increases cellular fatty acid levels. *Journal of Lipid Research*, Vol.40, No.5, (May 1999) pp. 967-972, PMID 10224167

Considine RV, Sinha MK, Heiman ML, Kriauciunas A, Stephens TW, Nyce MR, Ohannesian JP, Marco CC, McKee LJ, Bauer TL, Caro JF (1996). Serum immunoreative-leptin concentrations in normal-weight and obese humans. *The New England Journal of Medicine*, Vol.334, No.5, (February 1996) pp. 292-295, PMID 8532024

Corica F, Allegra A, Buemi M, Corsonello A, Bonanzinga S, Rubino F, Castagna L, Ceruso D (1997). Reduced plasma concentrations of transforming growth factor beta1 (TGF-beta1) in obese women. *International Journal of Obesity and Related Metabolic Disorders*, Vol.21, No.8, (August 1997) pp. 704-707, PMID 15481772

Cottam DR, Mattar SG, Barinas-Mitchell E, Eid G, Kuller L, Kelley DE, Schauer PR (2004). The chronic inflammatory hypothesis for the morbidity associated with morbid obesity: implications and effects of weight loss. *Obesity Surgery*, Vol.14, No.5, (May 2004) pp. 589-600, PMID 15186624

Dagogo-Jack S (2001). Human leptin regulation and promise in pharmacotherapy. *Current Drug Targets*, Vol.2, No.2, (June 2001) pp. 181-195, PMID 11469718

Dahlman I, Kaaman M, Olsson T, Tan GD, Bickerton AS, Wåhlén K, Andersson J, Nordström EA, Blomqvist L, Sjögren A, Forsgren M, Attersand A, Arner P (2005). A unique role of monocyte chemoattractant protein 1 among chemokines in adipose tissue of obese subjects. *The Journal of Clinical Endocrinology & Metabolism*, Vol.90, No.10, (October 2005) pp. 5834-5840, PMID 16091493

Dandona P, Aljada A, Ghanim H, Mohanty P, Tripathy C, Hofmeyer D, Chaudhuri A (2004). Increased plasma concentration of macrophage migration inhibitory factor (MIF) and MIF mRNA in mononuclear cells in the obese and the suppressive action of metformin. *The Journal of Clinical Endocrinology & Metabolism*, Vol.89, No.10, (October 2004) pp. 5043-5047, PMID 15472203

de Alba E, Tjandra N (2004). Structural studies on the Ca2+-binding domain of human nucleobindin (calnuc). *Biochemistry*, Vol.43, No.31, (August 2004) pp. 10039-10049, PMID 15287731

de Souza Batista CM, Yang RZ, Lee MJ, Glynn NM, Yu DZ, Pray J, Ndubuizu K, Patil S, Schwartz A, Kligman M, Fried SK, Gong DW, Shuldiner AR, Pollin TI, McLenithan JC (2007). Omentin plasma levels and gene expression are decreased in obesity. *Diabetes*, Vol.56, No.6., (June 2007) pp. 1655-1661, PMID 17329619

Despres JP, Lemieux I (2006). Abdominal obesity and metabolic syndrome. *Nature*, Vol.444, No.7121, (December 2006) pp. 881-887, PMID 17167477

Despres JP, Lemieux I, Bergeron J, Pibarot P, Mathieu P, Larose E, Rodes-Cabau J, Bertrand OF, Poirier P (2008). Abdominal obesity and the metabolic syndrome: contribution to global cardiometabolic risk. *Arteriosclerosis, Thrombosis, and Vascular Biology*, Vol.28, No.6, (June 2008) pp. 1039-1049, PMID 18356555

Dogru-Abbasoglu S, Kanbagli O, Bulur H, Babalik E, Ozturk S, Aykac-Toker G, Uysal M (1999). Lipid peroxides and antioxidant status in serum of patients with angiographically defined coronary atherosclerosis. *Clinical Biochemistry*, Vol.32, No.8, (November 1999) pp. 671-672, PMID 10638953

Donn RP, Ray DW (2004). Macrophage migration inhibitory factor: molecular, cellular and genetic aspects of a key neuroendocrine molecule. *Journal of Endocrinology*, Vol.182, No.1, (July 2004) pp. 1-9, PMID 15225126

Dutour A, Achard V, Sell H, Naour N, Collart F, Gaborit B, Silaghi A, Eckel J, Alessi MC, Henegar C, Clement K (2010). Secretory type II phospholipase A2 is produced and secreted by epicardial adipose tissue and overexpressed in patients with coronary artery disease. *The Journal of Clinical Endocrinology & Metabolism*, Vol. 95, No.2, (February 2010) pp. 963-967, PMID 20008021

Engeli S, Feldpausch M, Gorzelniak K, Hartwig F, Heintze U, Janke J, Mohlig M, Pfeiffer AF, Luft FC, Sharma AM (2003). Association between adiponectin and mediators of inflammation in obese women. *Diabetes*, Vol.52, No.4, (April 2003) pp. 942-947, PMID 12663465

Engeli S, Gorzelniak K, Kreutz R, Runkel N, Distler A, Sharma AM (1999). Co-expression of renin-angiotensin system genes in human adipose tissue. *Journal of Hypertension*, Vol.17, No.4, (April 1999) pp. 555-560, PMID 10404958

Esposito K, Pontillo A, Giugliano F, Giugliano G, Marfella R, Nicoletti G, Giugliano D (2003). Association of low interleukin-10 levels with the metabolic syndrome in obese women. *The Journal of Clinical Endocrinology & Metabolism*, Vol.88, No.3, (March 2003) pp. 1055-1058, PMID 12629085

Fain JN (2006). Release of interleukins and other inflammatory cytokines by human adipose tissue is enhanced in obesity and primarily due to the nonfat cells. *Vitamins and Hormones*, Vol.74, pp. 443-477, PMID 17027526

Fain JN (2010). Release of inflammatory mediators by human adipose tissue is enhanced in obesity and primarily by the nonfat cells: a review. *Mediators of Inflammation*, Vol.513948 (May 2010), PMID 20508843

Fain JN (2011). Correlative studies on the effects of obesity, diabetes and hypertension on gene expression in omental adipose tissue of obese women. *Nutrition and Diabetes*, in press

Fain JN, Bahouth SW (2000). Regulation of leptin release by mammalian adipose tissue. *Biochemical and Biophysical Research Communications*, Vol.274, No.3, (August 2000) pp. 571-575, PMID 10924319

Fain JN, Cheema PS, Bahouth SW, Hiler ML (2003). Resistin release by human adipose tissue explants in primary culture. *Biochemical and Biophysical Research Communications*, Vol. 300, No.3, (January 2003) pp. 674-678, PMID 12507502

Fain JN, Madan AK, Hiler ML, Cheema P, Bahouth SW (2004a). Comparison of the release of adipokines by adipose tissue, adipose tissue matrix, and adipocytes from visceral and subcutaneous abdominal adipose tissues of obese humans. *Endocrinology*, Vol.145, No.5, (May 2004) pp. 2273-2282, PMID 14726444

Fain JN, Bahouth SW, Madan AK (2004b). Haptoglobin release by human adipose tissue in primary culture. *Journal of Lipid Research*, Vol.45, No.3, (March 2004) pp. 536-542, PMID 14657203

Fain JN, Bahouth SW, Madan AK (2004c). TNFalpha release by the nonfat cells of human adipose tissue. *International Journal of Obesity and Related Metabolic Disorders*, Vol.28, No.4, (April 2004) pp. 616-622, PMID 14770194

Fain JN, Bahouth SW, Madan AK (2005a). Involvement of multiple signaling pathways in the post-bariatric induction of IL-6 and IL-8 mRNA and release in human visceral adipose tissue. *Biochemical Pharmacology*, Vol.69, No. 9, (May 2005) pp. 1315-1324, PMID 15826602

Fain JN, Tichansky DS, Madan AK (2005b). Transforming growth factor beta1 release by human adipose tissue is enhanced in obesity. *Metabolism*, Vol.54, No.11, (November 2005) pp. 1546-1551, PMID 16253647

Fain JN, Tichansky DS, Madan AK (2006). Most of the interleukin 1 receptor antagonist, cathepsin S, macrophage migration inhibitory factor, nerve growth factor, and interleukin 18 release by explants of human adipose tissue is by the non-fat cells, not by the adipocytes. *Metabolism*, Vol.55, No.8, (August 2006) pp. 1113-1121, PMID 16839849

Fain JN, Buehrer B, Bahouth SW, Tichansky DS, Madan AK (2008a). Comparison of messenger RNA distribution for 60 proteins in fat cells vs the nonfat cells of human omental adipose tissue. *Metabolism*, Vol.57, No.7, (July 2008) pp. 1005-1015, PMID 18555844

Fain JN, Sacks HS, Buehrer B, Bahouth SW, Garrett E, Wolf RY, Carter RA, Tichansky DS, Madan AK (2008b). Identification of omentin mRNA in human epicardial adipose tissue: comparison to omentin in subcutaneous, internal mammary artery periadventitial and visceral abdominal depots. *International Journal of Obesity (London)*, Vol 32, No. 5, (May 2008) pp. 810-815, PMID 18180782

Fain JN, Buehrer B, Tichansky DS, Madan AK (2008c). Regulation of adiponectin release and demonstration of adiponectin mRNA as well as release by the non-fat cells of human omental adipose tissue. *International Journal of Obesity (London)*, Vol.32, No.3, (March 2008) pp. 429-435, PMID 17895880

Fain JN, Cheema P, Tichansky DS, Madan AK (2008d). Stimulation of human omental adipose tissue lipolysis by growth hormone plus dexamethasone. *Molecular and Cellular Endocrinology*, Vol.295, No.1-2, (November 2008) pp. 101-105, PMID 18640775

Fain JN, Tagele BM, Cheema P, Madan AK, Tichansky DS (2010a). Release of 12 adipokines by adipose tissue, nonfat cells, and fat cells from obese women. *Obesity (Silver Spring)*, Vol.18, No.5, (May 2010) pp. 890-896, PMID 19834460

Fain JN, Cheema P, Madan AK, Tichansky DS (2010b). Dexamethasone and the inflammatory response in explants of human omental adipose tissue. *Molecular and Cellular Endocrinology*, Vol.315, No.1-2, (February 2010) pp. 292-298, PMID 19853017

Fernandez-Real JM, Broch M, Ricart W, Casamitjana R, Gutierrez C, Vendrell J, Richart C (1998). Plasma levels of the soluble fraction of tumor necrosis factor receptor 2 and insulin resistance. *Diabetes*, Vol.47, No.11, (November 1998) pp. 1757-1762, PMID 9792545

Fessler MB, Rudel LL, Brown JM (2009). Toll-like receptor signaling links dietary fatty acids to the metabolic syndrome. *Current Opinion in Lipidology*, Vol.20, No.5, (October 2009) pp. 379-385, PMID 19625959

Festa A, D'Agostino R Jr, Williams K, Karter AJ, Mayer-Davis EJ, Tracy RP, Haffner SM (2001). The relation of body fat mass and distribution to markers of chronic inflammation. *International Journal of Obesity and Related Metabolic Disorders*, Vol.25, No.10, (October 2001) pp. 1407-1415, PMID 11673759

Flaumenhaft R, Kojima S, Abe M, Rifkin DB (1993). Activation of latent transforming growth factor beta. *Advances in Pharmacology*, Vol.24, pp. 51-76, PMID 8504067

Forsblom C, Thomas MC, Moran J, Saraheimo M, Thorn L, Waden J, Gordin D, Frystyk J, Flyvbjerg A, Groop PH; on behalf of the FinnDiane Study Group (2011). Serum adiponectin concentration is a positive predictor of all-cause and cardiovascular mortality in type 1 diabetes. *Journal of Internal Medicine*, (May 2011) Epub ahead of print, PMID 21615808

Fowler JD, Krueth SB, Bernlohr DA, Katz SA (2009). Renin dynamics in adipose tissue: adipose tissue control of local renin concentrations. *American Journal of Physiology - Endocrinology Metabolism*, Vol.296, No.2, (February 2009) pp. E343-E350, PMID 19050177

Frangogiannis NG (2004). The role of the chemokines in myocardial ischemia and reperfusion. *Current Vascular Pharmacology*, Vol.2, No.2, (April 2004) pp. 163-174, PMID 15320517

Fukuhara A, Matsuda M, Nishizawa M, Segawa K, Tanaka M, Kishimoto K, Matsuki Y, Murakami M, Ichisaka T, Murakami H, Watanabe E, Takagi T, Akiyoshi M, Ohtsubo T, Kihara S, Yamashita S, Makishima M, Funahashi T, Yamanaka S, Hiramatsu R, Matsuzawa Y, Shimomura I (2005). Visfatin: a protein secreted by visceral fat that mimics the effects of insulin. *Science*, Vol.307, No.5708, (January 2005) pp. 426-430, PMID 15604363

Furuhashi M, Tuncman G, Gorgun CZ, Makowski L, Atsumi G, Vaillancourt E, Kono K. Babaev VR, Fazio S, Linton MF, Sulsky R, Robl JA, Parker RA, Hotamisligil GS (2007). Treatment of diabetes and atherosclerosis by inhibiting fatty-acid-binding protein aP2. *Nature*, Vol.447, No.7147, (June 2007) pp. 959-965, PMID 17554340

Furuhashi M, Fucho R, Gorgun CZ, Tuncman G, Cao H, Hotamisligil GS (2008). Adipocyte/macrophage fatty acid-binding proteins contribute to metabolic deterioration through actions in both macrophages and adipocytes in mice. *Journal of Clinical Investigation*, Vol.118, No.7, (July 2008) pp. 2640-2650, PMID 18551191

Gannage-Yared MH, Yaghi C, Habre B, Khalife S, Noun R, Germanos-Haddad M, Trak-Smayra V (2008). Osteoprotegerin in relation to body weight, lipid parameters insulin sensitivity, adipocytokines, and C-reactive protein in obese and non-obese young individuals: results from both cross-sectional and interventional study. *European Journal of Endocrinology*, Vol158, No.3, (March 2008) pp. 353-359, PMID 18299469

Gautron L, Elmquist JK (2011). Sixteen years and counting: an update on leptin in energy balance. *Journal of Clinical Investigation*, Vol.121, No.6, (June 2011) pp. 2087-2093, PMID 21633176

Giacchetti G, Faloia E, Mariniello B, Sardu C, Gatti C, Camilloni MA, Guerrieri M, Mantero F (2002). Overexpression of the renin-angiotensin system in human visceral adipose tissue in normal and overweight subjects. *American Journal of Hypertension*, Vol.15, No.5, (May 2002) pp. 381-388, PMID 12022238

Gogg S, Smith U, Jansson PA (2009). Increased MAPK activation and impaired insulin signaling in subcutaneous microvascular endothelial cells in type 2 diabetes: the role of endothelin-1. *Diabetes*, Vol.58, No.10, (October 2009) pp. 2238-2245, PMID 19581418

Goldbach-Mansky R (2009). Blocking interleukin-1 in rheumatic diseases. *Annals of the New York Academy of Sciences*, Vol. 1182, (December 2009) pp. 111-123, PMID 20074280

Gorzelniak K, Engeli S, Janke J, Luft FC, Sharma AM (2002). Hormonal regulation of the human adipose-tissue renin angiotensin system: relationship to obesity and hypertension. *Journal of Hypertension*, Vol.20, No.5, (May 2002) pp. 965-973, PMID 12011658

Graham TE, Yang Q, Bluher M, Hammarstedt A, Ciaraldi TP, Henry RR, Wason CJ, Oberbach A, Jansson PA, Smith U, Kahn BB (2006). Retinol-binding protein 4 and insulin resistance in lean, obese, and diabetic subjects. *The New England Journal of Medicine*, Vol.354, No.24, (June 2006) pp. 2552-2563, PMID 16775236

Haddad JJ, Harb HL (2005). L-gamma-Glutamyl-L-cysteinyl-glycine (glutathione; GSH) and GSH-related enzymes in the regulation of pro- and anti-inflammatory cytokines: a signaling transcriptional scenario for redox(y) immunologic sensor(s)? *Molecular Immunology*, Vol.42, No.9, (May 2005) pp. 987-1014, PMID 15829290

Hanusch-Enserer U, Cauza E, Spak M, Dunky A, Rosen HR, Wolf H, Prager R, Eibl MM (2003). Acute-phase response and immunological markers in morbid obese patients and patients following adjustable gastric banding. *International Journal of Obesity and Related Metabolic Disorders*, Vol.27, No. 3, (March 2003) pp. 355-361, PMID 12629563

Hasegawa G, Ohta M, Ichida Y, Obayashi H, Shigeta M, Yamasaki M, Fukui M, Yoshikawa T, Nakamura N (2005). Increased serum resistin levels in patients with type 2 diabetes are not linked with markers of insulin resistance and adiposity. *Acta Diabetologica*, Vol.42, No.2, (June 2005) pp. 104-109, PMID 15944845

Heinonen MV, Purhonen AK, Miettinen P, Paakkonen M, Pirinen E, Alhava E, Akerman K, Herzig KH (2005). Apelin, orexin-A and leptin plasma levels in morbid obesity and effect of gastric banding. *Regulatory Peptides*, Vol.130, No.1-2, (August 2005) pp. 7-13, PMID 15970339

Heinrich PC, Castell JV, Andus T (1990). Interleukin-6 and the acute phase response. *Biochemical Journal*, Vol.265, No.3, (February 1990) pp. 621-636, PMID 1689567

Herse F, Fain JN, Janke J, Engeli S, Kuhn C, Frey N, Weich HA, Bergmann A, Kappert K, Karumanchi SA, Luft FC, Muller DN, Staff AC, Dechend R (2011). Adipose tissue-derived soluble fms-like tyrosine kinase 1 is an obesity-relevant endogenous paracrine adipokine. *Hypertension*, Vol.58, No.1, (July 2011) pp. 37-42, PMID 21555675

Hida K, Wada J, Eguchi J, Zhang H, Baba M, Seida A, Hashimoto I, Okada T, Yasuhara A, Nakatsuka A, Shikata K, Hourai S, Futami J, Watanabe E, Matsuki Y, Hiramatsu R, Akagi S, Makino H, Kanwar YS (2005). Visceral adipose tissue-derived serine protease inhibitor: a unique insulin-sensitizing adipocytokine in obesity. *Proceedings of the National Academy of Sciences United States of America*, Vol. 102, No.30, (July 2005) pp. 10610-10615, PMID 16030142

Hoffstedt J, Arvidsson E, Sjolin E, Wahlen K, Arner P (2004). Adipose tissue adiponectin production and adiponectin serum concentration in human obesity and insulin resistance. *The Journal of Clinical Endocrinology & Metabolism*, Vol.89, No.3, (March 2004) pp. 1391-1396, PMID 15001639

Holecki M, Zahorska-Markiewicz B, Janowska J, Nieszporek T, Wojaczynska-Stanek K, Zak-Golab A, Wiecek A (2007). The influence of weight loss on serum osteoprotegerin concentration in obese perimenopausal women. *Obesity (Silver Spring)*, Vol.15, No.8, (August 2007) pp. 1925-1929, PMID 17712108

Hotamisligil GS, Shargill NS, Spiegelman BM (1993). Adipose expression of tumor necrosis factor-alpha: direct role in obesity-linked insulin resistance. *Science*, Vol.259, No.5091, (January 1993) pp. 87-91, PMID 7678183

Hotamisligil GS, Arner P, Caro JF, Atkinson RL, Spiegelman BM (1995). Increased adipose tissue expression of tumor necrosis factor-alpha in human obesity and insulin resistance. *Journal of Clinical Investigation*, Vol. 95, No.5, (May 1995) pp. 2409-2415, PMID 7738205

Hotamisligil GS, Johnson RS, Distel RJ, Ellis R, Papaioannou VE, Spiegelman BM (1996). Uncoupling of obesity from insulin resistance through a targeted mutation in aP2, the adipocyte fatty acid binding protein. *Science*, Vol.274, No.5291, (November 1996) pp. 1377-1379, PMID 8910278

Hotamisligil GS, Arner P, Atkinson RL, Spiegelman BM (1997). Differential regulation of the p80 tumor necrosis factor receptor in human obesity and insulin resistance. *Diabetes*, Vol.46, No.3, (March 1997) pp. 451-455, PMID 9032102

Hung J, McQuillan BM, Thompson PL, Beilby JP (2008). Circulating adiponectin levels associate with inflammatory markers, insulin resistance and metabolic syndrome independent of obesity. *International Journal of Obesity (London)* Vol.32, No.5, (May 2008) pp. 772-779, PMID 18253163

Hung WW, Hsieh TJ, Lin T, Chou PC, Hsiao PJ, Lin KD, Shin SJ (2011). Blockade of the renin-angiotensin system ameliorates apelin production in 3T3-L1 adipocytes. *Cardiovascular Drugs and Therapy*, Vol.25, No.1, (February 2011) pp. 3-12, PMID 21161354

Ishida J, Hashimoto T, Hashimoto Y, Nishiwaki S, Iguchi T, Harada S, Sugaya T, Matsuzaki H, Yamamoto R, Shiota N, Okunishi H, Kihara M, Umemura S, Sugiyama F, Yagami K, Kasuya Y, Mochizuki N, Fukamizu A (2004). Regulatory roles for APJ, a seven-transmembrane receptor related to angiotensin-type 1 receptor in blood pressure in vivo. *Journal of Biological Chemistry*, Vol.279, No.25, (June 2004) pp. 26274-26279, PMID 15087458

Janke J, Engeli S, Gorzelniak K, Luft FC, Sharma AM (2002). Resistin gene expression in human adipocytes is not related to insulin resistance. *Obesity Research*, Vol.10, No.1, (January 2002) pp. 1-5, PMID 11786595

Jobs E, Riserus U, Ingelsson E, Helmersson J, Nerpin E, Jobs M, Sundstrom J, Lind L, Larsson A, Basu S, Arnlov J (2010). Serum cathepsin S is associated with serum C-reactive protein and interleukin-6 independently of obesity in elderly men. *The Journal of Clinical Endocrinology & Metabolism*, Vol.95, No.9, (September 2010) pp. 4460-4464, PMID 20610597

Juge-Aubry CE, Somm E, Giusti V, Pernin A, Chicheportiche R, Verdumo C, Rohner-Jeanrenaud F, Burger D, Dayer JM, Meier CA (2003). Adipose tissue is a major source of interleukin-1 receptor antagonist: upregulation in obesity and inflammation. *Diabetes*, Vol.52, No.5, (May 2003) pp. 1104-1110, PMID 12716739

Jun LS, Siddall CP, Rosen ED (2011). A minor role for lipocalin 2 in high fat diet-induced glucose intolerance. *American Journal of Physiology Endocrinology Metabolism*, (July 2011), Epub ahead of print, PMID 21771968

Jung C, Gerdes N, Fritzenwanger M, Figulla HR (2010). Circulating levels of interleukin-1 family cytokines in overweight adolescents. *Mediators of Inflammation*, (February 2010), Epub, PMID 20169140

Kabon B, Nagele A, Reddy D, Eagon C, Fleshman JW, Sessler DI, Kurz A (2004). Obesity decreases perioperative tissue oxygenation. *Anesthesiology*, Vol.100, No.2, (February 2004) pp. 274-280, PMID 14739800

Karlsson C, Lindell K, Ottosson M, Sjostrom L, Carlsson B, Carlsson LM (1998). Human adipose tissue expresses angiotensinogen and enzymes required for its conversion to angiotensin II. *The Journal of Clinical Endocrinology & Metabolism*, Vol.83, No.11, (November 1998), pp. 3925-3929, PMID 9814470

Kawakami A, Urayama S, Yamasaki S, Hida A, Miyashita T, Kamachi M, Nakashima K, Tanaka F, Ida H, Kawabe Y, Aoyagi T, Furuichi I, Migita K, Origuchi T, Eguchi K (2004). Anti-apoptogenic function of TGFbeta1 for human synovial cells: TGFbeta1 protects cultured synovial cells from mitochondrial perturbation induced by several apoptogenic stimuli. *Annals of the Rheumatic Diseases*, Vol.63, No.1, (January 2004) pp.95-97, PMID 14672900

Kern PA, Saghizadeh M, Ong JM, Bosch RJ, Deem R, Simsolo RB (1995). The expression of tumor necrosis factor in human adipose tissue. Regulation by obesity, weight loss, and relationship to lipoprotein lipase. *Journal of Clinical Investigation*, Vol.95, No.5, (May 1995) pp. 2111-2119, PMID 7738178

Khaodhiar L, Ling PR, Blackburn GL, Bistrian BR (2004). Serum levels of interleukin-6 and C-reactive protein correlate with body mass index across the broad range of obesity. *Journal of Parenteral and Enteral Nutrition*, Vol. 28, No.6, (November-December 2004) pp. 410-415, PMID 15568287

Kim JH, Bachmann RA, Chen J (2009). Interleukin-6 and insulin resistance. *Vitamins and Hormones*, Vol.80, pp. 613-633, PMID 19251052

Kim SM, Cho GJ, Yannakoulia M, Hwang TG, Kim IH, Park EK, Mantzoros CS (2011). Lifestyle modification increases circulating adiponectin concentrations but does not change vaspin concentrations. *Metabolism*, Vol.60, No.9, (September 2011) pp. 1294-1299, PMID 21489569

Kirsch T, Woywodt A, Klose J, Wyss K, Beese M, Erdbruegger U, Grossheim M, Haller H, Haubitz M (2010). Endothelial-derived thrombospondin-1 promotes macrophage recruitment and apoptotic cell clearance. *Journal of Cellular and Molecular Medicine*, Vol.14, No.7, (July 2010) pp. 1922-1934, PMID 19508384

Kleeman R, Bucala R (2010). Macrophage migration inhibitory factor: critical role in obesity, insulin resistance, and associated comorbidities. *Mediators of Inflammation*, (February 2010) Epub, PMID 20169173

Kloting N, Berndt J, Kralisch S, Kovacs P, Fasshauer M, Schon MR, Stumvoll M, Bluher M (2006). Vaspin gene expression in human adipose tissue: association with obesity and type 2 diabetes. *Biochemical and Biophysical Research Communications,* Vol.339, No.1, (January 2006) pp. 430-436, PMID 16298335

Kobayashi J, Nakajima K, Nohara A, Kawashiri M, Yagi K, Inazu A, Koizumi J, Yamagishi M, Mabuchi H (2007). The relationship of serum lipoprotein lipase mass with fasting serum apolipoprotein B-48 and remnant-like particle triglycerides in type 2 diabetic patients. *Hormone and Metabolic Research,* Vol.39, No.8, (August 2007) pp. 612-616, PMID 17712727

Koistinen HA, Bastard JP, Dusserre E, Ebeling P, Zegari N, Andreelli F, Jardel C, Donner M, Meyer L, Moulin P, Hainque B, Riou JP, Laville M, Koivisto VA, Vidal H (2000). Subcutaneous adipose tissue expression of tumour necrosis factor-alpha is not associated with whole body insulin resistance in obese nondiabetic or in type-2 diabetic subjects. *European Journal of Clinical Investigation,* Vol.30, No.4, (April 2000) pp. 302-310, PMID 10759878

Korner A, Garten A, Bluher M, Tauscher R, Kratzsch J, Kiess W (2007). Molecular characteristics of serum visfatin and differential detection by immunoassays. *The Journal of Clinical Endocrinology & Metabolism,* Vol.92, No.12, (December 2007) pp. 4783-4791, PMID 17878256

Kotnik P, Fischer-Posovszky P, Wabitsch M (2011). RBP4 - a controversial adipokine. *European Journal of Endocrinology,*
(August 2011) Epub ahead of print, PMID 21835764

Kratchmarova I, Kalume DE, Blagoev B, Scherer PE, Podtelejnikov AV, Molina H, Bickel PE, Andersen JS, Fernandez MM, Bunkenborg J, Roepstorff P, Kristiansen K, Lodish HF, Mann M, Pandey A (2002). A proteomic approach for identification of secreted proteins during the differentiation of 3T3-L1 preadipocytes to adipocytes. *Molecular & Cellular Proteomics,* Vol.1, No.3, (March 2002) pp. 213-222, PMID 12096121

Kshatriya S, Liu K, Salah A, Szombathy T, Freeman RH, Reams GP, Spear RM, Villarreal D (2011). Obesity hypertension: the regulatory role of leptin. *International Journal of Hypertension,* (January 2011), PMID 21253519

Kugiyama K, Ota Y, Takazoe K, Moriyama Y, Kawano H, Miyao Y, Sakamoto T, Soejima H, Ogawa H, Doi H, Sugiyama S, Yasue H (1999). Circulating levels of secretory type II phospholipase A(2) predict coronary events in patients with coronary artery disease. *Circulation,* Vol.100, No.12, (September 1999) pp. 1280-1284, PMID 10491371

Lafarge JC, Naour N, Clement K, Guerre-Millo M (2010). Cathepsins and cystatin C in atherosclerosis and obesity. *Biochimie,* Vol.92, No. 11, (November 2010) pp. 1580-1586, PMID 20417681

Lan H, Cheng CC, Kowalski TJ, Pang L, Shan L, Chuang CC, Jackson J, Rojas-Triana A, Bober L, Liu L, Voigt J, Orth P, Yang X, Shipps GW Jr, Hedrick JA (2011). Small-molecule inhibitors of FABP4/5 ameliorate dyslipidemia but not insulin resistance in mice with diet-induced obesity. *Journal of Lipid Research,* Vol.52, No.4, (April 2011) pp. 646-656, PMID 21296956

Larsson A, Hansson LO (2003). High sensitivity CRP and serum amyloid A as expressions of low grade inflammation do not correlate with bFGF or VEGF. *Upsala Journal of Medical Sciences*, Vol.108, No.1, pp. 51-59, PMID 12903837

Leclerc P, Biarc J, St-Onge M, Gilbert C, Dussault AA, Laflamme C, Pouliot M (2008). Nucleobindin co-localizes and associates with cyclooxygenase (COX)-2 in human neutrophils. *Public Library of Science ONE*, Vol.3, No.5, (May 2008) pp. e2229, PMID 18493301

Lee MH, Song HK, Ko GJ, Kang YS, Han SY, Han KY, Kim HK, Han JY, Cha DR (2008a). Angiotensin receptor blockers improve insulin resistance in type 2 diabetic rats by modulating adipose tissue. *Kidney International*, Vol.74, No.7, (October 2008) pp. 890-900, PMID 18596725

Lee YS, Kim AY, Choi JW, Kim M, Yasue S, Son HJ, Masuzaki H, Park KS, Kim JB (2008b). Dysregulation of adipose glutathione peroxidase 3 in obesity contributes to local and systemic oxidative stress. *Molecular Endocrinology*, Vol.22, No.9, (September 2008) pp. 2176-2189, PMID 18562625

Lee YS, Choi JW, Hwang I, Lee JW, Lee JH, Kim AY, Huh JY, Koh YJ, Koh GY, Son HJ, Masuzaki H, Hotta K, Alfadda AA, Kim JB (2010). Adipocytokine orosomucoid integrates inflammatory and metabolic signals to preserve energy homeostasis by resolving immoderate inflammation. *Journal of Biological Chemistry*, Vol.285, No.29, (July 2010) pp. 22174-22185, PMID 20442402

Lehrke M, Reilly MP, Millington SC, Iqbal N, Rader DJ, Lazar MA (2004). An inflammatory cascade leading to hyperresistinemia in humans. *Public Library of Science Medicine*, Vol.1, No.2, (November 2004) pp. e45, PMID 15578112

Levinson SS, Miller JJ, Elin RJ (2004). Poor predictive value of high-sensitivity C-reactive protein indicates need for reassessment. *Clinical Chemistry*, Vol.50, No.10, (October 2004) pp. 1733-1735, PMID 15388655

Li S, Shin HJ, Ding EL, van Dam RM (2009). Adiponectin levels and risk of type 2 diabetes: a systematic review and meta-analysis. *Journal of the American Medical Association*, Vol.302, No.2, (July 2009) pp. 179-188, PMID 19584347

Lin Y, Rajala MW, Berger JP, Moller DE, Barzilai N, Scherer PE (2001). Hyperglyciemia-induced production of acute phase reactants in adipose tissue. *Journal of Biological Chemistry*, Vol.276, No.45, (November 2001) pp. 42077-42083, PMID 11546817

Lindeman JH, Pijl H, Toet K, Eilers PH, van Ramshorst B, Buijs MM, van Bockel JH, Kooistra T (2007). Human visceral adipose tissue and the plasminogen activator inhibitor type 1. *International Journal of Obesity* (*London*), Vol.31, No.11, (November 2007) pp. 1671-1679, PMID 17471294

Livingston EH, Ko CY (2005). Effect of diabetes and hypertension on obesity-related mortality. *Surgery*, Vol.137, No.1, (January 2005) pp. 16-25, PMID 15614276

Lo J, Bernstein LE, Canavan B, Torriani M, Jackson MB, Ahima RS, Grinspoon SK (2007). Effects of TNF-alpha neutralization on adipocytokines and skeletal muscle adiposity in the metabolic syndrome. *American Journal of Physiology Endocrinology and Metabolism*, Vol. 293, No.1, (July 2007) pp. E102-E109, PMID 17374698

Luc G, Empana JP, Morange P, Juhan-Vague I, Arveiler D, Ferrieres J, Amouyel P, Evans A, Kee F, Bingham A, Machez E, Ducimetiere P (2010). Adipocytokines and the risk of coronary heart disease in healthy middle aged men: the PRIME Study. *International*

Journal of Obesity (London), Vol.34, No.1, (January 2010), pp. 118-126, PMID 19823188

Maachi M, Pieroni L, Bruckert E, Jardel C, Fellahi S, Hainque B, Capeau J, Bastard JP (2004). Systemic low-grade inflammation is related to both circulating and adipose tissue TNFalpha, leptin and IL-6 levels in obese women. *International Journal of Obesity and Related Metabolic Disorders*, Vol.28, No.8, (August 2004) pp. 993-997, PMID 15211360

Madan AK, Tichansky DS, Coday M, Fain JN (2006). Comparison of IL-8, IL-6 and PGE(2) formation by visceral (omental) adipose tissue of obese Caucasian compared to African-American women. *Obesity Surgery*, Vol.16, No.10, (October 2006) pp. 1342-1350, PMID 17059745

Madani R, Karastergiou K, Ogston NC, Miheisi N, Bhome R, Haloob N, Tan GD, Karpe F, Malone-Lee J, Hashemi M, Jahangiri M, Mohamed-Ali V (2009). RANTES release by human adipose tissue in vivo and evidence for depot-specific differences. *American Journal of Physiology Endocrinology and Metabolism*, Vol.296, No.6, (June 2009) pp. E1262-E1268, PMID 19240255

Magkos F, Mohammed BS, Mittendorfer B (2009). Plasma lipid transfer enzymes in non-diabetic lean and obese men and women. *Lipids*, Vol.44, No.5, (May 2009) pp. 459-464, PMID 19198915

Malavazos AE, Cereda E, Morricone L, Coman C, Corsi MM, Ambrosi B (2005). Monocyte chemoattractant protein 1: a possible link between visceral adipose tissue-associated inflammation and subclinical echocardiographic abnormalities in uncomplicated obesity. *European Journal of Endocrinology*, Vol.153, No.6, (December 2005) pp. 871-877, PMID 16322393

Manco M, Fernandez-Real JM, Equitani F, Vendrell J, Valera Mora ME, Nanni G, Tondolo V, Calvani M, Ricart W, Castagneto M, Mingrone G (2007). Effect of massive weight loss on inflammatory adipocytokines and the innate immune system in morbidly obese women. *The Journal of Clinical Endocrinology & Metabolism*, Vol.92, No.2, (February 2007) pp. 483-490, PMID 17105839

Manigrasso MR, Ferroni P, Santilli F, Taraborelli T, Guagnano MT, Michetti N, Davi G (2005). Association between circulating adiponectin and interleukin-10 levels in android obesity: effects of weight loss. *The Journal of Clinical Endocrinology & Metabolism*, Vol.90, No.10, (October 2005) pp. 5876-5879, PMID 16030165

Masri B, Knibiehler B, Audigier Y (2005). Apelin signalling: a promising pathway from cloning to pharmacology. *Cellular Signalling*, Vol.17, No.4, (April 2005) pp. 415-426, PMID 15601620

Maury E, Ehala-Aleksejev K, Guiot Y, Detry R, Vandenhooft A, Brichard SM (2007). Adipokines oversecreted by omental adipose tissue in human obesity. *American Journal of Physiology Endocrinology and Metabolism*, Vol.293, No.3, (September 2007) pp. E656-E665, PMID 17578888

McGillicuddy FC, Harford KA, Reynolds CM, Oliver E, Claessens M, Mills KH, Roche HM (2011). Lack of interleukin-1 receptor 1 (IL-1RI) protects mice from high-fat diet-induced adipose tissue inflammation coincident with improved glucose homeostasis. *Diabetes*, Vol.60, No.6, (June 2011) pp. 1688-1698, PMID 21515850

Meier CA, Bobbioni E, Gabay C, Assimacopoulos-Jeannet F, Golay A, Dayer JM (2002). IL-1 receptor antagonist serum levels are increased in human obesity: a possible link to the resistance to leptin? *The Journal of Clinical Endocrinology & Metabolism*, Vol.87, No.3, (March 2002) pp. 1184-1188, PMID 11889184

Miller GE, Stetler CA, Carney RM, Freedland KE, Banks WA (2002). Clinical depression and inflammatory risk markers for coronary heart disease. *The American Journal of Cardiology*, Vol.90, No.12, (December 2002) pp. 1279-1283, PMID 12480034

Miyazawa-Hoshimoto S, Takahashi K, Bujo H, Hashimoto N, Saito Y (2003). Elevated serum vascular endothelial growth factor is associated with visceral fat accumulation in human obese subjects. *Diabetologia*, Vol.46, No.11, (November 2003) pp. 1483-1488, PMID 14534780

Mocellin S, Panelli MC, Wang E, Nagorsen D, Marincola FM (2003). The dual role of IL-10. *Trends in Immunology*, Vol.24, No.1, (January 2003) pp. 36-43, PMID 12495723

Mohamed-Ali V, Goodrick S, Rawesh A, Katz DR, Miles JM, Yudkin JS, Klein S, Coppack SW (1997). Subcutaneous adipose tissue releases interleukin-6, but not tumor necrosis factor-alpha, in vivo. *The Journal of Clinical Endocrinology & Metabolism*, Vol.82, No.12, (December 1997) pp. 4196-4200, PMID 9398739

Moschen AR, Molnar C, Enrich B, Geiger S, Ebenbichler CF, Tilg H (2011). Adipose and liver expression of interleukin (IL)-1 family members in morbid obesity and effects of weight loss. *Molecular Medicine*, Vol.17, No.7-8, pp. 840-845, PMID 21394384

Mracek T, Ding Q, Tzanavari T, Kos K, Pinkney J, Wilding J, Trayhurn P, Bing C (2010). The adipokine zinc-alpha2-glycoprotein (ZAG) is downregulated with fat mass expansion in obesity. *Clinical Endocrinology*, Vol.72, No.3, (March 2010) pp. 334-341, PMID 19549246

Nagaev I, Smith U (2001). Insulin resistance and type 2 diabetes are not related to resistin expression in human fat cells or skeletal muscle. *Biochemical and Biophysical Research Communications*, Vol.285, No.2, (July 2001) pp. 561-564, PMID 11444881

Nagasawa H, Yokota C, Toyoda K, Ito A, Minematsu K (2011). High level of plasma adiponectin in acute stroke patients is associated with stroke mortality. *Journal of the Neurological Sciences*, Vol.304, No.1-2, (May 2011) pp. 102-106, PMID 21377692

Naour N, Rouault C, Fellahi S, Lavoie ME, Poitou C, Keophiphath M, Eberle D, Shoelson S, Rizkalla S, Bastard JP, Rabasa-Lhoret R, Clement K, Guerre-Millo M (2010). Cathepsins in human obesity: changes in energy balance predominantly affect cathepsin s in adipose tissue and in circulation. *The Journal of Clinical Endocrinology & Metabolism*, Vol. 95, No.4, (April 2010) pp. 1861-1868, PMID 20164293

Napolitano A, Lowell BB, Damm D, Leibel RL, Ravussin E, Jimerson DC, Lesem MD, Van Dyke DC, Daly PA, Chatis P, White RT, Spiegelman BM, Flier JS (1994). Concentrations of adipsin in blood and rates of adipsin secretion by adipose tissue in humans with normal, elevated and diminished adipose tissue mass. *International Journal of Obesity and Related Metabolic Disorders*, Vol.18, No.4, (April 1994) pp. 213-218, PMID 8044195

Nilsson J (2005). CRP--marker or maker of cardiovascular disease? *Arteriosclerosis, Thrombosis, and Vascular Biology*, Vol.25, No.8, (August 2005) pp. 1527-1528, PMID 16055753

Pardina E, Lecube A, Llamas R, Catalan R, Galard R, Fort JM, Allende H, Vargas V, Baena-Fustegueras JA, Peinado-Onsurbe J (2009). Lipoprotein lipase but not hormone-sensitive lipase activities achieve normality after surgically induced weight loss in morbidly obese patients. *Obesity Surgery*, Vol.19, No.8, (August 2009) pp. 1150-1158, PMID 19455372

Pasarica M, Sereda OR, Redman LM, Albarado DC, Hymel DT, Roan LE, Rood JC, Burk DH, Smith SR (2009). Reduced adipose tissue oxygenation in human obesity: evidence for rarefaction, macrophage chemotaxis, and inflammation without an angiogenic response. *Diabetes*, Vol.58, No.3, (March 2009) pp. 718-725, PMID 19074987

Pischon T, Boeing H, Hoffmann K, Bergmann M, Schulze MB, Overvad K, van der Schouw YT, Spencer E, Moons KG, Tjonneland A, Halkjaer J, Jensen MK, Stegger J, Clavel-Chapelon F, Boutron-Ruault MC, Chajes V, Linseisen J, Kaaks R, Trichopoulou A, Trichopoulos D, Bamia C, Sieri S, Palli D, Tumino R, Vineis P, Panico S, Peeters PH, May AM, Bueno-de-Mesquita HB, van Duijnhoven FJ, Hallmans G, Weinehall L, Manjer J, Hedblad B, Lund E, Agudo A, Arriola L, Barricarte A, Navarro C, Martinez C, Quirós JR, Key T, Bingham S, Khaw KT, Boffetta P, Jenab M, Ferrari P, Riboli E (2008). General and abdominal adiposity and the risk of death in Europe. *The New England Journal of Medicine*, Vol.359, No.20, (November 2008) pp. 2105-2120, PMID 19005195

Platell C, Cooper D, Papadimitriou JM, Hall JC (2000). The omentum. *World Journal of Gastroenterology*, Vol.6, No.2, (April 2000) pp. 169-176, PMID 11819552

Poitou C, Viguerie N, Cancello R, De Matteis R, Cinti S, Stich V, Coussieu C, Gauthier E, Courtine M, Zucker JD, Barsh GS, Saris W, Bruneval P, Basdevant A, Langin D, Clement K (2005). Serum amyloid A: production by human white adipocyte and regulation by obesity and nutrition. *Diabetologia*, Vol.48, No.3, (March 2005) pp. 519-528, PMID 15729583

Poitou C, Coussieu C, Rouault C, Coupaye M, Cancello R, Bedel JF, Gouillon M, Bouillot JL, Oppert JM, Basdevant A, Clément K (2006). Serum amyloid A: a marker of adiposity-induced low-grade inflammation but not of metabolic status. *Obesity (Silver Spring)*, Vol.14, No.2, (February 2006) pp. 309-318, PMID 16571858

Pories WJ (2008). Bariatric surgery: risks and rewards. *The Journal of Clinical Endocrinology & Metabolism*, Vol.93, No.11, S1 (November 2008) pp. S89-S96, PMID 18987275

Premaratna SD, Manickam E, Begg DP, Rayment DJ, Hafandi A, Jois M, Cameron-Smith D, Weisinger RS (2011). Angiotensin-converting enzyme inhibition reverses diet-induced obesity, insulin resistance and inflammation in C57BL/6J mice. *International Journal of Obesity* (*London*) (May 2011) Epub ahead of print, PMID 21556046

Quaye IK (2008). Haptoglobin, inflammation and disease. *Transactions of the Royal Society of Tropical Medicine and Hygiene*, Vol.102, No.8, (August 2008) pp. 735-742, PMID 18486167

Ramanjaneya M, Chen J, Brown JE, Tripathi G, Hallschmid M, Patel S, Kern W, Hillhouse EW, Lehnert H, Tan BK, Randeva HS (2010). Identification of nesfatin-1 in human and murine adipose tissue: a novel depot-specific adipokine with increased levels in obesity. *Endocrinology*, Vol.151, No.7, (July 2010) pp. 3169-3180, PMID 20427481

Rana JS, Arsenault BJ, Despres JP, Cote M, Talmud PJ, Ninio E, Wouter Jukema J, Wareham NJ, Kastelein JJ, Khaw KT, Matthijs Boekholdt S (2011). Inflammatory biomarkers, physical activity, waist circumference, and risk of future coronary heart disease in healthy men and women. *European Heart Journal*, Vol.32, No.3, (February 2011) pp. 336-344, PMID 19224930

Reape TJ, Groot PH (1999). Chemokines and atherosclerosis. *Atherosclerosis*, Vol.147, No.2, (December 1999) pp. 213-225, PMID 10559506

Retnakaran R, Youn BS, Liu Y, Hanley AJ, Lee NS, Park JW, Song ES, Vu V, Kim W, Tungtrongchitr R, Havel PJ, Swarbrick MM, Shaw C, Sweeney G (2008). Correlation of circulating full-length visfatin (PBEF/NAMPT) with metabolic parameters in subjects with and without diabetes: a cross-sectional study. *Clinical Endocrinology*, Vol.69, No.6, (December 2008) pp. 885-893, PMID 18410550

Rodbell M (1964). Localization of lipoprotein lipase in fat cells of rat adipose tissue. *Journal of Biological Chemistry*, Vol. 239, No.3, (March 1964) pp. 753-755, PMID 14154450

Roncon-Albuquerque R Jr, Moreira-Rodrigues M, Faria B, Ferreira AP, Cerqueira C, Lourenço AP, Pestana M, von Hafe P, Leite-Moreira AF (2008). Attenuation of the cardiovascular and metabolic complications of obesity in CD14 knockout mice. *Life Sciences*, Vol. 83, No.13-14, (September 2008) pp. 502-510, PMID 18761356

Rosen BS, Cook KS, Yaglom J, Groves DL, Volanakis JE, Damm D, White T, Spiegelman BM (1989). Adipsin and complement factor D activity: an immune-related defect in obesity. *Science*, Vol.244, No.4911, (June 1989) pp. 1483-1487, PMID 2734615

Rosenson RS, Gelb MH (2009). Secretory phospholipase A2: a multifaceted family of proatherogenic enzymes. *Current Cardiology Reports*, Vol.11, No.6, (November 2009) pp. 445-451, PMID 19863869

Rupnick MA, Panigrahy D, Zhang CY, Dallabrida SM, Lowell BB, Langer R, Folkman MJ (2002). Adipose tissue mass can be regulated through the vasculature. *Proceedings of the National Academy of Sciences United States of America*, Vol.99, No.16, (August 2002) pp. 10730-10735, PMID 12149466

Sacks HS, Fain JN, Cheema P, Bahouth SW, Garrett E, Wolf RY, Wolford D, Samaha J (2011). Depot-specific overexpression of proinflammatory, redox, endothelial cell, and angiogenic genes in epicardial fat adjacent to severe stable coronary atherosclerosis. *Metabolic Syndrome and Related Disorders*, (June 2011) Epub ahead of print, PMID 21679057

Savage DB, Sewter CP, Klenk ES, Segal DG, Vidal-Puig A, Considine RV, O'Rahilly S (2001). Resistin / Fizz3 expression in relation to obesity and peroxisome proliferator-activated receptor-gamma action in humans. *Diabetes*, Vol.50, No.10, (October 2001) pp. 2199-2202, PMID 11574398

Scaglione R, Argano C, di Chiara T, Colomba D, Parrinello G, Corrao S, Avellone G, Licata G (2003). Central obesity and hypertensive renal disease: association between higher levels of BMI, circulating transforming growth factor beta1 and urinary albumin excretion. *Blood Pressure*, Vol.12, No.5-6, pp. 269-276, PMID 14763657

Schaffler A, Neumeier M, Herfarth H, Furst A, Scholmerich J, Buchler C (2005). Genomic structure of human omentin, a new adipocytokine expressed in omental adipose tissue. *Biochimica et Biophysica Acta*, Vol.1732, No.1-3, (December 2005) pp. 96-102, PMID 16386808

Scherzer R, Shen W, Bacchetti P, Kotler D, Lewis CE, Shlipak MG, Heymsfield SB, Grunfeld C; Study of Fat Redistribution Metabolic Change in HIV Infection (FRAM)(2008). Simple anthropometric measures correlate with metabolic risk indicators as strongly as magnetic resonance imaging-measured adipose tissue depots in both HIV-infected and control subjects. *The American Journal of Clinical Nutrition*, Vol.87, No.6, (June 2008) pp. 1809-1817, PMID 18541572

Scriba PC, Bauer M, Emmert D, Fateh-Moghadam A, Hofmann GG, Horn K, Pickardt CR (1979). Effects of obesity, total fasting and re-alimentation on L-thyroxine (T4), 3,5,3'-L-triiodothyronine (T3), 3,3',5'-L-triiodothyronine (rT3), thyroxine binding globulin (TBG), cortisol, thyrotrophin, cortisol binding globulin (CBG), transferrin, alpha 2-haptoglobin and complement C'3 in serum. *Acta Endocrinologica*, Vol.91, No.4, (August 1979) pp. 629-643, PMID 115194

Selva DM, Lecube A, Hernandez C, Baena JA, Fort JM, Simo R (2009). Lower zinc-alpha2-glycoprotein production by adipose tissue and liver in obese patients unrelated to insulin resistance. *The Journal of Clinical Endocrinology & Metabolism*, Vol.94, No.11, (November 2009) pp. 4499-4507, PMID 19622624

Shen W, Punyanitya M, Chen J, Gallagher D, Albu J, Pi-Sunyer X, Lewis CE, Grunfeld C, Heshka S, Heymsfield SB (2006). Waist circumference correlates with metabolic syndrome indicators better than percentage fat. Obesity *(Silver Spring)*, Vol. 14, No.4, (April 2006) pp. 727-736, PMID 16741276

Shi Y, Massague J (2003). Mechanisms of TGF-beta signaling from cell membrane to the nucleus. *Cell*, Vol.113, No.6, (June 2003) pp. 685-700, PMID 12809600

Shibata R, Takahashi R, Kataoka Y, Ohashi K, Ikeda N, Kihara S, Murohara T, Ouchi N (2011). Association of a fat-derived plasma protein omentin with carotid artery intima-media thickness in apparently healthy men. *Hypertension Research*, (August 2011) Epub ahead of print, PMID 21814208

Sjoholm K, Palming J, Olofsson LE, Gummesson A, Svensson PA, Lystig TC, Jennische E, Brandberg J, Torgerson JS, Carlsson B, Carlsson LM (2005). A microarray search for genes predominantly expressed in human omental adipocytes: adipose tissue as a major production site of serum amyloid A. *The Journal of Clinical Endocrinology & Metabolism*, Vol.90, Vol.4, (April 2005) pp. 2233-2239, PMID 15623807

Skurk T, Herder C, Kraft I, Muller-Scholze S, Hauner H, Kolb H (2005). Production and release of macrophage migration inhibitory factor from human adipocytes. *Endocrinology*, Vol.146, No.3, (March 2005) pp. 1006-1011, PMID 15576462

Smirnoff P, Almiral-Seliger D, Schwartz B (2001). Serum leptin levels in the elderly: relationship with gender and nutritional status. *The Journal of Nutrition, Health & Aging*, Vol.5, No.1, pp. 29-32, PMID 11250666

Sommer G, Garten A, Petzold S, Beck-Sickinger AG, Bluher M, Stumvoll M, Fasshauer M (2008). Visfatin/PBEF/Nampt: structure, regulation and potential function of a novel adipokine. *Clinical Science (London)*, Vol.115, No.1, (July 2008) pp. 13-23, PMID 19016657

Stejskal D, Karpisek M, Humenanska V, Hanulova Z, Stejskal P, Kusnierova P, Petzel M (2008). Lipocalin-2: development, analytical characterization, and clinical testing of a new ELISA. *Hormone and Metabolic Research*, Vol.40, No.6, (June 2008) pp. 381-385, PMID 18393169

Steppan CM, Bailey ST, Bhat S, Brown EJ, Banerjee RR, Wright CM, Patel HR, Ahima RS, Lazar MA (2001). The hormone resistin links obesity to diabetes. *Nature*, Vol.409, No.6818, (January 2001) pp. 307-312, PMID 11201732

Straczkowski M, Dzienis-Straczkowska S, Stepien A, Kowalska I, Szelachowska M, Kinalska I (2002). Plasma interleukin-8 concentrations are increased in obese subjects and related to fat mass and tumor necrosis factor-alpha system. *The Journal of Clinical Endocrinology & Metabolism*, Vol.87, No.10, (October 2002) p. 4602-4606, PMID 12364441

Sugarman HJ, Wolfe LG, Sica DA, Clore JN (2003). Diabetes and hypertension in severe obesity and effects of gastric bypass-induced weight loss. *Annals of Surgery*, Vol.237, No.6, (June 2003) pp. 751-756, PMID 12796570

Taes YE, De Bacquer D, De Backer G, Delanghe JR (2005). Haptoglobin and body mass index. *The Journal of Clinical Endocrinology & Metabolism*, Vol.90, No.1, (January 2005) pp. 594, PMID 15643024

Takagaki M, Honke K, Tsukamoto T, Higashiyama S, Taniguchi N, Makita A, Ohkubo I (1994). Zn-alpha 2-glycoprotein is a novel adhesive protein. *Biochemical and Biophysical Research Communications*, Vol.201, No.3, (June 1994) pp. 1339-1347, PMID 8024578

Takahashi K, Ghatei MA, Lam HC, O'Halloran DJ, Bloom SR (1990). Elevated plasma endothelin in patients with diabetes mellitus. *Diabetologia*, Vol.33, No.5, (May 1990) pp. 306-310, PMID 2198188

Taleb S, Clement K (2007). Emerging role of cathepsin S in obesity and its associated diseases. *Clinical Chemistry and Laboratory Medicine*, Vol.45, No.3, (2007) pp. 328-332, PMID 17378727

Tan BK, Adya R, Farhatullah S, Lewandowski KC, O'Hare P, Lehnert H, Randeva HS (2008). Omentin-1, a novel adipokine, is decreased in overweight insulin-resistant women with polycystic ovary syndrome: ex vivo and in vivo regulation of omentin-1 by insulin and glucose. *Diabetes*, Vol.57, No.4, (April 2008) pp. 801-808, PMID 18174521

Tan BK, Adya R, Chen J, Farhatullah S, Heutling D, Mitchell D, Lehnert H, Randeva HS (2009). Metformin decreases angiogenesis via NF-kappaB and Erk1/2/Erk5 pathways by increasing the antiangiogenic thrombospondin-1. *Cardiovascular Research*, Vol.83, No.3, (August 2009) pp. 566-574, PMID 19414528

Tan BK, Hallschmid M, Kern W, Lehnert H, Randeva HS (2011). Decreased cerebrospinal fluid/plasma ratio of the novel satiety molecule, nesfatin-1/NUCB-2, in obese humans: evidence of nesfatin-1/NUCB-2 resistance and implications for obesity treatment. *The Journal of Clinical Endocrinology & Metabolism*, Vol.96, No.4, (April 2011) pp. E669-E673, PMID 21252251

Terra X, Quintero Y, Auguet T, Porras JA, Hernández M, Sabench F, Aguilar C, Luna AM, Del Castillo D, Richart C (2011). Fatty acid binding protein 4 is associated with inflammatory markers and metabolic syndrome in morbidly obese women. *European Journal of Endocrinology*, Vol.164, No.4, (April 2011) pp. 539-547, PMID 21257725

Thomas T, Burguera B, Melton LJ 3rd, Atkinson EJ, O'Fallon WM, Riggs BL, Khosla S (2000). Relationship of serum leptin levels with body composition and sex steroid and insulin levels in men and women. *Metabolism*, Vol.49, No.10, (October 2000) pp. 1278-1284, PMID 11079816

Thorne A, Lonnqvist F, Apelman J, Hellers G, Arner P (2002). A pilot study of long-term effects of a novel obesity treatment: omentectomy in connection with adjustable gastric banding. *International Journal of Obesity and Related Metabolic Disorders*, Vol.26, No.2, (February 2002) pp. 193-199, PMID 11850750

Trujillo ME, Scherer PE (2005). Adiponectin--journey from an adipocyte secretory protein to biomarker of the metabolic syndrome. *Journal of Internal Medicine*, Vol.257, No.2, (February 2005) pp. 167-175, PMID 15656875

Tsuchiya T, Shimizu H, Yamada M, Osaki A, Oh-I S, Ariyama Y, Takahashi H, Okada S, Hashimoto K, Satoh T, Kojima M, Mori M (2010). Fasting concentrations of nesfatin-1 are negatively correlated with body mass index in non-obese males. *Clinical Endocrinology*, Vol.73, No.4, (October 2010) pp. 484-490, PMID 20550530

Tsuji S, Uehori J, Matsumoto M, Suzuki Y, Matsuhisa A, Toyoshima K, Seya T (2001). Human intelectin is a novel soluble lectin that recognizes galactofuranose in carbohydrate chains of bacterial cell wall. *Journal of Biological Chemistry*, Vol.276, No.26, (June 2001) pp. 23456-23463, PMID 11313366

van Dielen FM, van't Veer C, Schols AM, Soeters PB, Buurman WA, Greve JW (2001). Increased leptin concentrations correlate with increased concentrations of inflammatory markers in morbidly obese individuals. *International Journal of Obesity and Related Metabolic Disorders*, Vol.25, No.12, (December 2001) pp. 1759-1766, PMID 11781755

van Harmelen V, Elizalde M, Ariapart P, Bergstedt-Lindqvist S, Reynisdottir S, Hoffstedt J, Lundkvist I, Bringman S, Arner P (2000). The association of human adipose angiotensinogen gene expression with abdominal fat distribution in obesity. *International Journal of Obesity and Related Metabolic Disorders*, Vol.24, No.6, (June 2000) pp. 673-678, PMID 10878672

van Harmelen V, Eriksson A, Astrom G, Wahlen K, Naslund E, Karpe F, Frayn K, Olsson T, Andersson J, Ryden M, Arner P (2008). Vascular peptide endothelin-1 links fat accumulation with alterations of visceral adipocyte lipolysis. *Diabetes*, Vol.57, No.2, (February 2008) pp. 378-386, PMID 18025413

Varma V, Yao-Borengasser A, Bodles AM, Rasouli N, Phanavanh B, Nolen GT, Kern EM, Nagarajan R, Spencer HJ 3rd, Lee MJ, Fried SK, McGehee RE Jr, Peterson CA, Kern PA (2008). Thrombospondin-1 is an adipokine associated with obesity, adipose inflammation, and insulin resistance. *Diabetes*, Vol.57, No.2, (February 2008) pp. 432-439, PMID 18057090

Venuraju SM, Yerramasu A, Corder R, Lahiri (2010). Osteoprotegerin as a predictor of coronary artery disease and cardiovascular mortality and morbidity. *Journal of the American College of Cardiology*, Vol.55, No.19, (May 2010) pp. 2049-2061, PMID 20447527

Verschuren L, Kooistra T, Bernhagen J, Voshol PJ, Ouwens DM, van Erk M, de Vries-van der Weij J, Leng L, van Bockel JH, van Dijk KW, Fingerle-Rowson G, Bucala R, Kleemann R (2009). MIF deficiency reduces chronic inflammation in white adipose tissue and impairs the development of insulin resistance, glucose intolerance, and associated atherosclerotic disease. *Circulation Research*, Vol.105, No.1, (July 2009) pp. 99-107, PMID 19478200

Volanakis JE, Narayana SV (1996). Complement factor D, a novel serine protease. *Protein Science*, Vol.5, No.4, (April 1996) pp. 553-564, PMID 8845746

Vozarova B, Weyer C, Hanson K, Tataranni PA, Bogardus C, Pratley RE (2001). Circulating interleukin-6 in relation to adiposity, insulin action, and insulin secretion. *Obesity Research*, Vol.9, No.7, (July 2001) pp. 414-417, PMID 11445664

Wallenius V, Wallenius K, Ahren B, Rudling M, Carlsten H, Dickson SL, Ohlsson C, Jansson JO (2002). Interleukin-6-deficient mice develop mature-onset obesity. *Nature Medicine*, Vol.8, No.1, (January 2002) pp. 75-79, PMID 11786910

Wang H, Eckel RH (2009). Lipoprotein lipase: from gene to obesity. *American Journal of Physiology Endocrinology and Metabolism*, Vol.297, No.2, (August 2009) pp. E271-E288, PMID 19318514

Wang Y, Lam KS, Kraegen EW, Sweeney G, Zhang J, Tso AW, Chow WS, Wat NM, Xu JY, Hoo RL, Xu A (2007). Lipocalin-2 is an inflammatory marker closely associated with obesity, insulin resistance, and hyperglycemia in humans. *Clinical Chemistry*, Vol.53, No.1, (January 2007) pp. 34-41, PMID 17040956

Weisberg SP, McCann D, Desai M, Rosenbaum M, Leibel RL, Ferrante AW Jr (2003). Obesity is associated with macrophage accumulation in adipose tissue. *Journal of Clinical Investigation*, Vol.112, No.12, (December 2003), pp. 1796-1808, PMID 14679176

Weyer C, Yudkin JS, Stehouwer CD, Schalkwijk CG, Pratley RE, Tataranni PA (2002). Humoral markers of inflammation and endothelial dysfunction in relation to adiposity and in vivo insulin action in Pima Indians. *Atherosclerosis*, Vol.161, No.1, (March 2002) pp. 233-242, PMID 11882337

Wrackmeyer U, Hansen GH, Seya T, Danielsen EM (2006). Intelectin: a novel lipid raft-associated protein in the enterocyte brush border. *Biochemistry*, Vol.45, No.30, (August 2006) pp. 9188-9197, PMID 16866365

Wu H, Ghosh S, Perrard XD, Feng L, Garcia GE, Perrard JL, Sweeney JF, Peterson LE, Chan L, Smith CW, Ballantyne CM (2007). T-cell accumulation and regulated on activation, normal T cell expressed and secreted upregulation in adipose tissue in obesity. *Circulation*, Vol.115, No.8, (February 2007) pp. 1029-1038, PMID 17296858

Xu A, Tso AW, Cheung BM, Wang Y, Wat NM, Fong CH, Yeung DC, Janus ED, Sham PC, Lam KS (2007). Circulating adipocyte-fatty acid binding protein levels predict the development of the metabolic syndrome: a 5-year prospective study. *Circulation*, Vol.115, No.12, (March 2007) pp. 1537-1543, PMID 17389279

Xu H, Barnes GT, Yang Q, Tan G, Yang D, Chou CJ, Sole J, Nichols A, Ross JS, Tartaglia LA, Chen H (2003). Chronic inflammation in fat plays a crucial role in the development of obesity-related insulin resistance. *Journal of Clinical Investigation*, Vol.112, No.12, (December 2003) pp. 1821-1830, PMID 14679177

Yadav H, Quijano C, Kamaraju AK, Gavrilova O, Malek R, Chen W, Zerfas P, Zhigang D, Wright EC, Stuelten C, Sun P, Lonning S, Skarulis M, Sumner AE, Finkel T, Rane SG (2011). Protection from obesity and diabetes by blockade of TGF-β/Smad3 signaling. *Cell Metabolism*, Vol.14, No.1, (July 2011) pp. 67-79, PMID 21723505

Yan P, Liu d, Long M, Ren Y, Pang J, Li R (2011). Changes of serum omentin levels and relationship between omentin and adiponectin concentrations in type 2 diabetes mellitus. *Experimental and Clinical Endocrinology & Diabetes*, Vol.119, No.4, (April 2011) pp. 257-263, PMID 21374544

Yan QW, Yang Q, Mody N, Graham TE, Hsu CH, Xu Z, Houstis NE, Kahn BB, Rosen ED (2007). The adipokine lipocalin 2 is regulated by obesity and promotes insulin resistance. *Diabetes*, Vol.56, No.10, (October 2007) pp. 2533-2540, PMID 17639021

Yang Q, Graham TE, Mody N, Preitner F, Peroni OD, Zabolotny JM, Kotani K, Quadro L, Kahn BB (2005). Serum retinol binding protein 4 contributes to insulin resistance in obesity and type 2 diabetes. *Nature*, Vol.436, No.7049, (July 2005) pp. 356-362, PMID 16034410

Yang RZ, Lee MJ, Hu H, Pollin TI, Ryan AS, Nicklas BJ, Snitker S, Horenstein RB, Hull K, Goldberg NH, Goldberg AP, Shuldiner AR, Fried SK, Gong DW (2006a). Acute-phase serum amyloid A: an inflammatory adipokine and potential link between obesity and its metabolic complications. *Public Library of Science Medicine*, Vol.3, No.6, (June 2006), pp. 884-894, PMID 16737350

Yang RZ, Lee MJ, Hu H, Pray J, Wu HB, Hansen BC, Shuldiner AR, Fried SK, McLenithan JC, Gong DW (2006b). Identification of omentin as a novel depot-specific adipokine in human adipose tissue: possible role in modulating insulin action. *American Journal of Physiology Endocrinology and Metabolism*, Vol.290, No.6, (June 2006) pp. E1253-E1261, PMID 16531507

Yang X, Deignan JL, Qi H, Zhu J, Qian S, Zhong J, Torosyan G, Majid S, Falkard B, Kleinhanz RR, Karlsson J, Castellani LW, Mumick S, Wang K, Xie T, Coon M, Zhang C, Estrada-Smith D, Farber CR, Wang SS, van Nas A, Ghazalpour A, Zhang B, Macneil DJ, Lamb JR, Dipple KM, Reitman ML, Mehrabian M, Lum PY, Schadt EE, Lusis AJ, Drake TA (2009). Validation of candidate causal genes for obesity that affect shared metabolic pathways and networks. *Nature Genetics*, Vol.41, No.4, (April 2009) pp. 415-423, PMID 19270708

Yao-Borengasser A, Varma V, Bodles AM, Rasouli N, Phanavanh B, Lee MJ, Starks T, Kern LM, Spencer HJ 3rd, Rashidi AA, McGehee RE Jr, Fried SK, Kern PA (2007). Retinol binding protein 4 expression in humans: relationship to insulin resistance, inflammation, and response to pioglitazone. *The Journal of Clinical Endocrinology & Metabolism*, Vol.92, No.7, (July 2007) pp. 2590-2597, PMID 17595259

Yudkin JS (2007). Inflammation, obesity, and the metabolic syndrome. *Hormone and Metabolic Research*, Vol.39, No.10, (October 2007) pp. 707-709, PMID 17952830

Yudkin JS, Stehouwer CD, Emeis JJ, Coppack SW (1999). C-reactive protein in healthy subjects: associations with obesity, insulin resistance, and endothelial dysfunction: a potential role for cytokines originating from adipose tissue? *Arteriosclerosis, Thrombosis, and Vascular Biology*, Vol.19, No.4, (April 1999) pp. 972-978, PMID 10195925

Yudkin JS, Kumari M, Humphries SE, Mohamed-Ali V (2000). Inflammation, obesity, stress and coronary heart disease: is interleukin-6 the link? *Atherosclerosis*, Vol.148, No.2, (February 2000) pp. 209-214, PMID 10657556

Zeyda M, Farmer D, Todoric J, Aszmann O, Speiser M, Gyori G, Zlabinger GJ, Stulnig TM (2007). Human adipose tissue macrophages are of an anti-inflammatory phenotype but capable of excessive pro-inflammatory mediator production. *International Journal of Obesity (London)*, Vol.31, No.9, (September 2007) pp. 1420-1428, PMID 17593905

Zhang J, Wu Y, Zhang Y, Leroith D, Bernlohr DA, Chen X (2008). The role of lipocalin 2 in the regulation of inflammation in adipocytes and macrophages. *Molecular Endocrinology*, Vol.22, No.6, (June 2008) pp. 1416-1426, PMID 18292240

Zhang Y, Proenca R, Maffei M, Barone M, Leopold L, Friedman JM (1994). Positional cloning of the mouse obese gene and its human homologue. *Nature*, Vol.372, No.6505, (December 1994) pp. 425-432, PMID 7984236

Zhu N, Pankow JS, Ballantyne CM, Couper D, Hoogeveen RC, Pereira M, Duncan BB, Schmidt MI (2010). High-molecular-weight adiponectin and the risk of type 2 diabetes in the ARIC study. *The Journal of Clinical Endocrinology & Metabolism*, Vol.95, No.11, (November 2010) pp. 5097-5104, PMID 20719834

3

The Economic Impact of Bariatric Surgery

Anke-Peggy Holtorf[1,2], Harald Rinde[2], Frederic Rupprecht[3],
Henry Alder[3] and Diana Brixner[1]
[1]*University of Utah,*
[2]*BioBridge Strategies LLC,*
[3]*Ethicon Endosurgery*
[1, 3]*USA,*
[2]*Switzerland*

1. Introduction

It is estimated that 5.7% of American adults, or approximately 14.5 million people, are morbidly obese, defined as a body mass index (BMI) of >40 kg/m^2 and thus are eligible for bariatric surgery. (Flegal et al. 2010) If in one year, only 10% of these morbidly obese patients (approximately 1.45 Million) would undergo bariatric surgery, with an average expenditure of approximately $20,000, this would result in a total cost of US$ 29 billion. This amount is equivalent to about 1% of the total healthcare expenditure in the USA.(National Health Expenditure Data 2011) This estimate most likely underestimates the potential cost because the obesity epidemic is still growing in the USA, which has an obesity rate of over 30%.(Aasheim and Søvik 2011; Finucane et al. 2011; Flegal et al. 2010; Shao and Chin 2011) Because of the potentially significant impact on overall healthcare expenditures, policy makers and payers are very careful to allow free access to bariatric surgery for all severely or morbidly obese patients. In addition to appraising the impact on the future health status of morbidly obese patients, payers and decision makers want to be able to estimate the impact of bariatric surgery on their budgets and resources as well as to understand the potential return on such an investment. To determine the most recent knowledge on the economic consequences relating to bariatric surgery for payers in different healthcare settings, a literature review of economic or outcome publications was conducted and is summarized in this book chapter.

Short-term cost is often a major barrier to payers and other interested parties. Understanding the full cost consequences of bariatric surgery includes consideration and comparison of both conventional treatment and surgery for morbid obesity against the associated overall health outcome. This information is needed to make rational decisions. Nonsurgical approaches to weight loss, however, are often requested or even reimbursed before agreeing to surgery - despite the fact that the impact of these therapies has been shown to be modest and short term for most patients. (Bockelbrink et al. 2008; Picot et al. 2009; Li et al. 2005; Snow et al. 2005) To allow a rational decision, it is important to assess how bariatric surgery impacts health outcomes in comparison to the best existing alternatives and how much total expenditure is generated by bariatric surgery in comparison to the alternative approaches to weight loss.

1.1 Short introduction to health economics

This section gives a brief introduction to health economics relevant to this chapter. Those familiar with health economics can skip this introduction.

Cost-effectiveness analysis is an attempt to answer the question: *"How much more (than today) are we willing pay for an improvement in health outcomes?"* Improvements in health outcomes include a gain of life years, a reduction of disability or an improvement in the quality of life. In the cost-utility analysis, clinical and humanistic parameters are combined as quality adjusted life years (QALY) and the cost to improve the outcome by one QALY is calculated. (Berger and International Society for Pharmacoeconomics and Outcomes Research 2003)

A QALY is a measure of additional life-time gained by a medical intervention (which could be a drug, surgery, diagnostic, etc.) adjusted by the utility or quality of life of the patients. The utility is evaluated through standardized and validated questionnaires (which can be general quality of life questionnaires or tailored to specific diseases) and quantified by *health utilities* or *quality of life indices*. These range from 1, a perfect state of health, to 0, equivalent to death. QALYs are determined by multiplying the number of additional life years by the health utilities (for example, 4 years with a utility of 0.75 = 3 QALYs). Cost-utility analysis allows comparing a broad range of healthcare interventions for their cost-utility and consequently help setting healthcare investment priorities. The incremental cost-effectiveness or cost-utility ratios (ICER or ICUR) how much more has to be spent for a new technology over the comparator (usually the current standard of care) to achieve one additional QALY. (Berger and International Society for Pharmacoeconomics and Outcomes Research 2003)

Authorities in some countries, such as UK, Canada, Australia and Sweden, are using the incremental cost per QALY for making decisions on the degree of reimbursement for interventions. Theoretically, interventions achieving improved outcomes at lower total healthcare cost are dominant and should be used and reimbursed; interventions with a worse outcome at higher cost should never be reimbursed. For technologies which result in increased cost but produce better outcomes, there should be an agreed upon threshold of acceptable cost per QALY or cost-utility ratios. This threshold varies and is subject of many discussions, but usually lies around 1 to 3 times the gross domestic product per capita. (Landa 2008; Shiroiwa et al. 2010) Technologies with higher cost per QALY should not be reimbursed as a general rule. However, other factors are also taken into consideration when deciding whether to reimburse or not (e.g. local economy, culture, ethics, innovation factor, budget impact, others). In other countries, such as the USA, France or Germany, the cost per QALY is not generally considered a key decision criterion. In these countries, cost-effectiveness or budget impact over a limited time period might be considered more important by payer decision makers.

Another way to estimate the value of bariatric surgery is to calculate the return on investment (ROI). ROI is a measure used to evaluate the efficiency of the investment in the surgery and is calculated for a defined time span by dividing the net financial gain (dollars gained from surgery minus the cost of surgery) by the cost of surgery.

2. Economic outcomes of bariatric surgery

The general agreement is that patients with a BMI>40 kg/m^2, or with a BMI>35 kg/m^2 and a serious obesity-related comorbidity, who have failed to respond to conservative treatment (diet, exercise, pharmacology) are eligible for bariatric surgery. Despite this, less than 2% of these patients actually are offered or choose bariatric surgery. (Kim, White, and Buffington 2010) A core question to payers before extending access to bariatric surgery will be what impact the increased use of bariatric surgery will have on their overall budgets. (Powers, Rehrig, and Jones 2007)

2.1 Cost associated with obesity and bariatric surgery

The key cost components of obesity are:

- The need for ongoing dietary and behavioral interventions.
- Treatment of the health consequences of obesity such as type 2 diabetes and cardiovascular disease.
- Decreased work productivity.
- Increased overall cost of living (e.g., additional services needed because of decreased mobility, adaptation of articles of daily use or furniture, etc.).

The substantial health and quality of life benefits of decreased weight have been described in other chapters in this book. The question is whether the decreased costs of obesity listed above offset the cost of bariatric surgery, which is perceived as a costly procedure. The key cost components of surgery are (1) the surgical procedure and the associated hospital stay, (2) potentially serious short term and long term complications (e.g. surgical risk, food intolerance and micronutrient deficiencies, surgery related mortality), (3) supportive care services and treatments, and if necessary, potential reversal surgery.

2.1.1 Cost of obesity

Many studies have shown that obesity is associated with increased mortality, decreased quality of life, increased disability, and increased healthcare costs. (Finkelstein et al. 2009; Pendergast et al. 2010; Cawley 2010) The amount of this increase is different across different countries as shown by the following studies. Finkelstein et al estimated obesity-related diseases to account for $147 billion in the USA in 2006. The same study showed that the rate of obesity in the US increased by 37% from 1998 to 2006 with an increase of 89% in money spent on obesity-related diseases. This resulted in an increase from 6.5% to 9.1% of the total US healthcare budget spent on obesity and obesity related diseases. Finkelstein et al. calculated the adult annual per capita medical spending attributable to obesity (compared to a normal weight population) was $1,429 (42% higher than non-obese cost per capita). (Finkelstein et al. 2009) Significantly higher estimates of increased healthcare spending due to obesity were obtained by Pendergast et al. who calculated the annualized healthcare utilization costs for the US and Germany and found that in the US obese patients spent 73% more than non-obese people ($4,780 more) and 59% more in Germany ($1,035 more). (Pendergast et al. 2010) Cawley et al. estimated that obesity raises annual medical costs by $2,826 (2005 dollars) per obese patient and that the total annual cost of treating obesity in the US adult non-institutionalized population was $168 billion, or 16.5% of national spending on medical care. (Cawley 2010) Future trends exacerbate the problem.

2.1.2 Cost of bariatric surgery

2.1.2.1 Cost of surgery procedure

The cost of bariatric surgery has been estimated in several countries and from diverse perspectives. A summary of the cost estimates is listed in Table 1. For example for laparoscopic gastric banding (LAGB) the reported cost of surgery ranges from US$7,125 in the UK to US$25,000 in the US. The total short and long term cost of obesity or bariatric surgery is influenced by several factors, such as the cost of the intervention, the cost of adaptations (e.g. band adjustment) adverse events, reversals, nutritional supplements, secondary health-related cost such as treating the consequences of the fast and extensive weight loss, and cost of the general supportive care (e.g., dietary, educational, psychosocial). There is high variability amongst the existing studies as to which cost had been considered. A study in the UK estimated the immediate direct medical cost in the first year of LAGB to be £4,750 ($7,125). In this study, conventional obesity therapy was calculated to be £336 (US$500) in the first year. (Clegg et al. 2002) A year later, the same authors compared the direct medical cost of two types of surgery by calculating the direct medical cost over 20 years (£10,795 for LAGB and £9,627 for vertical gastric banding (VBG)[1]) with conventional care (£6,964). (Clegg et al. 2002)

Some cost factors that have strongly affected the surgery-related cost for gastric banding in the early years, e.g. regular readjustment of the gastric band in the hospital, have been decreasing with greater experience and further development of the technology. Increasingly, the adjustments can now be performed during the regular visits in the outpatient setting, without the need for high cost hospital interventions. (Jan et al. 2007)

2.1.2.2 Cost offset of usual care for those not receiving surgery

It is crucial to consider, in addition to the immediate intervention-related cost, the cost from the longer-term consequences of obesity, such as type 2 diabetes mellitus, hypertension, cardiovascular diseases and increased cancer risk, in addition to reduced work productivity. For example, Ackroyd et al. published a model for bariatric surgery projected over five years for patients with type 2 diabetes in UK, France or Germany. (Ackroyd et al. 2006) The five-year cost of adjustable gastric banding in Germany was €13,610, in UK €12,838 (£9,072) and in France €14,796. While in UK the five-year direct medical cost of conventional care was lower than the surgical interventions (£7,080 equivalent to €10,030), in both Germany and France the cost for usual care exceeded that of the surgical interventions (€17,197 and €19,267 respectively). This modelling study focused on patients with diabetes and incorporated all direct medical cost from third party payers' perspective. Thus, the conventional treatment cost not only included the cost for diet and exercise therapy but also the treatment of comorbidities and office visits during the five-year time frame in this patient segment (see Table 1). This model was based on the conservative assumption that the length of stay after LAGB would be five days. In newer research, this time is much shorter (Jan et al. 2007). This means that this study probably overestimates the cost of LAGB.

---

[1] £10,000 would be equivalent to €15'800 or US$15,000

Publication	Data Year	Cost	Country
Salem, 2008	2004	$16,200	USA
Paxton, 2005	Before 2005	$17,660 - $29,443	USA
Livingston, 2005	2001/2002	$19,794 - $23,355	USA
Ikramuddin, 2009	2007	$19,760	USA
Hoerger, 2010	2005	$15,536 - $20,326	USA
Chang, 2011	2010	$23,778 - $64,784	USA
Clegg, 2003	Before 2001	£9,627 - £10,795	UK
Ackroyd, 2006	1998-2003	£7,088 - £9,121	UK
Ackroyd, 2006	1998-2003	€12,166 - €17,197	GER
Ackroyd, 2006	1998-2003	€13,399 - €19,276	FRA

Table 1. Summary of publications reporting cost of bariatric surgery.

Salem et al calculated the three-year cost of LAGB at US$16,200 and for Roux-en-Y gastric bypass (RYGB) at US$27,560, based on 2004 hospital charges associated with the surgery, including procedural fees, treatment of postoperative complications, follow-up care, and treatment of obesity-related diseases, such as coronary heart disease, stroke, type 2 diabetes, hypercholesterolemia, and hypertension.

More recent publications estimate an additional cost of US$15,000 – US$20,000 over the 32-38 years after surgery. (Ikramuddin et al. 2009; Hoerger et al. 2010) Chang et al differentiated between patients with obesity related diseases (ORD) and those without ORDs and analyzed the cost for three BMI classes, BMI above 35 and below 40, BMI between 40 and 50, and BMI above 50kg/m^2. (Chang, Stoll, and Colditz 2011) Bariatric surgery in patients without ORDs incurred higher incremental cost over conventional therapy than in patient who had ORDs. In addition, the authors found that the incremental cost diminished with increasing BMI. This may be explained by the positive impact of bariatric surgery on ORDs, which lead to a prevention of costs related to the ORDs. On the other hand, higher BMI is a risk factor for developing ORDs and therefore, the total incremental cost of bariatric surgery as compared to non-surgery decreases with higher BMI.

2.2 Cost and outcomes of bariatric surgery depending on the hospital's experience

The more experienced the care team is the lower the cost of bariatric surgery. Nguyen et al compared bariatric surgery (Roux-en-Y gastric bypass) performed at low volume hospitals (less than 50 procedures per year) with high volume hospitals (more than 100 procedures per year). They found that high volume hospitals had shorter length of stay (3.8 days vs. 5.1 days for low volume hospitals), lower overall complications (10.2% vs. 14.5%) and lower cost ($10,292 vs. $13,908), (Nguyen 2004) which was driven to a large extent by the shorter hospital stay. The reduction of time in the hospital depends on the success rate of surgery and the avoidance of complications. (Encinosa 2009) Since hospital cost is a major driver in the overall cost of surgery, a reduction in the length of stay leads to an improved cost-effectiveness ratio.

Increased improvement in the efficiency of surgery will improve the cost-utility ratio. For example, Jan et al. found in their retrospective analysis of data of a US hospital (in the high volume or Center of Excellence category) an average length of stay for LAGB of 1.1 days, while the time assumed in earlier models, or in studies integrating both open and laparoscopic adjustable gastric bypass, was more than 3 times as much. (Jan et al. 2007) As in the example of Ackroyd's analysis of surgery for diabetic patients, better patient profiling may also improve the cost-effectiveness ratio with improved targeting of the intervention and consequently, improved outcomes. (Ayckrod 2006)

2.3 Cost-effectiveness of bariatric surgery

When assessing the cost impact of bariatric surgery, it is important to compare the surgery related cost versus the cost consequences of obesity over time. The resulting cost difference can be assessed in relation to the desired outcomes, such as the length of life and the health related quality of life of the patients.

Ikramuddin et al. prospectively collected outcomes data in a practical real-life setting from 567 obese patients with type 2 diabetes that underwent Roux-en-Y gastric by-pass surgery between 2001 and 2007 at the University of Minnesota Medical Center, Minneapolis. The data was entered into a health economic model (CORE Model). (Ikramuddin et al. 2009) In the model, the patient data was compared to a standard population of obese diabetic patients based on data obtained from the United Kingdom Prospective Diabetes Study (UKPDS), and the Framingham Heart Study. (Palmer et al. 2004a,b) At baseline, the patients were on average 50.1 years old, had a mean duration of diabetes or pre-diabetes of 8.7 years and 77.9% were female. The model projected cost and outcome over a time period of 35 years and predicted that, after discounting cost and outcomes, patients that had bariatric surgery would on average live 11.54 years (undiscounted 15.94 years), while those only treated with conservative medical intervention would survive on average 10.87 years (undiscounted 14.66 years). In addition, the patients undergoing bariatric surgery would experience a better quality of life as measured by standardized quality of life questionnaires. Therefore, the model estimated a significant increase in QALYs by 0.9 to 6.78 compared to 5.88 QALYs achieved by conservative medical treatment. The model projected cost savings from bariatric surgery in the areas of patient management of type 2 diabetes (screening procedures, medication), cardiovascular disease, renal complications, while additional costs were incurred by the surgery. The overall incremental cost-effectiveness was estimated to be US$ 21,973 per QALY, which would generally be accepted as cost-effective. The incremental cost per life year gained was US$ 29,676. It is important to note that the degree of cost-effectiveness was strongly dependent on the long-term perspective and on the estimated improvement in quality of life. The highest costs in both cohorts were those associated with cardiovascular disease (CVD), which were higher for the medical-management cohort ($37,824) than for the bariatric surgery cohort ($34,811) and represented an 8% decrease in CVD-related costs. Limitations of this study were that the model was extrapolated far beyond the time frame of the prospective data collection and that instead of collecting comparative control data these were extrapolated from previous UK studies. In sensitivity analyses, shortening the time horizon to 5 and 10 years and excluding the negative impact of increased body mass index on the patient's quality of life had the greatest adverse impact on the ICERs (i.e. higher cost per QALY). (Ikramuddin et al. 2009)

Chang and his collaborators used a model for a representative US population (National Health and Nutrition Examination Survey III/NHANES III) and retrieved clinical and quality of life outcomes data from a meta-analysis. They gave a preference to newer data because the outcomes of bariatric surgery have greatly improved over the last 20 years. (Chang, Stoll, and Colditz 2011) Bariatric surgery was cost-effective for obese people with BMI greater than 35 kg/m^2, with a cost per incremental QALY of less than US$4,000. It was also cost-saving for patients with a BMI greater than 50 kg/m^2 with one or more obesity-related comorbidity before surgery. Even for patients with a BMI above 30kg/m^2, the cost per incremental QALY was only US$1,222 for patients without comorbidities or US$2,926 if they had comorbidities. If the willingness-to-pay-threshold is assumed to be US$40-60,000 per QALY the results of this analysis support a broader use of bariatric surgery.

In all studies, bariatric surgery remained cost-effective in the eligible patient group. Differences could be seen among subgroups.

2.3.1 BMI level

Craig et al. showed decreasing cost per QALY with increasing BMI. (Craig and Tseng 2002) That means that the more obese patients are the more value they can get from the surgery. This is probably connected to the risk of comorbidities increasing with higher BMI. Similarly, Chang et al used a model to analyze the cost-utility ratio in different BMI groups. (Chang, Stoll, and Colditz 2011) While the surgery intervention was cost-effective for all levels of BMI above 35kg/m^2, the cost-utility ratio decreased with increasing BMI (over 35kg/m^2, over 40kg/m^2, over 50kg/m^2).

2.3.2 Gender

Salem et al. published an analysis of lifetime cost and incremental cost-utility for men and women from two laparoscopic bariatric surgery techniques as compared to conventional therapy. The incremental cost-utility for men aged 35 and a BMI of 40 or over was US$11,604 per incremental QALY for laparoscopic adjustable gastric banding (LAGB) while for women it was US$8,878. For Roux-en-Y gastric bypass (RYGB) the cost per incremental QALY was US$18,543 for men and US$14,680/QALY for women. (Salem et al. 2008)

2.3.3 Cost-effectiveness for obese patients with BMI over 35 and type 2 diabetes

As already mentioned in the previous discussion, a large proportion of the potential savings induced by bariatric surgery is due to the reduction in comorbidities. The reduction of medical needs and degree of remission in type 2 diabetes from bariatric surgery is best supported by data. It is, therefore, no surprise that the favourable cost-effectiveness of bariatric surgery becomes most apparent for morbidly obese patients with type 2 diabetes.

In a study conducted in Italy, Austria and Spain, a cost-effectiveness and budget impact model was used to estimate the resource utilization and cost of adjustable gastric banding and gastric bypass vs. conventional treatment in patients with a BMI ≥ 35 kg/m^2 and type 2 diabetes. (Anselmino et al. 2009) In all scenarios analyzed for Italy and Austria, over a time span of 5 years, both procedures turned out to be cost-saving versus conventional treatment. In Spain there was incremental overall cost associated with both surgical interventions when compared to conventional treatment, but remained cost-effective even in the worst case scenario. Ackroyd et al. showed savings in addition to improved outcomes (QALYs) from bariatric surgery in German and French patients with type 2 diabetes. (Ackroyd et al. 2006)

An American group used the Center of Disease Control (CDC)-RTI Diabetes Cost-Effectiveness Markov Simulation Model to estimate the overall cost of gastric bypass or gastric banding surgery relative to conventional therapy throughout disease progression (from diagnosis of type 2 diabetes to either death or age 95 years). (Hoerger et al. 2010) The model also simulated diabetes-related complications on three microvascular disease paths (nephropathy, neuropathy, and retinopathy) and two macrovascular disease paths (coronary heart disease and stroke) and of remission and relapse of type 2 diabetes. Both surgical alternatives remained cost-effective in all scenarios but did not achieve cost-saving in this US based model. Gastric bypass surgery resulted in US$7,000/QALY for patients with BMI > 35 and newly diagnosed type 2 diabetes and US$12,000/QALY for those with diabetes existing for a longer time. Similarly, gastric banding surgery resulted in US$11,000/QALY and US$13,000/QALY for the respective groups. With this cost-effectiveness range, both surgical alternatives remained below the typical cost-effectiveness of current anti-diabetic medications. (Hoerger et al. 2010) As an example, intensive glycemic and lipid control in comparison to conventional risk factor control have been shown to have incremental cost effectiveness ratio of US$41,384/QALY for patients with BMI > 35 and newly diagnosed diabetes and US$51,889/QALY for those with diabetes existing for a longer time. (CDC Diabetes Cost Effectiveness Group 2002)

A study was conducted in seven Blue Cross/Blue Shield health care plans. It was a retrospective time-series study of patients who had undergone bariatric surgery and had evidence of preoperative diabetes based on medication use. The authors concluded that bariatric surgery was associated with a reduction of 98% in the total use of medication and in a reduction of overall health care costs in patients with type 2 diabetes. They, therefore, recommended that health insurers should cover bariatric surgery because of its health and cost benefits. (Makary et al. 2010)

Another retrospective US database analysis by Klein and collaborators compared the economic impact between two matched cohorts of obese patients (BMI > 35) with type 2 diabetes with or without bariatric surgery. In this database all types of bariatric surgery before 2004 were recorded under the same code. (Klein et al. 2011) Between 2004 and 2007, 65% of the procedures were performed as laparoscopic interventions, and by 2007 they reached 94% of all bariatric surgeries. Approximately half of these were gastric banding procedures. The authors found that in the latter years, on average it took 29 months (range 21-38) to fully recoup the cost of open surgery (US$ 28,845) and 26 months (range 20-32) for the cost of laparoscopic procedures (US$ 19,124). While in the no surgery control group, the rate of diabetes diagnosis or prescription claims fell to approximately 80%, it dropped to around 25% in the surgery group. In addition, medication supply cost slightly increased in the control group and it dropped by 80% in the surgery group, and remained stable throughout 36 months after surgery. (Klein et al. 2011)

Because of the strong clinical evidence the International Diabetes Federation (IDF) in 2011 officially published a consensus statement supporting the positive impact of bariatric surgery on clinical and economic diabetes related outcomes. Consequently, IDF called for National guidelines for bariatric surgery in patients with type 2 diabetes and a BMI of 35 kg $/m^2$ or more to be developed and promoted. (J B Dixon et al. 2011)

In a recent discussion of existing evidence, Villamizar suggested that due to both the positive clinical and economic impact to extend the eligibility criteria for bariatric surgery in the diabetic population even further to include patients a BMI of 30 kg $/m^2$ or above. (Villamizar and Pryor 2011) Health plans and other budget holders would have to expect increased short term cost, with a negative impact on their short term financial resources, and savings would only be expected two to three years after surgery. This may be one reason why payer organizations hesitate to give better access to bariatric surgery for all patients eligible per guideline definitions.

2.4 Comparison of types of surgery

After conservative weight reduction attempts failed and a decision to perform bariatric surgery has been made, there are different methodological approaches to bariatric surgery, which have been presented and discussed in other chapters of this book. Each intervention has advantages or disadvantages for specific patient groups. The three currently most used methods are gastric bypass surgery[2], adjustable gastric banding[3], and sleeve gastrectomy[4]. The individual patient profile (e.g. eating habits, BMI, general health, readiness to assume risk, eagerness for fast results) should be considered when making the decision for the most suitable surgical type. From the patient's perspective, the surgery center's capabilities and historical success rates in the specific type of surgery are important factors to consider.

There is sufficient evidence to support offering a choice of procedures and making the decision together with the patient. The choice depends on his or her risk profile, eating habits, BMI, psychosocial situation, and personal preferences (Table 2 and Fig. 1). When performed in a surgical center experienced in obesity care, bariatric surgery usually achieves the goals of obesity therapy with acceptable low risk of surgery-related complications. In addition, Encinosa et al. were able to show in a retrospective insurance claims data analysis in the USA that the use of laparoscopy reduced total healthcare costs by 12%, while gastric banding decreased costs by 20%. Laparoscopy had no impact on readmissions; the increase in banding without bypass reduced readmissions. (Encinosa 2009).

In the USA, laparoscopic gastric bypass and laparoscopic gastric banding are currently the two most commonly performed operations for the treatment of morbid obesity, (Hinojosa et al. 2009) although sleeve gastrectomy is increasingly used as an effective method of bariatric

---

[2] Gastric bypass surgery involves the creation of a small gastric pouch and a shortcut of the remaining stomach and parts of the GI tract (bypass)

[3] A band placed around the upper part of the stomach to create a small pouch limits the amount of food intake at a time and can be adjusted regularly to maintain the effectiveness.

[4] The stomach is reduced to about 25% of its original size, by surgical removal of a large portion of the stomach, following the major curve. The open edges are then attached together to form a sleeve or tube. The procedure permanently reduces the size of the stomach.

surgery. Many cost-utility studies which evaluated various types of surgery methods in different patient groups have been published and are summarized in Table 2.

Nguyen et al. conducted a randomized controlled trial comparing gastric bypass and gastric banding with respect to short and long term clinical outcomes, cost, and quality of life impact with 111 patients undergoing gastric bypass surgery and 86 patients receiving gastric banding surgery. (Nguyen et al. 2009) The study showed that a higher complexity of gastric bypass surgery is reflected in a longer time needed for surgery and recovery (see Table 3). Increasing complexity was also associated with higher complication rates and higher total cost. On the other hand, gastric bypass surgery was more effective for weight loss in terms of the extent of weight loss and the response rate. The authors suggested considering the trade-offs of increased complexity, cost, and complications versus improved weight outcomes, when making the decision on which type of surgery is the best for the individual patient. They also argued that even the inferior weight loss after the gastric banding procedure is far better than any non-surgical intervention and led to the same improvement of quality of life for the patients as gastric bypass surgery.

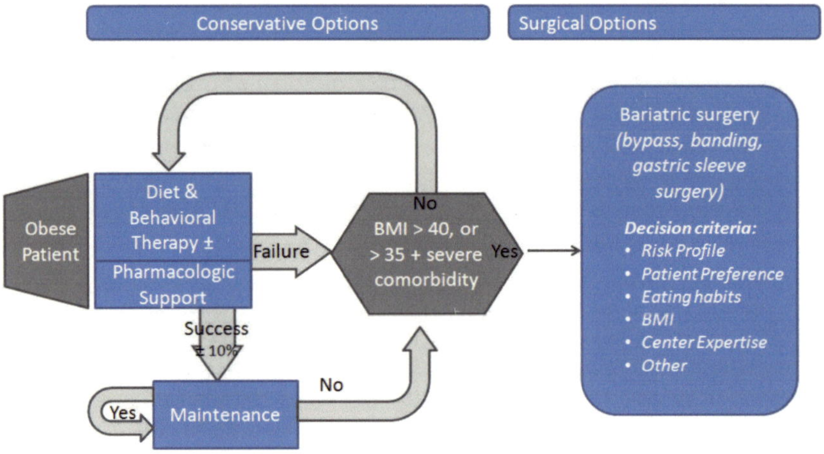

Fig. 1. Conceptual treatment path of obese patients

A smaller study was conducted by Ojo et al. in a hospital in New Haven, CT / USA and compared the cost of 83 laparoscopic adjustable gastric banding (LAGB) procedures with the cost of 59 laparoscopic vertical banded gastroplasty (LVBG) procedures. (Ojo and Valin 2009) This group found in their setting a cost advantage for LVBG (US$1,927 lower cost of surgery but a somewhat higher follow-up cost). The authors found however, that the excess weight loss in LVBG patients was realized more rapidly than in LAGB patients.

Another research group in the USA (Campbell et al. 2010) used the results of a five year European randomized clinical trial published in 2007 (Angrisani, Lorenzo, and Borrelli 2007) and base data from a systematic review of 36 English-language studies of weight loss outcomes following LAGB or laparoscopic RYGB (O'Brien et al. 2006). The authors conclusion was that both LAGB and LRYGB provided significant weight loss and were cost-effective compared to conventional treatment at accepted thresholds for medical interventions. (Campbell et al. 2010) In the base case of the overall eligible population the incremental cost per life year saved was US$9,300 for LAGB and US$10,200 for LRYGB versus conventional therapy. The cost-utility was US$5,400 for LAGB and US$5,600 for

LRYGB versus conventional therapy. Comparing the two methods, LRYGB had an ICER of US$12,900 / Life Year saved versus LAGB and an ICUR of US$6,200 per QALY. The cost utility ratio improved with increasing morbidity and was generally better for females. However, in all cases the ICUR remained below US$15,000/QALY and the surgical procedures both were cost saving and improved clinical outcomes for females with a BMI > 50 kg/m². (Campbell et al. 2010) Since the input data originated from data collected before 2006, it can be assumed that the rate of surgery related mortality and complications were overestimated in this model compared to today. Therefore the cost-effectiveness would be expected to be even more favourable for both types of surgery.

Table 2 summarizes studies that reported on cost-utility analyses of bariatric surgery.

	Data Year	Cost/ QALY	Method / Country	Patient Type	Limitations
Craig, Tseng 2002	1997-2001	$ 28,600 $ 10,700 $ 14,700 $ 5,700 $ 35,600 $ 13,300 $ 16,100 $ 5,400	GB /USA	M. BMI > 40, A 35 M, BMI > 50, A 35 W, BMI > 40, A 35 W, BMI > 50, A 35 M. BMI > 40, A 50 M, BMI > 50, A 50 W, BMI > 40, A 50 W, BMI > 50, A 50	Cost for treatment for many obesity-related diseases (such as gastro-esophageal reflux disease, sleep apnea, and degenerative joint disease) were not included
Clegg et al. 2003	< 2002	£ 6,289 £ 8,527 £ 10,237	GB/UK AGB/UK VBG/UK		Cost estimates after one year only based on expert opinion. Only diabetes as cost of comorbidity; no productivity considerations.
Ackroyd et al. 2006	< 2005	£ 3,251 £ 2,599 € (1,305) € (2,208) € (1,379) € (4,000)	AGB/UK GB/UK AGB/GER GB/GER AGB/FRA GB/FRA	Patients with T2DM	Payor perspective. No productivity data. 5-year time frame. Limited sensitivity analysis i.e. testing of extreme points
Salem et al. 2008*	2004	$ 11,604 $ 18,543 $ 8,878 $ 14,680	LAGB/USA RYGB/USA LAGB/USA RYGB/USA	M. A 35; BMI 40 W. A 35; BMI 40	Incremental cost effectiveness ratio (ICER) of LAGB or LRYGB as compared with medical interventions
Ikramuddin et al. 2009	2001 - 2007	$ 21,973 $ 122,001	GB/USA	35 year time horizon 10 year time horizon	CORE Diabetes Model for T2DM or pre-diabetes. Comparison GB surgery versus Medical Treatment.
Campbell et al. 2010	< 2006	$5,400 $ 5,600	LAGB/USA LRYGB		Input data from previous European or literature review
Chang et al. 2011	2010 price levels	$ 2,413 $ 3,872 $ 1,853 $ 3,770 dominant $ 1,904	all types	BMI >35<40, ORD BMI >35<40, no ORD BMI >40<50, ORD BMI >40<50, no ORD BMI >50, ORD BMI >50, no ORD	Model for a population (age ≥ 17), obtained from National Health and Nutrition Examination Survey (NHANES) III and data from meta-Analysis including RCT and non-RCT data
Hoerger et al. 2010	2005 price levels	$ 7,000 $ 1,000 $ 12,000 $ 13,000	GB/USA AGB/USA	Newly diag. T2DM Established T2DM Newly diag. T2DM Established T2DM	Centers for Disease Control and Prevention-RTI Diabetes Cost-Effectiveness Model extended to bariatric surgery

Table 2. List of studies reporting cost-utility ratios (Cost/QALY). M=Men; W=Women; ORD=Obesity Related Disease

	Gastric Bypass N=111	Gastric Banding N=86	P
Peri-surgery outcome			
Operative time (minutes)	136.9±31.9	68.21 ±24.7	<0.01
Estimated blood loss	4x	Reference (1)	<0.01
Length of hospital stay	3.1 ± 1.5	1.5 ± 1.1	<0.01
ICU use	2.7%	1.2%	N.S.
30 day mortality	0	0	N.S.
Recovery			
Return to daily living activities (d)	14.5 ± 12.7	10.4 ± 10.1	<0.02
Return to work (d)	21.0 ± 13.65	14.0 ± 10.1	<0.01
Complications			
Major early complications	6.3%	2.3%	N.S.
Minor early complications	15.3%	4.7%	0.02
Major late complications	26.1%	11.6%	0.01
Minor late complications	13.5%	0%	<0.01
30 day reoperation	5.4%	1.2%	N.S.
Late reoperation	7.2%	11.6%	N.S.
90 day mortality	0	0	N.S.
Weight Loss			
Excess weight loss 2 yrs	68.9%	41.8%	
Excess weight loss 4 yrs	68.4%	45.4%	
Treatment success and failure rate			
Treatment failure rate (excl. patients lost to follow-up)	0%	16.7%	
Treatment failure rate (incl. patients lost to follow-up)	15.3%	23.3%	
%age of patients with adequate or good weight loss	35.9%	67.9%	
%age of patients with excellent or exceptional weight loss	54.1%	15.3%	
Total Cost			
Total cost (US$)	12,310 ± 3,099	10,767 ± 1,631	<0.01
Quality of Life (SF 36)			
QoL after 1 month	Improved in 5 of 8 domains	Improved in 1 of 8 domains	
QoL after 1 year	Improved to normal in all domains	Improved to normal in all domains	

Table 3. Summary of study results of randomized controlled trial comparing laparoscopic gastric bypass surgery and laparoscopic gastric banding for clinical, economic, and quality of life outcomes

The evidence shows that both LAGB and RYGB are cost-effective. However, there is no clear evidence supporting superior cost-effectiveness of either surgical intervention compared to the other but there is a tendency that with increasing proficiency and experience LAGB may decrease cost by (1) requiring shorter time for surgery, hospitalization and recovery (2) lowering peri-surgical morbidity and mortality and (3) reducing severe surgery-related morbidity in the short and long term.

2.5 Budget impact, break-even or time to payback

A study by Cremieux et al., using a private insurer claims database, quantified the effect of bariatric surgery on direct medical costs in 3,651 US patients for up to five years after bariatric surgery. (Cremieux et al. 2008) Compared to a matched group of morbidly obese patients with similar comorbidity profile, but did not receive bariatric surgery, the authors found that the surgery group accrued incremental costs of approximately US$24,500 for all types of bariatric surgery combined (US$26,000 for open surgery, and US$17,000 for laparoscopic surgery) during the period from one month before surgery to two months following surgery. From month three onwards, cost savings associated with the bariatric surgery patients started accumulating. One and a half years after surgery the monthly savings associated with bariatric surgery reached more than US$500 for the whole sample. Monthly savings associated with laparoscopic bariatric surgery reached more than US$900 as early as 13 months following surgery ($P<0.01$). Open surgery between 2003 and 2005 achieved the break-even after 49 months (95% CI, -35 to 63 months), and the cost of laparoscopic surgery were fully recovered after 25 months (95% CI, -16 to 34 months). The savings came from reductions in prescription drug costs, physician visit costs and hospital costs (including emergency department visits and inpatient and outpatient visits). The reduced cost was associated with multiple major diagnosis categories, including type 2 diabetes, coronary artery disease, hypertension, and sleep apnea. This analysis had several conclusions:

- The cost of laparoscopic bariatric surgery could be recovered after a little over two years. The savings accrued came mainly from reduced use of medication and healthcare services originating from comorbidities.
- Laparoscopic interventions were more cost-effective than the open surgery alternatives.
- Outcomes from surgery improved over time as the surgical team gained more experience, especially during the first few years. When analyzing the accumulated cost in the surgery group before 2003, an average of 77 months was needed to recover the investment (95% CI, -48 to 106 months).
- Third-party payers should invest in bariatric surgery because it generally will pay for itself through decreased comorbidities within two to four years in addition to potential quality-of-life and length-of-life benefits, as well as reduction in disability and work loss.

To confirm the observation of effective reduction of comorbidities, Cremieux et al. conducted another study where they analyzed data from 5,502 patients in the same database for comorbidity related claims before and after surgery. (Cremieux et al. 2008) Compared to the period before surgery, significant decreases ($p<0.05$) were observed as early as 120 days after surgery and remained lower until three years after surgery. All cardiovascular disorders decreased from 43.6% pre-surgery to 14.2% post-surgery. The diagnosis of diabetes mellitus fell from 19.9% to 7.7%. Chronic obstructive pulmonary disease and other respiratory conditions also improved by over 40 percentage points (from 57.7% before to

16.2% after surgery). In addition, prevalence of diseases of the musculoskeletal system and connective tissue was reduced from 32.6% to 27.7%, and mental disorders were approximately halved with 30.7% before and 14.8% after surgery.

Simultaneously, the medication use dropped significantly for a number of conditions including infections, pain, respiratory disease, cardiovascular disease, gastroenterological diseases, and diabetes. In addition, there was an improvement in the lipid profile of the patients. Anemia, however, increased from 3.8% to 9.9% and use of nutritional supplements increased significantly. Both are known consequences of the surgery.

A similar analysis of claims data (US MarketScan Commercial Claims and Encounters Database from January 1, 2003 to March 31, 2008) of more than 7,000 patients having undergone laparoscopic adjustable gastric banding surgery was published in 2011. (Finkelstein et al. (a) 2011) They determined that the average cost of surgery was approximately US$20,000 and that this investment was recouped within two years for the diabetic population and within four years for the non-diabetic patient group due to decreased utilization of healthcare services and medication.

A subsequent study used data from the US Medical Expenditure Panel Survey (MEPS) and data from the US National Health and Wellness Survey (NHWS) to calculate the time needed to recoup the cost of bariatric surgery when including direct medical cost (hospital, drugs, clinical services, etc.) and indirect cost (absenteeism and presenteeism) of obese patients who were eligible for bariatric surgery. (Finkelstein et al. (b) 2011) They concluded that it takes nine quarters to recoup the cost of surgery. The improvement in absenteeism or presenteeism balanced the time of lost work when the patients underwent the surgery. Beyond the break-even time horizon there are additional indirect benefits that accrue to employers as a result of the procedure.

Perry et al. analyzed 11,903 surgery patients matched to 11,901 controls selected from 190,448 Medicare patients matched for age, sex and comorbidity in the USA. (Perry et al. 2008) Throughout two years, the incidence of several obesity related diseases were reduced when compared to the control group (all results were statistically highly significant):

- Diabetes fell by 21%
- Sleep apnoea by 10%
- Hypertension by 21%
- Hyperlipidemia by 30%
- Coronary artery disease by 32%.

In contrast to the above studies, an analysis of long-term health care utilization and expenditures among veterans in the USA that underwent bariatric surgery in 12 Veteran Affairs (VA) medical centers from 2000 to 2006 did not reveal a reduction in overall health expenditures by the end of three years. The data indicated a significant decrease in outpatient health expenditures, but this reduction was offset by a significant increase in inpatient health expenditures. (Maciejewski et al. 2010) Several factors may have contributed to this result, including the fact that the analysis targeted a special subset of patients usually older than average patients undergoing bariatric surgery, had a higher degree of long established comorbidities and were male. In addition, none of the patients received laparoscopic banding procedures and only a minority of the surgeries used laparoscopic or less invasive methods.

More studies and models have attempted to calculate the time to break-even, or the time needed until an intervention starts to generate more savings than it cost.

Table 4 lists the results from several studies and, depending on the point of view, these authors expected the break-even in one to ten years. It depends on the type of cost and the comparators considered when the break-even point is reached – or even if it is reached. Employers paying for the healthcare of their employees would be interested in improved productivity and reduced absenteeism. From their point of view productivity and absenteeism should be included in the beak-even or time to pay-back calculations. On the other hand, insurers or national health systems might only be interested in the direct medical cost.

Publikacation	Country	Break-even or time to pay-back
Finkelstein; Brown 2005	USA	5-10 years for employer to recover cost
Snow et al. 2004	USA	Break-even after 2-3 years
Narbro et al. 2002	Sweden	Total cost similar
Christou et al. 2004	Canada	2-3 years
Sampalis et al. 2004	Canada	2-3 years
Gallagher et al. 2003	USA	Cost is off set in year 1 through reduction of outpatient visits in Veteran's Affairs population
Maciejewski et al. 2010	USA	No break-even in Veteran's Affairs population
Mullen; Marr 2010	USA	3.5 years after gastric baypass
Cremieux et al. 2008	USA	53 months for bariatric surgery overall 25 months for laparoscopic bariatric surgery
Finkelstein et al. 2011(a)	USA	2 years for diabetic patients 4 years for non-diabetic patients
Finkelstein et al. 2011(b)	USA	2.25 years for all patients, including direct and indirect cost & savings

Table 4. Summary of studies, which report a 'break-even' time for bariatric surgery cost

Several studies find that LAGB and RYGB are cost saving and improve clinical outcomes when compared to conventional therapy. Both procedures also have a relatively short time before reaching break-even (two to 10 years). (Cremieux et al. 2008)

2.6 Geographic areas

Most of the evidence on economic impact of bariatric surgery has been generated in the United States and in Europe. Several European countries as well as Canadian authorities and some US payer organizations have assessed the technology systematically by looking at the clinical and the economic evidence. The conclusions were not always consistent and depended on the evidence reviewed, the perspective of the evaluation, and the time frame assessed. Therefore, many assessments remain indecisive in their final conclusion and requested further evidence to be generated.

2.6.1 Europe

The recent health technology assessment in the UK, performed in 2009, included a literature review of the key published clinical studies and cost-effectiveness analysis. In addition, the cost-effectiveness of bariatric surgery was further analyzed in two models. (Picot et al. 2009) The incremental cost-effectiveness ratios (ICERs) ranged between £2,000 and £4,000 per QALY gained. The results were generally robust to changes in assumptions in the sensitivity analysis, and in all cases the ICERs remained within the range conventionally regarded as cost-effective from an NHS decision-making perspective. Surgical management (with AGB) of moderate to severe obesity (BMI ≥ 30 and < 40) in patients with type 2 diabetes was more costly than nonsurgical management, but resulted in improved clinical outcomes. The ICER was reduced with a longer time horizon, from £18,930 at two years to £1,367 at 20 years. The authors also analyzed the cost effectiveness of the intervention for the patients with a BMI between 30 and 35. Based on data from two clinical trials, the QALY gain at two years was small (0.08). The ICER was again reduced with a longer time horizon, from £60,754 at two years to £12,763 at 20 years. (Picot et al. 2009) The general conclusion was that bariatric surgery was a clinically effective and cost-effective intervention for moderately to severely obese people compared with non-surgical interventions.

The UK National Institute for Health and Clinical Excellence (NICE) guidelines state that bariatric surgery should be offered to patients with a BMI of 35 - 40 who have other conditions caused by being overweight, such as diabetes and obstructive sleep apnea or hypertension and all appropriate non-surgical measures have been tried but have failed to achieve or maintain adequate, clinically beneficial weight loss for at least 6 months or for those with a BMI of 40-50 with no other weight related conditions. For those with a BMI of 50 and over bariatric surgery can be offered as a first-line treatment (NICE Guideline CG43, 2010).

A health technology assessment conducted by a German expert group came to the conclusion that bariatric surgery seemed to be clinically effective and cost-effective, based on an extensive literature analysis. (Bockelbrink et al. 2008) At this time, no specific German cost-effectiveness analysis has been conducted.

Finland's health technology assessment agency (FINOHTA) included a cost-utility analysis for the most commonly used surgical techniques from the healthcare provider perspective over a ten year time frame. They concluded that bariatric surgery in Finland was more effective and less costly than the conventional therapy for morbid obesity and was the dominant technology. (Mäklin et al. 2009)

2.6.2 Canada

A recent health technology assessment from the Canadian authorities concluded that over a time period of 20 years, bariatric surgery for morbidly obese patients appeared to be cost-effective with an ICER of US$5,000 to US$30,000 / QALY. (Padwal et al. 2011; Klarenbach et al. 2010) For patients with type 2 diabetes, the intervention was recognized as cost saving and with improved outcomes. A retrospective data analysis performed in Quebec found cost savings after 3.5 years from bariatric surgery due to reduced health care utilization for a variety of obesity related disorders. (Sampalis et al. 2004) A new analysis is currently ongoing, where three patient groups are compared for clinical, quality of life, and cost outcomes for one year retrospectively and two years prospectively after referral or surgery.

The study will include 150 surgical cases, 200 medically treated controls, and 150 wait-listed controls. (APPLES study; (Padwal et al. 2010)). Final results for the APPLES analysis are anticipated by late 2012 or early 2013.

2.6.3 Australia

Keating and colleagues compared the cost to achieve diabetic remission in 60 morbidly obese patients through LAGB or conventional treatment in a two year randomized clinical trial in Australia. (Keating et al. 2009a) The study showed that in the time frame of the two-year study period, AU$16,000 additional expenditure for the surgical intervention was needed per additional remission of diabetes. The highest cost difference was detected in the first six months of the study period including the cost of the surgery and the short-term complications. Savings were subsequently demonstrated for the surgery group in the consumption of anti-diabetic medicine, with increasing consumption by the patients without bariatric surgery.

Subsequently, the same group of researchers extended the study results into an incremental cost-effectiveness Markov model and extrapolated the intervention costs based on the observed resource utilization during the trial. (Keating et al. 2009b) In this lifetime model, the mean discounted cost per patient was AU$98,900 for surgical therapy and AU$101,400 for conventional therapy. Over a lifetime, the health-care cost to treat type 2 diabetes became the overwhelming cost driver and cost differential between the two intervention groups. The researchers found a 57% chance of surgery to be cost saving, a 98% chance to be very cost-effective (below AU$7,000/QALY) and even in the worst-case scenario, surgery remained cost-effective with AU$39,700/QALY. The authors concluded that based on this trial in the Australian setting the cost of bariatric surgery (LAGB) for patients with BMI > 35 and type 2 diabetes should be recovered within 10 years after surgery.

2.6.4 Latin America

There is limited literature available for the use and cost-effectiveness of bariatric surgery in Latin America. One publication by Salgado et al. calculated the actual cost of bariatric surgery in the hospital setting and contrasted it with the very low standard reimbursed rate by the public health insurance (R$3,260 in 2004; R$4,615 after August 2007). (Salgado Júnior et al. 2010) The calculation was only based on 9 patients treated in 2004 (average cost of R$6,845/surgery) and 7 patients treated in 2007 (average cost of R$7,525/surgery) and no outcomes or cost-effectiveness were reported.

2.7 Effect on productivity (paid work)

Obesity tends to lead to reduced income. (Flum et al. 2005; Martin et al. 2010) It was estimated in New Mexico that the total labor income impact of obesity was nearly US$200 million, representing US$1,660 of output income and US$245 of labor income per household. Obesity may cost New Mexico more than 7,300 jobs and cuts state and local tax revenues by more than US$48 million. (Frezza and Wachtel 2009)

Few studies have examined the impact of bariatric surgery on productivity. According to a US analysis, obese workers eligible for bariatric surgery have 5.1 ($P < 0.01$) additional days of absenteeism and US$2,230 (in 2004 dollars) ($P < 0.01$) higher annual medical costs than persons of a BMI of less than 25. (Finkelstein and Brown 2005) Given that bariatric surgery has been shown to increase life expectancy and to reduce the impact of overweight and comorbidities an increase in productivity would be expected. (Frezza and Wachtel 2009)

A retrospective analysis in the Duke Health and Safety Surveillance System compared data of morbidly obese workers (BMI ≥ 40) with workers with a BMI 18.5 to 24.9 and revealed that the obese workers generated twice the amount of claims with 6.8 times higher medical claims cost and 11 times higher indemnity claims cost. In addition they lost 12.9 times more workdays than the non-obese workers. (Ostbye et al. 2007)

A UK study followed 59 patients for 14 months after bariatric surgery. (Hawkins et al. 2007) Before the surgery 58% of the patients worked, with an average work week of 30.1 hours, and 32% claimed some sort of incapacity benefits. After surgery 76% of the patients worked, with an average work week of 35.8 hours, and only 10% claimed benefits. The work or productivity profile of the patients after bariatric surgery looked very similar to that of the average population. Taking both the increase in percentage of people that worked and the increase in average number of hours worked per week, there was a 57% total increase in number of hours worked per week.

In a Dutch study the employment level was 53% before bariatric surgery and after surgery rose to 80%. (van Gemert et al. 1998) Since 1998, when the Dutch study was published, the outcome of bariatric surgery has improved significantly and it can be assumed that the impact on productivity would be even higher today.

2.8 The cost impact of full reimbursement of bariatric surgery

As was outlined in the beginning of this paper, payers are concerned with the potential high short-term cost as a consequence of broader access to bariatric surgery according to the clinical guidelines. There is, however, evidence that the utilization might not grow at a very high rate. In 2010, Kim et al. published their analysis of frequency of bariatric surgery in an employer insurance setting, which had decided to give free access to bariatric surgery to those who were eligible. The data showed that one year before the new policy 18 persons had a bariatric surgery with a utilization rate of 1.71%. In the year after the policy change, 16 people elected surgery with a utilization rate of 1.42%.(Kim, White, and Buffington 2010) The frequency of bariatric surgery in the United States may even have levelled at around 110-120,000 procedures per year despite an increasing prevalence of obesity and a prominent decrease in complication rates. (Livingston 2010) This indicates that there is a considerable barrier for patients to elect this intervention and it may not be the preferred solution for all morbidly obese patients. Fears connected to the perceived risk of the procedure and the perceived negative impact on quality of life after the intervention may be a reason for the barrier.

It may appear that the utilization of bariatric surgery will only increase slowly and the additional short term burden on payer budgets will remain a relatively controlled level. In addition, the evidence is strong that the number of bariatric surgeries might increase short term cost, but can be expected to generate mid- to long-term benefits at acceptable costs or even savings.

3. Conclusions on the value of bariatric surgery

Based on currently available clinical evidence, bariatric surgery is an effective method to decrease the long-term risk of obesity for morbidly obese patients. Bariatric surgery can effectively reduce disease sequelae of obesity such as diabetes, hypertension, sleep apnea, cancer and cardiovascular disease and reduces mortality from these diseases.

The different types of bariatric surgery have all been effective in reducing weight and diseases related to obesity. They do, however, have different levels of intervention risk as conceptualized in Fig. 2.

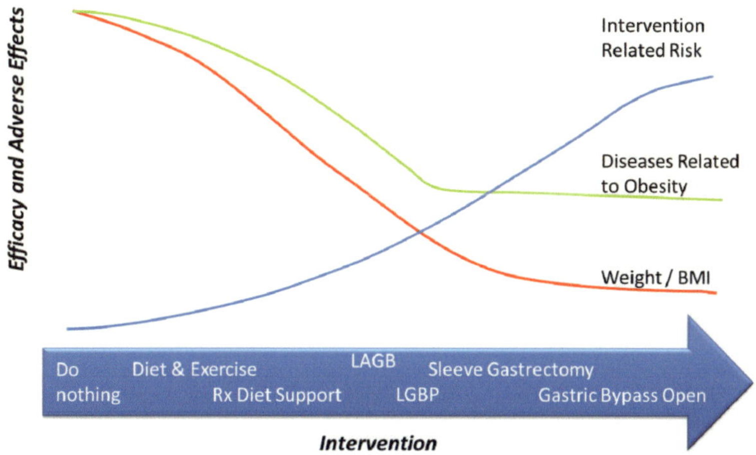

Fig. 2. Conceptual summary of clinical outcomes of treatment alternatives for morbidly obese patients. LAGB: Laparoscopic Adjustable Gastric Banding; LGBP: Laparoscopic Gastric Bypass

The investment in bariatric surgery is generally considered relatively high (US$7,000 to US$25,000) and there is reluctance to reimburse this kind of surgery. When a longer timeframe is considered, which would include reduction in cost of comorbidities, bariatric surgery for eligible obese patients is cost effective or even cost saving for many patients. For obese patients with existing obesity related comorbidities, like type 2 diabetes, bariatric surgery becomes even more cost effective and some studies have shown it to be cost saving. Evidence has also shown that the more experience the surgeons and the care team have, the more clinical outcomes are improved and bariatric surgery becomes more cost-effective. Despite the evidence supporting the cost-effectiveness or even cost savings for bariatric surgery, it seems that there are only a limited number of patients willing to elect this type of intervention. This may be due to the risk perceived by the patients and the fear of the behavioural consequences of the surgery and their impact on the subsequent lifestyle.

In conclusion: Bariatric surgery is cost-effective or cost saving for eligible patients, usually with a relatively short payback time. It can be even more cost-effective or often cost saving, for patients with obesity related comorbidities, especially when they are treated by experienced surgical and care teams. Given the positive impact on length of life and quality of life and considering the increasingly efficient and reliable methodologies and care process used today, bariatric surgery has become an attractive investment for eligible obese patients.

4. Appendix - methods (review of health economic publications on bariatric surgery)

The English-language literature was searched with Medline, PubMedCentral and the National Library of Medicine Catalog in 2008, 2009 and 2011. A search for relevant articles was conducted by entering the terms "bariatric surgery", "obesity surgery" or "morbid obesity" and "outcomes". For relevant article that were found, a "related article" search was performed. Additionally a search was based on MESH terms as listed below.

- MESH Terms:
- Gastric Bypass + Treatment Outcome
- Gastric Bypass/economics
- Gastroplasty + Treatment Outcome
- Gastroplasty /economics
- Treatment Outcome + Obesity,
- Morbid Obesity/ complications,
- Morbid Obesity + Treatment Outcome
- Obesity, Morbid
- Obesity, Morbid/complications
- Obesity, Morbid/complications
- Obesity, Morbid + Cost, Cost Analysis
- Obesity, Morbid/diet therapy
- Obesity, Morbid/drug therapy
- Obesity/economics/*surgery
- Obesity, Morbid + Health Care Cost
- Obesity, Morbid/*surgery
- Obesity, Morbid + Treatment Outcome

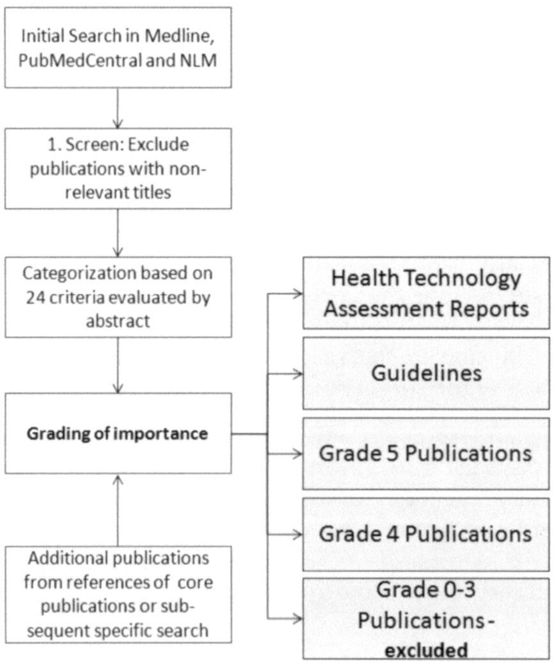

Fig. 3. Search strategy for review

The search strategy is outlined in Fig. 3 and screening and the assessment were performed by 2 evaluators.

All titles for potential interest to the subject of 'value of bariatric surgery' were screened for relevance. This excluded approximately 30%. Throughout the work process additional articles were added either from reference lists of core articles or as result of targeted subsequent search.

The remaining list was analyzed based on the abstracts, where available, and were then categorized. The categories were created before this second screen to help to differentiate the articles. The categories are: Economic or cost focus, HTA, Guideline, Outcomes Assessment, Geography (supportive if from Europe), Patient numbers, Length of study, Risk & complications, Comparison of surgery vs. Drug or diet / behavioral therapy, Study Type (Prospective/Retrospective, RCT etc.) Comparisons of surgery techniques were only considered if they reported relevant overall outcomes criteria but not if the comparison seemed to be limited to 1 or few specific factors.

The remaining publications were ranked from 1 (not relevant) to 5 (highly relevant; key publication) for relevance based on the categories.

Those were graded as 5 and used for the report.

Throughout the process original articles were consulted case of doubt and availability.

5. References

Aasheim, Erlend T, and Torgeir T Søvik. 2011. "Global trends in body-mass index." Lancet 377 (9781) (June 4): 1916-1917; author reply 1917-1918. doi:10.1016/S0140-6736(11)60804-0.

Ackroyd, Roger, Jean Mouiel, Jean-Marc Chevallier, and Frederic Daoud. 2006. "Cost-effectiveness and budget impact of obesity surgery in patients with type-2 diabetes in three European countries." Obesity surgery 16 (11) (November): 1488-503.

Ananthapavan, Jaithri, Marjory Moodie, Michelle Haby, and Robert Carter. 2010. "Assessing cost-effectiveness in obesity: laparoscopic adjustable gastric banding for severely obese adolescents." Surgery for Obesity and Related Diseases 6 (4) (August): 377-385. doi:10.1016/j.soard.2010.02.040.

Angrisani, Luigi, Michele Lorenzo, and Vincenzo Borrelli. 2007. "Laparoscopic adjustable gastric banding versus Roux-en-Y gastric bypass: 5-year results of a prospective randomized trial." Surgery for obesity and related diseases 3 (2) (February): 127-32; discussion 132-3.

Anonymous. 1991. "NIH conference. Gastrointestinal surgery for severe obesity. Consensus Development Conference Panel." Annals of internal medicine 115 (12) (December 15): 956-61

Anselmino, Marco, Tanja Bammer, José Maria Fernández Cebrián, Frederic Daoud, Giuliano Romagnoli, and Antonio Torres. 2009. "Cost-effectiveness and budget impact of obesity surgery in patients with type 2 diabetes in three European countries(II)." Obesity Surgery 19 (11) (November): 1542-1549. doi:10.1007/s11695-009-9946-z.

Berger, Marc L, and International Society for Pharmacoeconomics and Outcomes Research. 2003. Health care cost, quality, and outcomes : ISPOR book of terms. Lawrenceville, NJ: International Society for Pharmacoeconomics and Outcomes Research.

Bockelbrink, Angelina, Yvonne Stöber, Stefanie Roll, Cristoph Vauth, Stefan N Willich, and Johann-Matthias von der Schulenburg. 2008. "Evaluation of medical and health economic effectiveness of bariatric surgery (obesity surgery) versus conservative strategies in adult patients with morbid obesity." GMS Health Technology Assessment 4: Doc06.

Campbell, Joanna, Lisa A McGarry, Scott A Shikora, Brent C Hale, Jeffrey T Lee, and Milton C Weinstein. 2010. "Cost-effectiveness of laparoscopic gastric banding and bypass for morbid obesity." The American Journal of Managed Care 16 (7) (July): e174-187.

Cawley, John, and Chad Meyerhoefer. 2010. The medical care costs of obesity: an instrumental variables approach. Working Paper. National bureau of economic research.

CDC Diabetes Cost Effectiveness Group. 2002. "Cost-effectiveness of intensive glycemic control, intensified hypertension control, and serum cholesterol level reduction for type 2 diabetes." JAMA 287 (19) (May 15): 2542-2551. http://jama.ama-assn.org/content/287/19/2542.long.

Chang, Su-Hsin, Carolyn R T Stoll, and Graham A Colditz. 2011. "Cost-effectiveness of bariatric surgery: Should it be universally available?" Maturitas 69 (3) (July): 230-238. doi:10.1016/j.maturitas.2011.04.007.

Clegg, A J, J Colquitt, M K Sidhu, P Royle, E Loveman, and A Walker. 2002. "The clinical effectiveness and cost-effectiveness of surgery for people with morbid obesity: a systematic review and economic evaluation." Health technology assessment (Winchester, England) 6 (12): 1-153. http://www.hta.ac.uk/execsumm/summ612.htm.

Clegg, A, J Colquitt, M Sidhu, P Royle, and A Walker. 2003. "Clinical and cost effectiveness of surgery for morbid obesity: a systematic review and economic evaluation." International journal of obesity and related metabolic disorders 27 (10) (October): 1167-77. http://www.nature.com/ijo/journal/v27/n10/pdf/0802394a.pdf.

Craig, Benjamin M, and Daniel S Tseng. 2002. "Cost-effectiveness of gastric bypass for severe obesity." The American journal of medicine 113 (6) (October 15): 491-8.

Cremieux, Pierre-Yves, Henry Buchwald, Scott A Shikora, Arindam Ghosh, Haixia Elaine Yang, and Marric Buessing. 2008. "A study on the economic impact of bariatric surgery." The American Journal of Managed Care 14 (9) (September): 589-96. doi:10708. http://www.ajmc.com/article.cfm?ID=10708.

Dixon, J B, P Zimmet, K G Alberti, and F Rubino. 2011. "Bariatric surgery: an IDF statement for obese Type 2 diabetes." Diabetic Medicine 28 (6) (June): 628-642. doi:10.1111/j.1464-5491.2011.03306.x.

Encinosa, William E, Didem M Bernard, Dongyi Du, and Claudia A Steiner. 2009. "Recent improvements in bariatric surgery outcomes." Medical Care 47 (5) (May): 531-535. doi:10.1097/MLR.0b013e31819434c6.

Finkelstein, Eric A, Benjamin T Allaire, Somali M Burgess, and Brent C Hale. 2011. "Financial implications of coverage for laparoscopic adjustable gastric banding." Surgery for Obesity and Related Diseases 7 (3) (June): 295-303. doi:10.1016/j.soard.2010.10.011.

Finkelstein, Eric A, and Derek S Brown. 2005 (a). "A cost-benefit simulation model of coverage for bariatric surgery among full-time employees." The American journal of managed care 11 (10) (October): 641-6.

http://www.ajmc.com/article.cfm?ID=2959.

Finkelstein, Eric A, Benjamin T Allaire, Marco Dacosta Dibonaventura, and Somali M Burgess. 2011 (b). "Direct and Indirect Costs and Potential Cost Savings of Laparoscopic Adjustable Gastric Banding Among Obese Patients With Diabetes." Journal of Occupational and Environmental Medicine. doi: 10.1097/JOM.0b013e318229aae4.

Finkelstein, Eric A, Justin G Trogdon, Joel W Cohen, and William Dietz. 2009. "Annual medical spending attributable to obesity: payer-and service-specific estimates." Health Affairs (Project Hope) 28 (5) (October): w822-831. doi:10.1377/hlthaff.28.5.w822.

Finucane, Mariel M, Gretchen A Stevens, Melanie J Cowan, Goodarz Danaei, John K Lin, Christopher J Paciorek, Gitanjali M Singh, et al. 2011. "National, regional, and global trends in body-mass index since 1980: systematic analysis of health examination surveys and epidemiological studies with 960 country-years and 9•1 million participants." Lancet 377 (9765) (February 12): 557-567. doi:10.1016/S0140-6736(10)62037-5.

Flegal, Katherine M, Margaret D Carroll, Cynthia L Ogden, and Lester R Curtin. 2010. "Prevalence and trends in obesity among US adults, 1999-2008." JAMA 303 (3) (January 20): 235-241. doi:10.1001/jama.2009.2014. http://jama.ama-assn.org/content/303/3/235.full.pdf+html.

Flum, David R, Leon Salem, Jo Ann Broeckel Elrod, E Patchen Dellinger, Allen Cheadle, and Leighton Chan. 2005. "Early mortality among Medicare beneficiaries undergoing bariatric surgical procedures." JAMA 294 (15) (October 19): 1903-8.

Frezza, Eldo E, and Mitchell S Wachtel. 2009. "The economic impact of morbid obesity." Surgical Endoscopy 23 (4) (April): 677-679. doi:10.1007/s00464-008-0325-y.

Van Gemert, W G, E M Adang, J W Greve, and P B Soeters. 1998. "Quality of life assessment of morbidly obese patients: effect of weight-reducing surgery." The American Journal of Clinical Nutrition 67 (2) (February): 197-201. http://www.ajcn.org/content/67/2/197.long.

Hawkins, Simon C, Alan Osborne, Ian G Finlay, Swethan Alagaratnam, Janet R Edmond, and Richard Welbourn. 2007. "Paid work increases and state benefit claims decrease after bariatric surgery." Obesity Surgery 17 (4) (April): 434-7. doi:17608252.

Hinojosa, Marcelo W, J Esteban Varela, Dhavan Parikh, Brian R Smith, Xuan-Mai Nguyen, and Ninh T Nguyen. 2009. "National trends in use and outcome of laparoscopic adjustable gastric banding." Surgery for Obesity and Related Diseases 5 (2) (April): 150-155. doi:10.1016/j.soard.2008.08.006.

Hoerger, Thomas J, Ping Zhang, Joel E Segel, Henry S Kahn, Lawrence E Barker, and Steven Couper. 2010. "Cost-effectiveness of bariatric surgery for severely obese adults with diabetes." Diabetes Care 33 (9) (September): 1933-1939. doi:10.2337/dc10-0554.

Ikramuddin, Sayeed, David Klingman, Therese Swan, and Michael E Minshall. 2009. "Cost-effectiveness of Roux-en-Y gastric bypass in type 2 diabetes patients." The American Journal of Managed Care 15 (9) (September): 607-615.

Jan, Jay C, Dennis Hong, Sergio Jose Bardaro, Laura V July, and Emma J Patterson. 2007. "Comparative study between laparoscopic adjustable gastric banding and laparoscopic gastric bypass: single-institution, 5-year experience in bariatric surgery." Surgery for obesity and related diseases 3 (1) (January): 42-50; discussion 50-1.

Keating, Catherine L (a), John B Dixon, Marjory L Moodie, Anna Peeters, Liliana Bulfone, Dianna J Maglianno, and Paul E O'Brien. 2009. "Cost-effectiveness of surgically induced weight loss for the management of type 2 diabetes: modeled lifetime analysis." Diabetes Care 32 (4) (April): 567-574. doi:10.2337/dc08-1749.

Keating, Catherine L (b), John B Dixon, Marjory L Moodie, Anna Peeters, Julie Playfair, and Paul E O'Brien. 2009. "Cost-efficacy of surgically induced weight loss for the management of type 2 diabetes: a randomized controlled trial." Diabetes Care 32 (4) (April): 580-584. doi:10.2337/dc08-1748.

Kim, Keith, White, Vickie and Buffington, Cynthia K. 2010. "Utilization rate of bariatric surgery in an employee-based healthcare system following surgery coverage." Obesity Surgery 20 (11) (November): 1575-1578. doi:10.1007/s11695-010-0193-0.

Klarenbach, Scott, Raj Padwal, Natasha Wiebe, Maureen Hazel, Daniel Birch, Braden Manns, Shahzeer Karmali, Arya M Sharma, and Marcello Tonelli. 2010. Bariatric surgery for severe obesity: a systematic review and economic evaluation. Canada: Canadian Agency for Drugs and Technologies in Health. http://www.cadth.ca/index.php/en/hta/reportspublications/search/publication/2667.

Klein, Samuel, Arindam Ghosh, Pierre Y Cremieux, Sara Eapen, and Tamara J McGavock. 2011. "Economic impact of the clinical benefits of bariatric surgery in diabetes patients with BMI ≥35 kg/m2." Obesity (Silver Spring, Md.) 19 (3) (March): 581-587. doi:10.1038/oby.2010.199.

Landa, Krzysztof. 2008 Central & Eastern European Society of Technology Assessment in Health Care.

Li, Zhaoping, Margaret Maglione, Wenli Tu, Walter Mojica, David Arterburn, Lisa R. Shugarman, Lara Hilton, et al. 2005. "Meta-Analysis: Pharmacologic Treatment of Obesity." Ann Intern Med 142 (7) (April 5): 532-546. http://www.annals.org/cgi/content/abstract/142/7/532.

Livingston, Edward H. 2005. "Hospital costs associated with bariatric procedures in the United States." American journal of surgery 190 (5) (November): 816-20.

———. 2010. "The incidence of bariatric surgery has plateaued in the U.S." American Journal of Surgery 200 (3) (September): 378-385. doi:10.1016/j.amjsurg.2009.11.007.

Maciejewski, Matthew L, Valerie A Smith, Edward H Livingston, Andrew L Kavee, Leila C Kahwati, William G Henderson, and David E Arterburn. 2010. "Health care utilization and expenditure changes associated with bariatric surgery." Medical Care 48 (11) (November): 989-998. doi:10.1097/MLR.0b013e3181ef9cf7.

Makary, Martin A, Jeanne M Clarke, Andrew D Shore, Thomas H Magnuson, Thomas Richards, Eric B Bass, Francesca Dominici, Jonathan P Weiner, Albert W Wu, and Jodi B Segal. 2010. "Medication utilization and annual health care costs in patients with type 2 diabetes mellitus before and after bariatric surgery." Archives of Surgery (Chicago, Ill.: 1960) 145 (8) (August): 726-731. doi:10.1001/archsurg.2010.150.

Mäklin, Suvi, Antti Malmivaara, Miika Linna, Mikael Victorzon, Vesa Koivukangas, and Harri Sintonen. 2009. "[Cost-utility of bariatric surgery in the treatment for morbid obesity in Finland]." Duodecim; Lääketieteellinen Aikakauskirja 125 (20): 2265-2273.

Martin, Matthew, Alec Beekley, Randy Kjorstad, and James Sebesta. 2010. "Socioeconomic disparities in eligibility and access to bariatric surgery: a national population-based analysis." Surgery for Obesity and Related Diseases 6 (1) (February): 8-15. doi:10.1016/j.soard.2009.07.003.

National Health Expenditure Data, Department of Health & Human Services 2011

Nguyen, Ninh T, Mahbod Paya, C Melinda Stevens, Shahrzad Mavandadi, Kambiz Zainabadi, and Samuel E Wilson. 2004. "The relationship between hospital volume and outcome in bariatric surgery at academic medical centers." Annals of surgery 240 (4) (October): 586-93; discussion 593-4. http://www.pubmedcentral.nih.gov/articlerender.fcgi? tool=pubmed&pubmedid=15383786.

Nguyen, Ninh T, Johnathan A Slone, Xuan-Mai T Nguyen, Jaimee S Hartman, and David B Hoyt. 2009. "A prospective randomized trial of laparoscopic gastric bypass versus laparoscopic adjustable gastric banding for the treatment of morbid obesity: outcomes, quality of life, and costs." Annals of Surgery 250 (4) (October): 631-641. doi:10.1097/SLA.0b013e3181b92480.

NICE Guideline CG43: Obesity guidance on the prevention, identification, assessment and management of overweight and obesity in adults and children. 29 January 2010.

O'Brien, Paul E, Tracey McPhail, Timothy B Chaston, and John B Dixon. 2006. "Systematic review of medium-term weight loss after bariatric operations." Obesity Surgery 16 (8) (August): 1032-40. doi:10.1381/096089206778026316.

Ojo, Peter, and Elmer Valin. 2009. "Cost-effective restrictive bariatric surgery: laparoscopic vertical banded gastroplasty versus laparoscopic adjustable gastric band." Obesity Surgery 19 (11) (November): 1536-1541. doi:10.1007/s11695-008-9771-9.

Ostbye, Truls, John M Dement, and Katrina M Krause. 2007. "Obesity and workers' compensation: results from the Duke Health and Safety Surveillance System." Archives of Internal Medicine 167 (8) (April 23): 766-73. doi:167/8/766.

Padwal, Raj, Scott Klarenbach, Natasha Wiebe, Maureen Hazel, Daniel Birch, Shahzeer Karmali, Arya M Sharma, Braden Manns, and Marcello Tonelli. 2011. "Bariatric Surgery: A Systematic Review of the Clinical and Economic Evidence." Journal of General Internal Medicine (May 3). doi:10.1007/s11606-011-1721-x.

Palmer, Andrew J, Stéphane Roze, William J Valentine, Michael E Minshall, Volker Foos, Francesco M Lurati, Morten Lammert, and Giatgen A Spinas. 2004a. "The CORE Diabetes Model: Projecting long-term clinical outcomes, costs and cost-effectiveness of interventions in diabetes mellitus (types 1 and 2) to support clinical and reimbursement decision-making." Current Medical Research and Opinion 20 Suppl 1 (August): S5-26. doi:10.1185/030079904X1980.

———. 2004b. "Validation of the CORE Diabetes Model against epidemiological and clinical studies." Current Medical Research and Opinion 20 Suppl 1 (August): S27-40. doi:10.1185/030079904X2006.

Paxton, James H, and Jeffrey B Matthews. 2005. "The cost effectiveness of laparoscopic versus open gastric bypass surgery." Obesity surgery 15 (1) (January): 24-34.

Pendergast, Karen, Anne Wolf, Beth Sherrill, Xiaolei Zhou, Louis J Aronne, Ian Caterson, Nicholas Finer, et al. 2010. "Impact of waist circumference difference on health-care cost among overweight and obese subjects: the PROCEED cohort." Value in Health 13 (4) (July): 402-410. doi:10.1111/j.1524-4733.2009.00690.x.

Perry, Cynthia D, Matthew M Hutter, Daniel B Smith, Joseph P Newhouse, and Barbara J McNeil. 2008. "Survival and changes in comorbidities after bariatric surgery." Annals of Surgery 247 (1) (January): 21-7. doi:10.1097/SLA.0b013e318142cb4b.

Picot, J, J Jones, J L Colquitt, E Gospodarevskaya, E Loveman, L Baxter, and A J Clegg. 2009. "The clinical effectiveness and cost-effectiveness of bariatric (weight loss) surgery for obesity: a systematic review and economic evaluation." Health Technology Assessment (Winchester, England) 13 (41) (September): 1-190, 215-357, iii-iv. doi:10.3310/hta13410.

Powers, Kinga A, Scott T Rehrig, and Daniel B Jones. 2007. "Financial impact of obesity and bariatric surgery." The Medical clinics of North America 91 (3) (May): 321-38, ix.

Salem, Leon, Allison Devlin, Sean D Sullivan, and David R Flum. 2008. "Cost-effectiveness analysis of laparoscopic gastric bypass, adjustable gastric banding, and nonoperative weight loss interventions." Surgery for Obesity and Related Diseases 4 (1): 26-32. doi:S1550-7289(07)00672-7.

Salgado Júnior, Wilson, Karoline Calfa Pitanga, José Sebastião dos Santos, Ajith Kumar Sankarankutty, Orlando de Castro e Silva Jr, and Reginaldo Ceneviva. 2010. "Costs of bariatric surgery in a teaching hospital and the financing provided by the Public Unified Health System." Acta Cirúrgica Brasileira / Sociedade Brasileira Para Desenvolvimento Pesquisa Em Cirurgia 25 (2) (April): 201-205.

Sampalis, John S, Moishe Liberman, Stephane Auger, and Nicolas V Christou. 2004. "The impact of weight reduction surgery on health-care costs in morbidly obese patients." Obesity surgery 14 (7) (August): 939-47.

Shao, Qin, and Khew-Voon Chin. 2011. "Survey of American food trends and the growing obesity epidemic." Nutrition Research and Practice 5 (3) (June): 253-259. doi:10.4162/nrp.2011.5.3.253. http://www.ncbi.nlm.nih.gov/pmc/articles/PMC3133759/pdf/nrp-5-253.pdf.

Hiroiwa, Takeru, Yoon-Kyoung Sung, Takashi Fukuda, Hui-Chu Lang, Sang-Cheol Bae, and Kiichiro Tsutani. 2010. "International survey on willingness-to-pay (WTP) for one additional QALY gained: what is the threshold of cost effectiveness?" Health Economics 19 (4) (April 1): 422-437. doi:10.1002/hec.1481

Snow, Vincenza, Patricia Barry, Nick Fitterman, Amir Qaseem, Kevin Weiss, and for the Clinical Efficacy Assessment Subcommittee of the American College of Physicians*. 2005. "Pharmacologic and Surgical Management of Obesity in Primary Care: A Clinical Practice Guideline from the American College of Physicians." Ann Intern Med 142 (7) (April 5): 525-531. http://www.annals.org/cgi/reprint/142/7/525.pdf.

Villamizar, Nestor, and Aurora D Pryor. 2011. "Safety, effectiveness, and cost effectiveness of metabolic surgery in the treatment of type 2 diabetes mellitus." Journal of Obesity 2011: 790683. doi:10.1155/2011/790683.

4

Medical Assessment and Preparation of Patients Undergoing Bariatric Surgery

Wen Bun Leong[1] and Shahrad Taheri[2]
[1]*Specialist Registrar in Diabetes and Endocrinology and Honorary Research Fellow, Heart of England NHS Foundation Trust, University of Birmingham,*
[2]*Senior Lecturer and Consultant Physician, Lead in Weight Management, Co-Director Heartlands Biomedical Research Centre, Heart of England NHS Foundation Trust, University of Birmingham, UK*

1. Introduction

Bariatric surgery is an important option for patients with extreme obesity and co-morbidities. Bariatric surgery, however, has risks and complications involved. Obesity is associated with many health related complications such as cardiovascular disease, type 2 diabetes mellitus, dyslipidaemia, hypertension, and obstructive sleep apnoea (Avenell, Broom et al. 2004; Tsigos, Hainer et al. 2008; Mechanick, Kushner et al. 2009; Scottish Intercollegiate Guidelines and Scotland 2010). It is important to prepare patients to be at their best medical status prior to surgery to prevent adverse outcomes (Mechanick, Kushner et al. 2009). Detailed medical, nutritional and psychological assessments are crucial to improve patients' outcomes post surgery. This usually involves a multidisciplinary team working hand in hand with individual patients guiding them through the whole process as well as continuing lifelong follow up care. A multidisciplinary team usually includes a physician with interest in metabolism, nutrition and bariatric medicine, dietitian with special interest in obesity, a bariatric surgeon, a bariatric specialist nurse and psychologist, and finally a bariatric coordinator (Mechanick, Kushner et al. 2009). Additional expertise includes a psychiatrist, endocrinologist, sleep medicine specialist, cardiologist, gastroenterologist, physician nutrition specialist and certified nutrition support clinician (Mechanick, Kushner et al. 2009). However, the most important factor in the entire process is the individual patient and therefore it is important to individualise each patient's care. Good medical assessment with appropriate information provided for patients will help ease progress through bariatric surgery.

2. Patients' motivation and expectations

Patients undergo bariatric surgical procedures for different reasons. It is important to understand each patient's expectations prior to surgery. Studies have shown improvements in psychological or physical health, better quality of life and self esteem as well as better emotional satisfaction in relation with food post operatively (Wolfe and Terry 2006).

However, there is no gain in romantic and professional relationships post surgery (Wolfe and Terry 2006) and patients should be warned and be prepared for this.

Bariatric surgery offers reduction in body weight of between 20-32% within 2 years and between 10-25% after 10 year (Sjostrom, Narbro et al. 2007), or a reduction of 55.9% in excess weight within 2 years(Buchwald, Estok et al. 2009). Studies have shown of the discrepancies in opinion between medical professionals of a successful surgical outcome and patients' expectations (Foster, Wadden et al. 2001; Wee, Jones et al. 2006; Mechanick, Kushner et al. 2009; Heinberg, Keating et al. 2010). One study showed that the average patient 'dream' weight loss is 55kg, attributing to 94% of excess weight loss or losing 43% of their pre-surgical weight. About 90% of the patients in the study were willing to risk death in order achieve their 'dream' weight and almost all patients were willing to risk dying to have a perfect health and their 'dream' weight (Wee, Jones et al. 2006). Younger, Caucasian females with higher body mass index are more likely to have unrealistic expectations (Heinberg, Keating et al. 2010). The team will need to work with patients and provide clear understanding and information regarding realistic outcomes (Tsigos, Hainer et al. 2008) prior to surgery. The team will need to work with patients to negotiate achievable end points and set small feasible goals during the short term period. Providing good education and developing good relationships with patients are vital as this enhances compliance in the future.

Apart from patients' expectation, patients' attitude towards weight loss is also important. It has been shown that 2 years post bariatric surgery, dietary changes and physical activity become lax and patients start to gain weight (Sjostrom, Lindroos et al. 2004). The team will need to assess their likelihood and willingness to make life long changes in their eating habits and engagement in physical activities (National Heart, Blood et al. 1998; UK 2007; Tsigos, Hainer et al. 2008; Scottish Intercollegiate Guidelines and Scotland 2010) to prevent further weight gain pre or post surgery. Motivation could change over time due to various influences (UK 2007). Understanding the medical consequences of obesity will help motivate patients. Other areas to assess motivation are the likelihood to attend follow up appointments, potential barriers to initiate weight loss such as lack of self esteem or confidence in themselves and potential support from family and friends (National Heart, Blood et al. 1998).

3. Medical assessment

3.1 Clinic set up

Clinic set up is important to provide a safe and friendly environment for patients. Entrances and rooms should be spacious enough for bariatric wheel chair access. Chairs in the waiting area and in clinic rooms should provide armless bariatric chair (Mechanick, Kushner et al. 2009). Wheelchairs availability in hospital should accommodate both the weight and size of patients (Barr and Cunneen 2001). Other essential patient care equipments such as suitable examination table in the clinic room, appropriate weighing scales and stadiometer should be available (Mechanick, Kushner et al. 2009). Facilities such as toilets should not be overlooked and fixtures to help individuals with mobility problems may need to be adapted for bariatric patients (Barr and Cunneen 2001).

3.2 Medical history

A thorough medical history and good physical examination will help identify potential health problems. The most important history will be the patient's eating behaviour covering their history of weight gain and previous attempts for weight loss (Tsigos, Hainer et al. 2008; Mechanick, Kushner et al. 2009). History of weight gain, detailed food history and amount of physical activity is also important. Onset of weight gain could be a consequence of various factors including marriage, pregnancy, and smoking cessation, stress or drug induced. Eating patterns and dietary habits are useful to help exclude eating disorders (Tsigos, Hainer et al. 2008) and this will be covered in the nutritional and psychological section.

History should be holistic, including respiratory, cardiovascular, neurological, gastrointestinal, endocrine, musculoskeletal and genital urinary systems including sexual history. Medication and drug histories are also important as many drugs causes weight gain. It is also important to include usage of illegal drugs and over the counter medication. All past medical history must include mood disorders or other mental health illness (Mechanick, Kushner et al. 2009) as well as family history.

Apart from medical history, it is also essential to obtain the patient's functional status including activities of daily living. It is also important to ask about social history including support available either by family members or friends if patient is deemed suitable for surgery (Mechanick, Kushner et al. 2009). Occupation, alcohol and smoking histories should not be missed (Mechanick, Kushner et al. 2009). The patient should be advised to stop smoking but this should be monitored closely as quitting smoking is associated with weight gain. This holistic approach will paint a better picture of how obesity is affecting the patient. Patients with excessive alcohol intake need to be advised to return to recommended levels.

3.3 Physical examination

Physical examination should be thorough including all anthropometric measurement of height and weight to obtain body mass index (Mechanick, Kushner et al. 2009), and waist circumference. Cardiovascular, respiratory, neurology and abdominal systems should be assessed. Neck circumference is an important assessment for obstructive sleep apnoea (Scottish Intercollegiate Guidelines 2003; Epstein, Kristo et al. 2009). Acanthosis nigricans is a sign for insulin resistance (Tsigos, Hainer et al. 2008; Mechanick, Kushner et al. 2009). Other signs include striae distensae (stretch mark), lymphoedema, stasis pigmentation of the lower limbs, intertrigo, hidradenitis suppurativa and acrochordon (Mechanick, Kushner et al. 2009). In patients with history of uncontrolled hypertension and insulin resistance, Cushing's syndrome should be excluded. Signs of Cushing's syndrome are moon facies, posterior cervical fat pads, easy bruisability and purple striae on the abdomen. These signs are, however, rarely seen in clinical bariatric practice.

3.4 Investigations

All patients should have routine blood tests to screen for any potential health problems and treat accordingly prior to surgery (Mechanick, Kushner et al. 2009).

• Full blood count	Anaemia
• Renal function	Kidney disease, hypo or hyperkalaemia
• Liver function test	Hepatitis, non alcoholic induced fatty liver (see lower section)
• Coagulation profile	Coagulopathy, bleeding disorder
• Fasting glucose	Diabetes mellitus (see lower section)
• $HbA1_c$	Diabetes mellitus (see lower section)
• Fasting lipid profile	Dyslipidaemia
• Urine pregnancy test	Pregnancy

If secondary causes of obesity are suspected, patient should be evaluated for primary endocrine disorder such as hypothyroidism and Cushing's syndrome (Tsigos, Hainer et al. 2008; Mechanick, Kushner et al. 2009). Screening tests for these are as below (Mechanick, Kushner et al. 2009):

• Hypothyroidism	Thyroid function test
• Cushing's syndrome	Bedtime salivary cortisol level or 1mg low dose dexamethasone suppression test or 24 hour urine cortisol excretion

Interpretation of tests for Cushing's syndrome can be difficult and more detailed tests may be required. There is no indication for routine testing in this patient population. Only patients with indicative signs, history (including relevant metabolic and cardiovascular abnormalities) and where there is an inability to lose weight despite maximal effort, should be investigated.

Any patients undergoing malabsorptive procedure should have their micronutrients status checked prior to surgery and any deficiencies should be corrected (Mechanick, Kushner et al. 2009). If there is an indication of celiac disease based on these investigations, specific coeliac disease investigations should be carried out.

• Iron status (total iron binding capacity, ferritin, iron, transferring receptor)	Iron deficiency anaemia
• Vitamin B_{12} level	Pernicious anaemia, Vitamin B_{12} deficiency
• 25-OH Vitamin D	Vitamin D deficiency
• Parathyroid hormone (PTH)	Vitamin D deficiency
• Folate levels	Folic acid deficiency, hyperhomocysteinaemia
• Bone profile	Hypocalcaemia, hypophosphataemia
• Magnesium	Hypomagnesaemia

Testing for PTH can be costly and should only be undertaken if there are indications based on other test results.

4. Review of systems

4.1 Respiratory status

Chest x-ray has been recommended to be done for all patients to exclude any pulmonary disorders (Mechanick, Kushner et al. 2009). Chest X-ray, and indeed any imaging investigations are difficult to conduct and interpret in this patient population and may not provide any additional information. Any patients with previous history of respiratory disorder should have arterial blood gas and undergo pulmonary function tests (Mechanick, Kushner et al. 2009). Arterial gases are also useful for assessment of the obesity hypoventilation syndrome. Advising patient to quit smoking will help reduce peri-operative respiratory complications (Mechanick, Kushner et al. 2009).

4.1.1 Lung function in obesity

Breathlessness is a very common symptom among obese patients. It is shown that obesity could affect respiratory physiology including reduction in respiratory compliance and respiratory muscle strength (McClean, Kee et al. 2008; Sood 2009). In fact, many obese patients have problems with their respiratory function. If cardiac causes have been excluded and the patient is complaining of breathlessness, lung function and exercise tests are useful investigations to assess and rule out other significant respiratory problems such as chronic obstructive airway disease or asthma.

At baseline, pulmonary function tests are different between an obese patient and one with normal body mass index. The most significant difference in an obese patient is the reduction in functional residual capacity (FRC) and expiratory reserve volume (ERV) (Gibson 2000; Jones and Nzekwu 2006; Sood 2009). The higher the body mass index, the greater the effect of reduction (Jones and Nzekwu 2006) hence increasing the work of breathing at rest leading to dyspnoea. This can be explained by the effects of abdominal distension from visceral fat on the diaphragm (Gibson 2000; Rabec, de Lucas Ramos et al. 2011) as well as the reduction in chest wall distensibility (Jones and Nzekwu 2006; Rabec, de Lucas Ramos et al. 2011). There may also be an association in the reduction of forced expiratory volume in 1 second (FEV_1) (McClean, Kee et al. 2008; Sood 2009; Rabec, de Lucas Ramos et al. 2011).

4.1.2 Obstructive sleep apnoea (OSA)

Obstructive sleep apnoea (OSA) is a condition characterised by episodic complete or partial obstruction of the upper airway during sleep (Rabec, de Lucas Ramos et al. 2011). Obesity is one of the major risk factor for developing OSA. There is an increased in subcutaneous and periluminal fat causing narrowing of the pharynx leading to obstruction (Epstein, Kristo et al. 2009). This could cause difficulties during peri-operative airway management (Mechanick, Kushner et al. 2009) and presence of OSA has been shown in LABS study to increase 30 day operative mortality (Flum, Belle et al. 2009) hence the importance of the diagnosis leading to more stringent perioperative care of these individuals. About 40% of obese patients suffer with OSA (Sood 2009) and the prevalence can be as high as 98% in the morbidly obese patients (Valencia-Flores, Orea et al. 2000).

Excessive daytime somnolence, snoring at night, feeling unrefreshed on waking, restless sleep, impaired concentration, irritability and apnoeic episodes during sleep are some of the common symptoms of OSA. It has been recommended that all obese patients should be assessed to exclude OSA either by respiratory physician or use the validated questionnaires such as the Epworth's Sleepiness Score (ESS) (Johns 1991) or the Berlin Questionnaire (Netzer, Stoohs et al. 1999) The ESS should be completed by both the patient and the partner if possible. ESS has a maximum score of 24 and a score of > 18 is suggestive of severe subjective daytime somnolence, score of between 15 and 18 is moderate while score of between 11 and 14 is mild (Scottish Intercollegiate Guidelines 2003). Berlin questionnaire looked at 3 different categories; which are snoring, wake time sleepiness or drowsy driving and hypertension or obesity. High risk for OSA is defined as persistent symptoms in at least 2 of the categories with a sensitivity of 86% and specificity of 77% (Netzer, Stoohs et al. 1999). In our experience, the Berlin and Epworth questionnaires are not good indicators of OSA and we recommend formal evaluation for OSA in all bariatric patients.

All patients should undergo sleep studies depending on facilities available. Polysomnography is the investigation of choice to assess OSA and it consists of electroencephalogram (EEG), electroculogram (EOG), chin electromyogram, oxygen saturation, respiratory airflow, thoracic movements and electrocardiography (ECG) (Scottish Intercollegiate Guidelines 2003; Epstein, Kristo et al. 2009). Body position and snoring is monitored as well (Scottish Intercollegiate Guidelines 2003; Epstein, Kristo et al. 2009). Overnight monitoring is ideal and results will then be interpreted. If a full polysomnography is not available, then the sleep study usually consists of respiratory assessment, thoraco-abdominal movement, and monitor for snoring episodes (Scottish Intercollegiate Guidelines 2003). In-laboratory polysomnography may not be routinely available to all patients due to high cost and technical complexity (Collop, Anderson et al. 2007). In that case, unattended portable monitors could be alternative choice. American Academy of Sleep Medicine guideline stated the use of portable monitors should be 'in conjunction with a comprehensive sleep evaluation' for 'patients with high pretest probability of or moderate to severe OSA' who do not have significant co-morbidies such as severe pulmonary disease, neuromuscular disease or congestive heart failure (Collop, Anderson et al. 2007).

The aim of polysomnography is to measure apnoea or hypopnoea episodes. These episodes are reported as apnoea/hypopnoea index (AHI) or respiratory disturbance index (RDI) and can be divided into (Scottish Intercollegiate Guidelines 2003; Epstein, Kristo et al. 2009):

- Mild OSA AHI/RDI 5 - 14 per hour
- Moderate OSA AHI/RDI 15-30 per hour
- Severe OSA AHI/RDI > 30 per hour

Treatment for OSA is weight reduction hence bariatric surgery could help the condition. Non surgical treatment of OSA includes continuous positive airway pressures. Positive airway pressure can be continuous (CPAP), autotitrating (APAP) or bilevel (BPAP) (Scottish Intercollegiate Guidelines 2003; Epstein, Kristo et al. 2009). Sedatives and alcohol should be avoided in the evenings and at night as they reduce airway dilator function hence worsening of OSA (Scottish Intercollegiate Guidelines 2003). Post-operatively, these patients need to be monitored closely and to continue to use their positive airway pressure appliances (Mechanick, Kushner et al. 2009). There is debate regarding duration of CPAP use prior to operation (some centres recommending 3 months), peri-operatively (theoretical potential to disturb anastomoses in non gastric band operations), and post-operatively.

4.1.3 Obesity hypoventilation syndrome (OHS)

Obesity hypoventilation syndrome is a diagnosis of exclusion. The definition of OHS is a condition of consists of daytime hypercapnia and hypoxemia, sleep disordered breathing and obese patient (Mokhlesi 2010). The majority of OHS patients will also have OSA. Other respiratory conditions including intrinsic respiratory disorders, central hypoventilation syndromes and neuromuscular disorders should be excluded (Mokhlesi, Kryger et al. 2008).

Clinical features of OHS are similar to OSA consisting of hypersomnia and headache when awake, snoring and disturbed sleep (Casey, Cantillo et al. 2007). Pathogenesis is likely to be multifactorial. Reduction in respiratory compliance and lung volume, effects of leptin on central ventilatory drive, inspiratory muscle fatigue and depressed central ventilator control from sleep disturbances and raised PaCO2 on central ventilation are likely to play a role in this condition (Casey, Cantillo et al. 2007). Non-invasive positive pressure ventilation is effective and well tolerated in treating this condition (Mokhlesi and Tulaimat 2007; Priou, Hamel et al. 2010).

4.1.4 Smoking

Smoking causes adverse effects on health. The most common respiratory diseases associated with smoking are increased risk of chronic obstructive pulmonary disease and bronchogenic carcinoma. Smoking also increases risk of cardiovascular disease leading to myocardial infarction and peripheral vascular disease. Obese patients are already at higher risk of developing various health problems so these patients should be encouraged and assisted to stop smoking to help improve life expectancy (Scottish Intercollegiate Guidelines and Scotland 2010). It is recommended that patients should quit smoking at least 8 weeks prior to surgery to help reduce risk of respiratory complications (Mechanick, Kushner et al. 2009). Unfortunately, smoking cessation is associated with weight gain (Williamson, Madans et al. 1991; Flegal, Troiano et al. 1995; Wise, Enright et al. 1998; Scottish Intercollegiate Guidelines and Scotland 2010) and patients might be reluctant to quit (McClean, Kee et al. 2008).

Weight gain from smoking cessation is more pronounced in females compared to males (Williamson, Madans et al. 1991; Wise, Enright et al. 1998). Mean weight gain is between 2.8kg (Williamson, Madans et al. 1991) to 5kg (Flegal, Troiano et al. 1995; Wise, Enright et al. 1998) with females gaining approximately 1kg more than males (Williamson, Madans et al. 1991). A proportion of patients will gain more than 13kg in weight (Williamson, Madans et al. 1991). Weight gain from quitting smoking has been associated with increased in prevalence in overweight population (Flegal, Troiano et al. 1995) and this could lead to obesity in the future. Although there is risk of weight gain, the benefits from smoking cessation is greater in improvement in lung function in particular FEV_1 and FVC (Wise, Enright et al. 1998). The Framingham Heart Study found that obese smokers have almost doubled the reduction in life expectancy as compared to obese non smokers (Peeters, Barendregt et al. 2003).

Patient should be given advice to seek help for smoking cessation. The reasons for weight gain might be due to various mechanisms. An increased in food consumption (2010) of up to 250 to 300 kilocalories a day after stopping smoking, reduction in physical activity (Chiolero, Faeh et al. 2008), changes in fat metabolism e.g. lipoprotein activity (Williamson, Madans et al. 1991; Chiolero, Faeh et al. 2008) and changes in insulin homeostasis (Williamson, Madans et al. 1991) could all contribute to weight gain. Patients should be advised have low calorie diet, reduce in portion sizes during meal times and avoid second helpings (2008). Chewing gum or nicotine gum helps to prevent snacking. Dietary advice on healthy balanced diet and increase in physical activities, getting new hobbies to relieve boredom are some simple advice for patients to stop smoking (2008). Individualised treatment plan with dietary and cognitive behavioural intervention will help potential quitters prevent weight gain (Scottish Intercollegiate Guidelines and Scotland 2010). Buproprion helps with weight loss (Davtyan and Ma 2008) and this could be use along side with nicotine replacement therapy. Smokers tend to have a longer hospital stay and smoking cessation should be recommended well in advance of bariatric surgery.

4.2 Cardiovascular status

Obesity increases risk for cardiovascular disorder (Hubert, Feinleib et al. 1983; Jonsson, Hedblad et al. 2002; Wilson, D'Agostino et al. 2002; Wolk, Berger et al. 2003) and premature death (Jonsson, Hedblad et al. 2002; Peeters, Barendregt et al. 2003) but is not a risk factor for post-operative cardiac complication (Mechanick, Kushner et al. 2009). Blood pressure monitoring to assess for hypertension and electrocardiography are basic investigations to assess cardiovascular function. Cardiac sounding chest pain or angina episodes should be investigated further, but investigations are limited given body habitus and lack of resolution of diagnostic tests. Difficulties lie with patient complaining of dyspnoea as this could present as cardiac disease or obesity related dyspnoea. Exercise tolerance will be useful to assess cardiac risk. Presence of other metabolic risk factors especially diabetes mellitus increases the patient's risk for coronary artery disease (Fox, Coady et al. 2007).

4.2.1 Electrocardiogram (ECG)

Obesity may cause changes in ECG readings. Some common changes include left axis deviation likely due to displacement of the heart from raised diaphragm due to abdominal visceral fat and small voltages (Eisenstein, Edelstein et al. 1982; Frank, Colliver et al. 1986; Alpert, Terry et al. 2000; Poirier, Giles et al. 2006) from the increased distance between the heart and the chest wall (Poirier, Giles et al. 2006). Cardiac work load is also increased (Lavie, Milani et al. 2009) and this could lead to left ventricular hypertrophy (Lauer, Anderson et al. 1991; Poirier, Giles et al. 2006; Avelar, Cloward et al. 2007; Lavie, Milani et al. 2009; Movahed, Martinez et al. 2009). Pulmonary diseases such as obstructive sleep apnoea could cause cor pulmonale changes. Other possible ECG changes are increased in heart rate (Frank, Colliver et al. 1986; Poirier, Giles et al. 2006), prolonged PR interval (Frank, Colliver et al. 1986; Poirier, Giles et al. 2006; Seyfeli, Duru et al. 2006), prolonged QRS interval (Frank, Colliver et al. 1986; Poirier, Giles et al. 2006), prolonged QTc interval (Frank, Colliver et al. 1986; Alpert, Terry et al. 2000; Pontiroli, Pizzocri et al. 2004; Poirier, Giles et al. 2006; Arslan, Yiginer et al. 2010), ST-T wave abnormalities (Frank, Colliver et al. 1986; Poirier, Giles et al. 2006) and flattening of the T wave especially in the inferolateral leads (Eisenstein, Edelstein et al. 1982; Alpert, Terry et al. 2000; Lopez-Jimenez and Cortes-Bergoderi 2011).

4.2.2 Echocardiography

Technical difficulty in echocardiography is common in obese patients due to the size as well as the distance between chest wall and heart. Obesity increases the risk of left ventricular hypertrophy (LVH) (Lauer, Anderson et al. 1991; de la Maza, Estevez et al. 1994; Poirier,

Giles et al. 2006; Avelar, Cloward et al. 2007; Lavie, Milani et al. 2009; Movahed, Martinez et al. 2009) and this could be assessed using echocardiography. Presence of LVH increase risk of mortality as it is associated with coronary heart disease and stroke(Benjamin and Levy 1999). Other potential abnormality include left atrial enlargement (Lavie, Milani et al. 2009; Arslan, Yiginer et al. 2010), difficulty in the assessment of pericardial fluid due to thickened epicardial tissue (Poirier, Giles et al. 2006). Dobutamine stress echocardiography is probably more useful than conventional echocardiogram to assess cardiac function (Mechanick, Kushner et al. 2009).

4.2.3 Hypertension

Hypertension is a well-recognised risk factor for coronary artery disease (Kannel 1996; Diaz 2002; I 2010). Prevalence of hypertension is higher among overweight and obese population(Stamler, Stamler et al. 1978; Brown, Higgins et al. 2000) and is not associated with ethnicity or socioeconomic status (Diaz 2002). Indeed, increased in visceral abdominal fat in obesity increases the risk of hypertension (Narkiewicz 2006). Uncontrolled hypertension with blood pressure levels above 180/110mmHg should be corrected as this could lead to perioperative ischaemic events (Mechanick, Kushner et al. 2009).

Many mechanisms have been postulated for the causation of hypertension and this includes changes in substances released from adipose tissue (Benjamin and Levy 1999; I 2010), increased in sympathetic activity (Narkiewicz 2006; Poirier, Giles et al. 2006, Wilcox 2010) and presence of obstructive sleep apnoea (Diaz 2002; Avelar, Cloward et al. 2007). Increase in body weight leads to increase in sympathetic activity (Narkiewicz 2006; Poirier, Giles et al. 2006; Wilcox 2010); and this could be explained by the activation of renin-angiotensin-aldosterone system (Narkiewicz 2006; Wilcox 2010). Hypoxaemia and hypercapnic episodes as well as changes in the intrathoracic pressure in obstructive sleep apnoea has been found to increase blood pressure (Diaz 2002; Avelar, Cloward et al. 2007).

Adipose tissue releases several adipokines (Maenhaut and Van de Voorde 2011). One adipokine is the hormone leptin (Wilcox 2010; Maenhaut and Can de Voorde 2011). Leptin levels are elevated in hypertension and its effect could be via the activation of the sympathetic nervous system or dysfunction of the endothelium causing vasoconstriction leading to increase in peripheral vascular resistance (Maenhaut and Van de Voorde 2011).

Apart from increased risk in coronary heart disease, hypertension also increases the risk of developing renal failure (Narkiewicz 2006; Wilcox 2010). It is important to treat this condition vigilantly to prevent perioperative ischaemic event (Mechanick, Kushner et al. 2009). Many guidelines are available as references for the treatment of hypertension such as the JNC VII report (Chobanian, Bakris et al. 2003) and British Hypertension Society guidelines (Williams, Poulter et al. 2004).

4.2.4 Coronary heart disease

Obesity increases the risk of myocardial infarction and coronary heart disease and is an independent risk factor for cardiovascular disease (Hubert, Feinleib et al. 1983; Wilson, D'Agostino et al. 2002). Given that there is increasing prevalence in hypertensive patients and obesity related obstructive sleep apnoea as well as increased risk of dyslipidaemia and insulin resistance, these factors most likely contribute to the cumulative risks for obese patients (Poirier, Giles et al. 2006; Lopez-Jimenez and Cortes-Bergoderi 2011). Apart from this, it has been found that in young men, obesity could accelerate the development of atherosclerosis (McGill, McMahan et al. 2002). Patients with cardiac sounding chest pain or any previous history of cardiac disease should not be taken lightly prior to surgery and should be investigated thoroughly by a cardiologist and treated accordingly to minimise risk during surgery. Prophylactic beta-blocker therapy has been recommended for patients who have high risk of cardiac disease (Mechanick, Kushner et al. 2009).

4.3 Metabolic control

A high proportion of patients with obesity suffer from metabolic syndrome. Diagnosis of metabolic syndrome is based on the presence of insulin resistance, obesity, dyslipidaemia, and hypertension. Both International Diabetes Federation (IDF) (Alberti, Zimmet et al. 2005) and National Cholesterol Education Program Adult Treatment Panel (NCEP ATP III)(2002) have their own criteria for metabolic syndrome as summarized below:

	Obesity	Lipid	Blood pressure	Glucose
IDF – Obesity plus 2 factors	Waist circumference (ethnic specific) > 94cm (M) or > 80cm (F)	Raised Tg ≥ 150mg/dl or HDL < 50 (M) or < 40mg/dl (F) or on therapy	≥130/85 mmHg or on therapy	Fasting glucose > 100mg/dl or known diabetes mellitus
NCEP ATP III -any 3 criteria	Waist circumference > 102cm/40 inches (M) or > 88cm/35 inches (F)	Raised Tg ≥ 150mg/dl or HDL < 40mg/dl (M) or < 50mg/dl (F) or on therapy	≥130/85mmHg or on therapy	Fasting glucose > 110mg / dl or known diabetes mellitus

M=Male; F=Female

Table 1. Criteria for metabolic syndrome

4.3.1 Diabetes mellitus

Obesity can cause insulin resistance due to changes in adipokines, inflammatory mechanisms and intrinsic cell mechanisms (Qatanani and Lazar 2007). Insulin resistance could in turn lead to development of diabetes mellitus (Chan, Rimm et al. 1994; Koh-Banerjee, Wang et al. 2004). Raised visceral or waist to hip ratios (Chan, Rimm et al. 1994; Koh-Banerjee, Wang et al. 2004) and duration of obesity (Wannamethee and Shaper 1999) are good predictors of diabetes mellitus. Many individuals might already have diagnoses of diabetes mellitus and the rest needs to be screened with either fasting plasma glucose, $HbA1_c$ or a formal oral glucose tolerance test.

Diagnosis of diabetes could be made by the presence of either one of the following based on the American Diabetes Association criteria (ADA) (2011):

- $HbA1_c \geq$ 48mmol/mol or 6.5%
- Fasting plasma glucose ≥ 126mg/dl or 7.0mmol/l
- Oral glucose tolerance test after 75g of oral glucose with a result of fasting plasma glucose of ≥ 126mg/dl or 7.0mmol/l or 2 hour post-prandial reading of ≥200 mg/dl or 11.1mmol/l.
- Random plasma glucose of ≥ 200mg/dl or 11.1mmol/l with classical symptoms of hyperglycaemia or hyperglycaemia crisis such as hyperglycaemic hyperosmolar state or diabetic ketoacidosis.

Newly diagnosed patients with diabetes mellitus should be managed appropriately. Lifestyle measures are usually the first step (Nathan, Buse et al. 2009; National Institute for et al. 2009). ADA and European Association of Study of Diabetes (EASD) (Nathan, Buse et al. 2009) as well as National Institute for Health and Clinical Excellence (NICE) (2009) have published guidelines for the management of type 2 diabetes mellitus. There are various different medications for diabetes mellitus and are associated with their own adverse effects including drug induced weight gain (Makimattila, Nikkila et al. 1999). A summary of the medications with effects on $HbA1_c$, weight and adverse effects is as below (Nathan, Buse et al. 2009; Dicker 2011):

Anti-diabetic medications	Reduction in $HbA1_c$ (%)	Effects on weight	Other adverse side effects
Biguanides Eg. Metformin	1.0 – 2.0	Weight neutral	Gastrointestinal side effects, rarely lactic acidosis
Sulphonylureas Eg. gliclazide, glipizide, glibenclamide	1.0 – 2.0	Weight gain	Hypoglycaemia
α-glucosidase inhibitors Eg. Acarbose	0.5 - 0.8	Weight neutral	Gastrointestinal side effects
Glucagon like peptide (GLP)-1 Eg. exenatide, liraglutide	0.5 - 1.0	Weight loss	Nausea, vomiting
Pramlintide	0.5 - 1.0	Weight loss	Gastrointestinal side effects
Glinides Eg. repaglinide and nateglinide	0.5 – 1.5	Weight gain	Gastrointestinal side effects
Insulin	1.5 - 3.5	Weight gain	Hypoglycaemia
Thiazolidinediones Eg. pioglitazone, rosiglitazone*	0.5 - 1.4	Weight gain	Fluid retention, *increased cardiovascular risk
Dipeptidyl peptidase 4 (DPP-4) inhibitor(Dicker 2011) Eg. sitagliptin, saxagliptin, vildagliptin	0.43 - 1.4	Weight neutral	Upper respiratory tract infection, nasopharyngitis, headache

*Rosiglitazone is associated with increased cardiovascular risk and is withdrawn in the United Kingdom (2010) and in europe (2010). United States Food and Drug Administration (FDA) have issued restriction on its usage (2011).

Table 2. HbA1c, weight and adverse effects of anti-diabetic medications (Nathan, Buse et al. 2009; Dicker 2011)

It is recommend to have a $HbA1_c$ level of < 53mmol/mol or 7.0% (Mechanick, Kushner et al. 2009; 2011), fasting plasma glucose of < 110mg/dl or 6.1mmol/l (2011) preoperatively to ensure good outcome. This, however, is unrealistic in many patients who are having bariatric surgery to treat their poor diabetes control. There is a greater propensity for day case and short stay bariatric surgery which allows patients with less well-controlled diabetes to have bariatric surgery.

4.3.2 Dyslipidaemia

Increased in visceral adipose tissue in obesity is associated with raised triglyceride levels, raised small dense low density lipoprotein (sdLDL) and reduction in high density lipoprotein cholesterol (HDL) levels (Ginsberg and Maccallum 2009; Athyros, Tziomalos et al. 2011). In addition, presence of insulin resistance as previously described can further increased free fatty acids availability to other organs (Athyros, Tziomalos et al. 2011). Guidelines such as the National Cholesterol Education Program on adult treatment panel III (NCEP ATP III) (2002) and NICE guidelines on lipid modifications (2010) are useful to help treat and reduce cardiovascular risk.

4.4 Gastrointestinal (GI) status

Presence of any gastrointestinal (GI) symptoms should warrant further evaluation with additional investigations (Mechanick, Kushner et al. 2009). Gastroenterology referral is appropriate and endoscopy could be performed to rule out serious diseases. It is important to note that obesity is associated with a number of cancers. Physicians should be vigilant to distinguish between healthy planned weight loss and weight loss due to sinister reasons such as cancer.

4.4.1 Common gastrointestinal problems in obesity

There appears to be a positive correlation between obesity and gastrointestinal symptoms especially abdominal pain, vomiting and diarrhoea (Delgado-Aros, Locke et al. 2004; Talley, Howell et al. 2004). It is still unclear as to the mechanisms causing these symptoms (Delgado-Aros, Locke et al. 2004; Talley, Howell et al. 2004). Other upper GI symptoms could be caused by gastroesophageal reflux disease (GERD). GERD is a common disorder and patients present with different symptoms including heartburn, acid regurgitation, chest pain, dysphagia and dyspepsia (Locke, Talley et al. 1997). One of the major risk factor for GERD is obesity (El-Serag, Graham et al. 2005; Corley and Kubo 2006). Oesophageal erosions are also more prevalent in obese patients (El-Serag, Graham et al. 2005). This is important as symptomatic GERD is associated with future development of Barrett's oesophagus and oesophageal adenocarcinoma (Lagergren, Bergstrom et al. 1999). Therefore it is important to treat this condition adequately either through medical therapies or weight loss through surgery.

4.4.2 Gallstones

Gallstones disease is common in obese population and could cause abnormality in liver enzyme levels. Rapid weight loss post bariatric surgery especially with Roux-en-Y gastric bypass surgery is associated with biliary stasis and lithiasis (Caruana, McCabe et al. 2005;

Quesada, Kohan et al. 2010). Patients could have concomitant cholecystectomy during surgery with disadvantage of increased in intrasurgical time or treat with prophylactic ursodeoxycholic acid post surgery for 6 months (Quesada, Kohan et al. 2010).

4.4.3 Non-alcoholic fatty liver disease

Obesity is one of the major risk factor for non-alcoholic fatty liver disease (NAFLD) (Clain and Lefkowitch 1987; Salgado Junior, Santos et al. 2006; Scaglioni, Ciccia et al. 2011) and is often asymptomatic (Salgado Junior, Santos et al. 2006). Abnormal liver function test results especially with raised aspartate transaminase (AST) and AST/ALT (alanine transaminase) ratio are some predictors of this disease (Liew, Lee et al. 2006; Salgado Junior, Santos et al. 2006). Viral, autoimmune and other rare causes such as Wilson's disease and alpha-1 antitrypsin deficiency should be ruled out in the presence of abnormal test results. Other laboratory abnormalities are raised γ- glutamyltransferease (γGT) and alkaline phosphatase (ALP), dyslipidaemia and hyperglycaemia (Salgado Junior, Santos et al. 2006). Liver biopsy is the gold standard for diagnosing this condition (Salgado Junior, Santos et al. 2006; Vuppalanchi and Chalasani 2009). Ultrasound scan of the liver (Mechanick, Kushner et al. 2009) or liver biopsy(Salgado Junior, Santos et al. 2006)is recommended in the presence of 2-3 folds increased in the liver enzymes. Transient elastography (Lupsor, Badea et al. 2010) including using XL probe for obese patients (Myers, Pomier-Layrargues et al. 2011) is an alternative method in assessing liver stiffness hence able to detect liver fibrosis. Hepatotoxic medications should be avoided in these patients (Salgado Junior, Santos et al. 2006) and bariatric surgery can potentially reverse the condition (Srivastava and Younossi 2005; De Ridder, Schoon et al. 2007; Kaila and Raman 2008).

4.4.4 Alcohol

Alcohol is another common cause for abnormal liver function test results and excessive intake could potentially cause liver problems including cirrhosis. In a study, it is found that overweight and obese individuals have higher risk of raised liver enzymes with only 2 alcohol drinks per day (Ruhl and Everhart 2005). Current history of excess alcohol use is contraindicated for bariatric surgery (Snyder 2009) and these patients should be referred to other services to help quit. Patients undergoing bariatric surgery need to be counselled regarding alcohol. Total abstinence is not necessary as in gastric band patients, those who are teetotal appear to lose less weight (Dixon, Dixon et al. 2001). Alcohol absorption is greater in malabsorptive type operations and patients should be warned that there are risks of rapid intoxication and greater liver damage by alcohol.

4.5 Endocrine disorders causing obesity

A small proportion of patients' weight problem might be due to endocrine disorders especially for patients with history of recent weight gain. The common disorders include hypothyroidism, Cushing's syndrome and prolactinoma. Hypothyroidism is associated with weight gain through reduction in metabolic rate and thermogenesis (Reinehr 2010). Associations have been found between obesity and thyroid function especially elevation in thyroid stimulating hormone (TSH) (Knudsen, Laurberg et al. 2005; Nyrnes, Jorde et al. 2006). This is likely to help in increasing energy expenditure leading to reduction in fat deposition (Reinehr 2010). Furthermore, obesity is associated with reduced tissue conversion of T4 to T3. It should be noted that in up to 30% of patients with thyroid overactivity, weight gain may occur rather than weight loss.

Hyperprolactinaemia could lead to increase in weight as shown in patients with prolactinomas. When prolactin levels fall after treatment so does patients' weight (Greenman, Tordjman et al. 1998). The relationship between prolactin level and weight could be due to the changes within central dopaminergic pathway and reduction in serotonin secretion(Kopelman 2000). Prolactin level has been found to be elevated in obese females (Kok, Roelfsema et al. 2004) and levels falls after weight loss (Kok, Roelfsema et al. 2006). Raised prolactin level in obesity might be a result of hyperinsulinaemic state or alterations in doperminergic and serotoninergic activities centrally (Kopelman 2000).

Cushing's syndrome is a condition of chronic excessive glucocorticoid production. This condition causes weight gain amongst other clinical features as described above. In patients with morbid obesity, mild hypercortisolaemia could be found with increased urinary free cortisol level (Nieman, Biller et al. 2008). Other conditions mimicking Cushing's syndrome are chronic alcoholism, major depressive disorder (Orth 1995), poorly controlled diabetes mellitus, and pregnancy (Nieman, Biller et al. 2008). One should always keep in mind these potential endocrine abnormalities causing obesity and investigate further in suspicious cases.

4.6 Reproductive status

In males, increased in BMI is associated with fertility problems (Nguyen, Wilcox et al. 2007) and this could be related to reduction in testosterone, sex hormone binding globulin (SHBG) and free testosterone as weight increases (MacDonald, Herbison et al. 2010). Oestradiol level on the other hand is increased (Hammoud, Gibson et al. 2009) and this is likely caused by aromatisation of adipose tissue. Hormonal changes are likely to cause problems with sexual quality of life and this can be reversed with bariatric surgery (Hammoud, Gibson et al. 2009).

In females, high body mass index could cause problem with menstrual irregularities (Jones, Srinivasan et al. 2007; Wei, Schmidt et al. 2009; Kulie, Slattengren et al. 2011). The underlying cause could be due to polycystic ovarian syndrome, oligomenorrhoea or amenorrhoea (Jones, Srinivasan et al. 2007) leading to issues with ovulation. Links have been found between increased abdominal fat with anovulation (Kuchenbecker, Groen et al. 2010) likely due to insulin resistance (Pasquali, Pelusi et al. 2003). These problems in turn lead to sub- or infertility by disrupting spontaneous ovulation and can reduced efficacy of assisted fertility treatment (Pasquali, Pelusi et al. 2003; Balen 2007; Farquhar 2007; Pasquali, Patton et al. 2007). However, fertility is improved post bariatric surgery due to weight loss (Guelinckx, Devlieger et al. 2009; Shah and Ginsburg 2010; Hezelgrave and Oteng-Ntim 2011; Kulie, Slattengren et al. 2011). Early pregnancy post surgery might be associated with increased risk of miscarriages and possibility of preterm birth (Guelinckx, Devlieger et al. 2009). Therefore, patients suitable for surgery are generally advised not to seek pregnancy at least 1 year after surgery (Guelinckx, Devlieger et al. 2009; Mechanick, Kushner et al. 2009). This is especially important in patients receiving malabsorptive surgeries as there are potentially severe nutritional deficiencies that could be exacerbated in pregnancy (Guelinckx, Devlieger et al. 2009; Hezelgrave and Oteng-Ntim 2011).

Contraception advice is vital. Obesity is a risk factor for venous thromboembolism (Stein, Beemath et al. 2005) and can cause recurrent thromboses (Eichinger, Hron et al. 2008). Oestrogen therapy is recommended to be stopped a month prior to surgery to avoid this complication (Mechanick, Kushner et al. 2009). Individuals going for malabsorptive procedures should be advice to avoid oral contraception as post operative as there is a risk of failure to absorb leading to failure of treatment (2010; Paulen, Zapata et al. 2010). There are concerns as well regarding risk of fractures due to effects on bone mineral density from usage of depot medroxyprogesterone acetate (DMPA) after malabsorptive surgery (Paulen, Zapata et al. 2010).

4.7 Medications causing weight gain

The commonest cause of weight gain is due to adverse effect from drug therapy and patients should be advised on weight gain when these medications are prescribed (Scottish Intercollegiate Guidelines and Scotland 2010). Common medications causing weight gain are as follows (Kulkarni and Kaur 2001; Ness-Abramof and Apovian 2005; Leslie, Hankey et al. 2007; Davtyan and Ma 2008; Scottish Intercollegiate Guidelines and Scotland 2010; Nihalani, Schwartz et al. 2011):

- Anti-convulsants (sodium valproate, carbamazepine, gabapentin)
- Anti-psychotics (clozapine, olanzapine, risperidone, quetiapine, clopromazine, ziprasidone, aripiprazole)
- Anti-depressants (tricyclic anti-depressants (TCA), selective serotonin reuptake inhibitors (SSRI), mirtazapine)
- Mood stabilisers (lithium)
- Anti-hypertensives (beta blockers, calcium channel blockers)
- Anti-diabetic medications (insulin, sulphonylurea, thiazolidinedione)
- Steroid
- Anti-neoplastic agents (tamoxifen)
- Anti-histamines

Mechanisms of medications causing weight gain could be due to their effects on appetite through receptors at the central nervous system or effects on the body's metabolism. Anti-histaminergic effect by most psychotropic medications including anti-depressants and anti-psychotics causes cravings for carbohydrate (Davtyan and Ma 2008; Nihalani, Schwartz et al. 2011). Antipsychotics cause inhibitory effect on serotonin and epinephrine receptors thus stimulating appetite (Davtyan and Ma 2008). These effects could cause 2 to 17kg of weight gain during treatment (Nihalani, Schwartz et al. 2011). Lithium is used as mood stabilisers and might cause weight gain through increasing level of serum leptin (Atmaca, Kuloglu et al. 2002) or changes in thyroid function. As many obese patients suffer from depression, medications to treat the condition could be a cause of obesity or exacerbate the problem. Venlafaxine is weight neutral while bupropion causes weight loss so could be treatment of choice if patient is not contraindicated to these medications (Davtyan and Ma 2008).

Anticonvulsants cause weight gain through the effects on endocrine system and body metabolism. Sodium valproate causes increase in insulin and leptin levels with reduction in gluconeogenesis and metabolic rate (Davtyan and Ma 2008). Alternative medication using weight neutral anticonvulsants such as lamotrigine (Kulkarni and Kaur 2001) and levetiracetam (Davtyan and Ma 2008) could help prevent the problem, and topiramate may help induce weight loss (Kulkarni and Kaur 2001; Davtyan and Ma 2008).

Beta adrenergic receptors are present in adipose tissue and when stimulated by noradrenaline, help to metabolize fat into energy source (Nihalani, Schwartz et al. 2011). Beta blocker not only reverses this effect, it also causes reduction in resting metabolic rate (Davtyan and Ma 2008). Verapamil might cause weight gain through inhibition in dopaminergic receptor while clonidine reduces sympathetic activity via central nervous system thus decreasing the metabolic rate (Davtyan and Ma 2008). Angiotensin converting enzyme (ACE) inhibitors and diuretics are other possibilities as treatment for hypertension (Davtyan and Ma 2008).

Obesity is associated with metabolic syndrome and this causes insulin resistance leading to diabetes mellitus. Some anti-diabetic medications causes weight gain mostly through effect on metabolism. Correction of catabolic state of diabetes causing retention of calories, endogenous or exogenous insulin causing inhibition of lipolysis, reduction in leptin production and appetite stimulation from hypoglycaemic episodes contributes towards weight gain (Davtyan and Ma 2008). One of the side effects of thiazolidinediones is fluid retention (Davtyan and Ma 2008). Medications helping in weight loss is glucagon-like peptite-1 (GLP-1) (Nathan, Buse et al. 2009) while dipeptidyl-peptidase (DPP)-4 inhibitor (Dicker 2011), gliclazide modified release (Zoungas, Chalmers et al. 2010) and metformin(Nathan, Buse et al. 2009) are weight neutral . These might be better choice for obese patients if there are no contraindications. It is important to recognise drug induced weight gain and sometimes changing medications could enhance potential weight lost post surgery.

5. Psychological assessment

All patients who undergo surgery will need long term behavioural and eating habit changes. Indeed, some view bariatric surgery as a forced behavior modification (van Hout and van Heck 2009). Psychological and psychiatric disorders could lead to a negative outcome post operatively (Pull 2010). These include those who have active psychosis, current illicit drug users or alcohol abuse and personality disorders(Susan F. Franks 2008). Surgery is contraindicated in patients who are currently abusing drugs or alcohol (Susan F. Franks 2008; Snyder 2009). Patients with previous history of sexual abuse, found in a significant percentage of bariatric patients, will need more support as they might find difficulties with attention gained post surgery due to change in body image and thus risk regaining weight(Snyder 2009). Psychological disorders can include depression, anxiety, eating disorders and low self esteem (Abiles, Rodriguez-Ruiz et al. 2010). Patients known or suspected to have psychological or psychiatric disorders should be referred for further mental health assessment (Susan F. Franks 2008; Mechanick, Kushner et al. 2009) by a psychologist or psychiatrist. The assessment usually contains one or two parts: a clinical interview and psychological testing (Mechanick, Kushner et al. 2009; Snyder 2009).

5.1 Depression and anxiety

Depression is very common (Susan F. Franks 2008; Snyder 2009; Abiles, Rodriguez-Ruiz et al. 2010) and prevalence is highly variable depending on the use of a choice of structured clinical interview for diagnostic and statistical manual of mental disorders (SCID) or clinical based diagnosis (Susan F. Franks 2008). Mild depressive disorder is relatively benign and might improve post surgery (Snyder 2009). On the other hand, severe depression with or without suicidal ideation could have adverse effects towards patients as they might have difficulty adhering with dietary or other advice provided(Snyder 2009). Patients will need these addressed prior to surgery (Mechanick, Kushner et al. 2009).

Anxiety is present in 15 to 37.5% of patients (Susan F. Franks 2008). Most patients' distress levels are reduced with weight loss post surgery (Ryden, Karlsson et al. 2003) but this could potentially cause problems with adaptability or ability to cope perioperatively (Snyder 2009).

5.2 Eating disorder

Eating disorder is common. This can include comfort eating from emotional stress or distress, binge eating, snacking (Mechanick, Kushner et al. 2009; Snyder 2009) and night time eating (Snyder 2009). Binge eating is characterised by subjective loss of control and consumed a large quantity of food within a short period (Snyder 2009). About 10-25% of patients have problems with binge eating (Snyder 2009). Psychologists could help alleviate the symptoms and reinforce the behaviour modification needed (Snyder 2009).

Night eating syndrome (NES) is characterised with night time hyperphagia, which is intake of 25% of total daily calories after evening meal, awaking from sleep to eat at night (Allison, Wadden et al. 2006; Howell, Schenck et al. 2009; Stunkard, Allison et al. 2009) and morning anorexia (Gluck, Geliebter et al. 2001). It is more common in women, and is associated with higher rate of depression, lower self-esteem and less day time hunger with poorer outcome in weight loss (Gluck, Geliebter et al. 2001). Patients with this condition should be considered for a referral to a psychologist for further evaluation and treatment. Sertraline has been shown to be useful in patients with night eating syndrome (O'Reardon, Allison et al. 2006).

Psychological assessments will help to distinguish patient who are contraindicated for surgery, improve patient's emotional well being and motivation as well as enhances patient's ability to cope with bariatric surgery (Snyder 2009).

6. Dietary and nutrition assessment

Food can be measured based on amount of calories. Weight is maintained when intake of calories equals expenditure. Obesity occurs when there is a chronic surplus of intake. Therefore, nutritional assessment by a specialist dietitian or nutritionist is essential. Assessment should again be holistic and this includes patient's lifestyle, eating habits, positive and negative influences on behaviour (Detitians in obesity management 2007). Practitioners should have specialist skills in nutritional assessment. Time recommended to evaluate lifestyle habits is initially is between 45 minutes and an hour with follow up appointments between 20 to 30 minutes (Detitians in obesity management 2007).

The patient's weight history could help identify onset of weight problem either since childhood indicating a genetic contribution (Farooqi and O'Rahilly 2007) or any important life events causing initiation of weight problem such as pregnancy (Smith, Lewis et al. 1994). Assessment should also include previous efforts and outcomes of weight loss attempts. Gibbons et al showed that on average, individuals had 4.7 attempts in losing weight before seeking surgery (Gibbons, Sarwer et al. 2006). This enables positive factors to be identified and maintained and previous failures addressed (Detitians in obesity management 2007).

Bariatric surgery will help in weight loss but Swedish Obese Subjects (SOS) study has shown that after maximum weight loss at 1 year, patients start to regain some of the excess weight loss after 2 years and weight gain stabilized after 8 to 10 years (Sjostrom, Narbro et al. 2007). Lifestyle modifications which include changes in diet, physical activity and behavioural therapy are paramount in preventing this problem post surgery and assist in weight maintenance (National Heart, Blood et al. 1998; Wadden, Butryn et al. 2007; Tsigos, Hainer et al. 2008).

Apart from these, it is also important to look at cultural, religious and personal beliefs or preferences in different type of food and eating behaviour. The use of a food diary is an important tool to assess quantity and type of food intake as well as able to provide practical suggestions on changes (Detitians in obesity management 2007; Scottish Intercollegiate Guidelines and Scotland 2010). However, obese patients tend to under-report their dietary intake (Detitians in obesity management 2007; Scottish Intercollegiate Guidelines and Scotland 2010).

6.1 Eating habits

There are different dietary behaviours within the obese population. Some patients eat for comfort especially during stress or negative emotions (Elfhag and Rossner 2005). There are many different eating habits and detailed assessment of dietary intake is vital in providing specific action plans for different patients. Binge eating and night eating syndrome are eating disorders as described above (Allison, Wadden et al. 2006; Tsigos, Hainer et al. 2008). It is important to identify patients who have this problem and referred to psychologist for further treatment prior to proceeding for bariatric surgery (Detitians in obesity management 2007).

Skipping meals especially breakfast is a common habit (Ruxton and Kirk 1997; Wyatt, Grunwald et al. 2002). Breakfast especially with cereal is low in fat, high in carbohydrate, fibre and micronutrients (Ruxton and Kirk 1997). Researchers have shown breakfast consumption is associated with lower body weight (Ruxton and Kirk 1997) and better success with future maintenance of weight loss (Wyatt, Grunwald et al. 2002; Elfhag and Rossner 2005; Wing and Phelan 2005; Grief and Miranda 2010). Nevertheless, it is common for patients to not feel hungry in the morning after bariatric surgery. Other erratic eating habits include periods of fasting, snacking or grazing food (Detitians in obesity management 2007). Sometimes the spouse or partner provides excessive feeding towards the patient causing excessive eating. It is important to address these behaviours and educate patients to have a balanced three meals per day to maintain good nutritional status prior to surgery (Tsigos, Hainer et al. 2008).

6.2 Dietary treatment

There are various types of food in the shelves of supermarkets and consumers have many different choices. Most food packaging now carry nutritional information on their labels for consumers to read. Educating patients to choose their food can help increase further awareness of label reading. Furthermore, it is also a good opportunity to educate patient to have a more balanced diet consisting of more fruits and vegetables, and less fat, salt and sugar ((FDA) 2004; NHS Choices 2011).

Nutritional requirements are different for each person depending on gender, height, weight, amount of physical activity and age. Dietitians could help to calculate the daily requirement while patients need to be taught how to read food label and perform their own calorie counting for their recommended daily caloric intake.

There are many dietary interventions available. The Dietary Approaches to Stop Hypertension (DASH) for obese patient with hypertension gives priority to a diet high in grain products, fruits, vegetables, low in fat and non dairy food. It has proven to lower blood pressure (Appel, Moore et al. 1997; Svetkey, Simons-Morton et al. 1999; Miller, Erlinger et al. 2006) and cholesterol (Miller, Erlinger et al. 2006). Other interventions that has shown success in weight loss include carbohydrate restriction diet including commercial weight loss programme (Nordmann, Nordmann et al. 2006; Gardner, Kiazand et al. 2007), the low glycaemic index diet (Thomas, Elliott et al. 2007), Mediterranean diet (Shai, Schwarzfuchs et al. 2008) and low fat diet(Nordmann, Nordmann et al. 2006).

6.3 Six hundred calorie deficit diet

It is recommended for patient to aim to lose weight of no more than 0.5 - 1kg (1 - 2Ib) per week (Heart, Blood et al. 1997; 2006; Scottish Intercollegiate Guidelines and Scotland 2010) and this equivalent to a calorie deficit of 500 to 1000kcal per day for 6 months (National Heart, Blood et al. 1998; Scottish Intercollegiate Guidelines and Scotland 2010); hence the 600kcal deficit approach (Detitians in obesity management 2007; Tsigos, Hainer et al. 2008; Scottish Intercollegiate Guidelines and Scotland 2010). Dietician will calculate the patient's estimated energy requirement and subtract it by 600kcal per day resulting in a negative balance (Detitians in obesity management 2007). This could be individualised to each patients' needs and preferences in food but should still maintain a healthy and balanced diet.

6.3.1 Low energy and very low energy diets

Patients who need to achieve a more rapid weight loss could try the more restricted calorie diet (Detitians in obesity management 2007; Tsigos, Hainer et al. 2008; Scottish Intercollegiate Guidelines and Scotland 2010). Low energy diet consists of total daily calories of between 800 to 1,500kcal and very low energy diet consists of less than 800kcal per day (National Heart, Blood et al. 1998; Detitians in obesity management 2007; Tsigos, Hainer et al. 2008; Scottish Intercollegiate Guidelines and Scotland 2010) or <50% reduction of the patient's predicted resting energy expenditure (Tsai and Wadden 2006). Low energy diet is associated with 5-8% of weight loss (National Heart, Blood et al. 1998; Scottish Intercollegiate Guidelines and Scotland 2010) over 12 months and this could be individualised to the patient's food preference (National Heart, Blood et al. 1998). Micronutrient supplementations are occasional necessary.

Very low energy diet (VLED) is usually a liquid diet consisting of a large amount of protein, up to 80g of carbohydrate and 15g of fat per day and fortified with micronutrients (Tsai and Wadden 2006). This intervention need to be done under close medical supervision (1993; Detitians in obesity management 2007; Tsigos, Hainer et al. 2008; Scottish Intercollegiate Guidelines and Scotland 2010). Maximum recommended duration of this intervention is 12 weeks (Detitians in obesity management 2007). The patient needs to consume a minimum of 2 litre of non-caloric fluid per day while on this diet (Tsai and Wadden 2006). Cambridge Weight Plan previously known as the Cambridge Diet uses VLED intervention. Adverse effects during this treatment include cholelithiasis, cold intolerance, hair loss, headache, fatigue, dizziness, muscle cramps, constipation, volume depletion and rarely cardiac complications causing death if unsupervised (1993; Tsai and Wadden 2006). Total weight loss at 12 months for VLED is similar to low calorie diet (National Heart, Blood et al. 1998; Tsai and Wadden 2006; Scottish Intercollegiate Guidelines and Scotland 2010). During first 3 to 4 months, initial weight loss with VLED is about 25-50% but patient regained 40–50% of the weight lost within 1–2 years while on VLED (Tsai and Wadden 2006) hence it is suitable for rapid weight loss. One study showed remission of type 2 diabetes in obese patient after 8 weeks of VLED (Lim, Hollingsworth et al. 2011).

VLED with liquid diet or low energy diet substituted with one or two of the three daily main meals and this intervention is called meal replacement intervention (Tsigos, Hainer et al. 2008). As the liquid diet consists of necessary micronutrients, this may help in weight loss while maintaining a balanced nutrition (Tsigos, Hainer et al. 2008); the low energy diet replacement needed to be fortified with the necessary vitamins and minerals (Heymsfield, van Mierlo et al. 2003). It is shown that meal replacement intervention induce between 6.97 to 7.31kg of weight loss at 1 year follow up as compared to 2.61-4.35kg with low energy diet alone (Heymsfield, van Mierlo et al. 2003).

7. Lifestyle intervention

After dietary changes in reducing calorie intake, the next step would be to increase in physical activity and finally help in engaging the patient for a more permanent change in lifestyle. Physical activity for about 30–60 min per day for at least 5 days a week of moderate intensity such as brisk walking has been recommended by various guidelines (National Heart, Blood et al. 1997; 2006; Tsigos, Hainer et al. 2008; Scottish Intercollegiate Guidelines and Scotland 2010). Increased physical activity has added effect on weight loss compared to just dietary interventions alone (Jakicic 2009; Goodpaster, Delany et al. 2010). It also improves cardiorespiratory fitness (National Heart, Blood et al. 1998), reduces cardiovascular risks (National Heart, Blood et al. 1998; Tsigos, Hainer et al. 2008; Goodpaster, Delany et al. 2010; Vetter, Faulconbridge et al. 2010), reduces abdominal fat (Jones, Wilson et al. 2007), improves anxiety and depression and helps with long term weight management(Jones, Wilson et al. 2007; Tsigos, Hainer et al. 2008; Jakicic 2009). Patients should also be encouraged to avoid sedentary lifestyle by choosing to use the stairs rather than elevators, walking or cycling to nearby places rather than driving and doing gardening (Vetter, Faulconbridge et al. 2010).

It has been shown by the Diabetes Prevention Programme (Knowler, Barrett-Connor et al. 2002) and the Finnish Diabetes Prevention studies (Tuomilehto, Lindstrom et al. 2001) that intensive lifestyle interventions promote weight loss of between 3.5-5.6kg. The Look AHEAD trial reported 6.15% weight loss after 4 years of interventions (Wing 2010). Most of the academic centres provide initial weekly interventions for a period of 16 to 26 weeks (Wadden, Butryn et al. 2007; Vetter, Faulconbridge et al. 2010). The entire treatment programme should be well structured along the lines of the Diabetes Prevention Programme. It is also more cost effective to have group sessions. Moreover, group sessions provide additional benefits on greater initial weight loss, better social support and healthy competition between members (Wadden, Butryn et al. 2007; Vetter, Faulconbridge et al. 2010).

Even after successful initial weight loss, weight regain could occur prior to surgery. Reasons behind weight regain are likely to be multifactorial including behavioural fatigue (Tsai and Wadden 2006), leaving from highly supportive care and return to initial 'damaging' environment or influence (Vetter, Faulconbridge et al. 2010). Hence health care professionals and patients should aim for long term behavioural change and it is the key in preventing weight regain prior and post surgery.

8. Final steps prior to surgery

After medical, psychological and nutritional assessments, the team will need to meet together to provide insight of the patients' conditions and discuss suitability of surgical interventions in them. Some centres propose a minimum 5 - 10% weight loss prior to surgery as some studies have shown this decreases length of hospital stay (Still, Benotti et al. 2007), reduces operative time (Huerta, Dredar et al. 2008) and less complications (Liu, Sabnis et al. 2005). As most of the dietary advice post surgery advises patients to have a liquid diet first, it is also important to review all patients' medications pre-surgery and change medications into liquid or soluble form prior to surgery.

9. Conclusion

Assessing and preparing patients for bariatric surgery is a complex process requiring input from a multi-disciplinary team. The primary aim is to optimise treatment of patients' pre-existing conditions hence minimising peri and post-operative complications and mortality. The surgery itself is only the first step. Post operatively, bariatric team members as well as patients' general practitioners need to continue to encourage patients' adherence to lifestyle changes including dietary energy restriction and increase in physical activity to help in long-term weight maintenance.

10. Acknowledgement

The views expressed in this publication are not necessarily those of the NIHR, the Department of Health, NHS South Birmingham, University of Birmingham or the CLAHRC-BBC Theme 8 Management/Steering group.

This work was funded by the National Institute for Health Research (NIHR) through the Collaborations for Leadership in Applied Health Research and Care for Birmingham and Black Country (CLAHRC-BBC) programme

11. References

"Cambridge weight plan." from http://www.cambridgeweightplan.com/

"The DASH diet eating plan." from http://dashdiet.org/default.asp.

(1993). "Very low-calorie diets. National Task Force on the Prevention and Treatment of Obesity, National Institutes of Health." JAMA 270(8): 967-974.

(2002). "Third Report of the National Cholesterol Education Program (NCEP) Expert Panel on Detection, Evaluation, and Treatment of High Blood Cholesterol in Adults (Adult Treatment Panel III) final report." Circulation 106(25): 3143-3421.

(2006). Obesity [electronic resource]: the prevention, identification, assessment and management of overweight and obesity in adults and children : NICE clinical guidance 43. [London], NICE.

(2008). Worried about gaining weight when you stop smoking? . Scottish nutrition and diet resources initiative (SNDRi). UK, Scottish Government. 1005 05/05.

(2009). Management of type 2 diabetes: NICE guidelines, Royal College of Physicians.

2010). You can control your weight as you quit smoking. U.S. Department of Health and Human Services. N. I. o. D. a. D. a. K. Diseases. United States, National Institute of Health. 03-4159: 1-7.

(2010). "European Medicines Agency recommends suspension of Avandia, Avandamet and Avaglim." from http://www.ema.europa.eu/ema/index.jsp?curl=pages/news_and_events/news/2010/09/news_detail_001119.jsp&mid=WC0b01ac058004d5c1&murl=menus/news_and_events/news_and_events.jsp&jsenabled=true.

(2010). "Rosiglitazone: recommended withdrawal from clinical use." from http://www.mhra.gov.uk/Safetyinformation/Safetywarningsalertsandrecalls/Safetywarningsandmessagesformedicines/CON094121

(2010). "U S. Medical Eligibility Criteria for Contraceptive Use, 2010." MMWR Recomm Rep 59(RR-4): 1-86.

(2011). "Executive summary: standards of medical care in diabetes--2011." Diabetes Care 34 Suppl 1: S4-10.

(2011). "Updated risk evaluation and mitigation strategy (REMS) to restrict access to rosiglitazone-containing medicines including Avandia, Avandamet and Avandaryl." from http://www.fda.gov/Drugs/DrugSafety/ucm255005.htm

NICE CG 67, (2010, March 2010). "Lipid Modification: cardiovascular risk assessment and the modification of blood lipids for the primary and secondary prevention of cardiovascular disease." Retrieved 20/08/2011, from http://www.nice.org.uk/nicemedia/live/11982/40689/40689.pdf

FDA, (2004, November 2004). "How to understand and use the nutrition facts label." Retrieved 26/8/2011, from http://www.fda.gov/food/labelingnutrition/consumerinformation/ucm078889.htm.

(WIN), W. C. N. (2010). You can control your weight as you quit smoking. N. I. o. D. a. D. a. K. Diseases. United States, National Institute of Health. 03-4159: 1-7.

Abiles, V., S. Rodriguez-Ruiz, et al. (2010). "Psychological characteristics of morbidly obese candidates for bariatric surgery." Obes Surg 20(2): 161-167.

Alberti, K. G., P. Zimmet, et al. (2005). "The metabolic syndrome--a new worldwide definition." Lancet 366(9491): 1059-1062.

Allison, K. C., T. A. Wadden, et al. (2006). "Night eating syndrome and binge eating disorder among persons seeking bariatric surgery: prevalence and related features." Obesity (Silver Spring) 14 Suppl 2: 77S-82S.

Alpert, M. A., B. E. Terry, et al. (2000). "The electrocardiogram in morbid obesity." Am J Cardiol 85(7): 908-910, A910.

Appel, L. J., T. J. Moore, et al. (1997). "A clinical trial of the effects of dietary patterns on blood pressure. DASH Collaborative Research Group." N Engl J Med 336(16): 1117-1124.

Arslan, E., O. Yiginer, et al. (2010). "Effect of uncomplicated obesity on QT interval in young men." Pol Arch Med Wewn 120(6): 209-213.

Athyros, V. G., K. Tziomalos, et al. (2011). "Dyslipidaemia of obesity, metabolic syndrome and type 2 diabetes mellitus: the case for residual risk reduction after statin treatment." Open Cardiovasc Med J 5: 24-34.

Atmaca, M., M. Kuloglu, et al. (2002). "Weight gain and serum leptin levels in patients on lithium treatment." Neuropsychobiology 46(2): 67-69.

Avelar, E., T. V. Cloward, et al. (2007). "Left ventricular hypertrophy in severe obesity: interactions among blood pressure, nocturnal hypoxemia, and body mass." Hypertension 49(1): 34-39.

Avenell, A., J. Broom, et al. (2004). "Systematic review of the long-term effects and economic consequences of treatments for obesity and implications for health improvement." Health Technol Assess 8(21): iii-iv, 1-182.

Balen, A. (2007). Polycystic ovarian syndrome, obesity and reproductive function. London, RCOG press.

Barr, J. and J. Cunneen (2001). "Understanding the bariatric client and providing a safe hospital environment." Clin Nurse Spec 15(5): 219-223.

Benjamin, E. J. and D. Levy (1999). "Why is left ventricular hypertrophy so predictive of morbidity and mortality?" Am J Med Sci 317(3): 168-175.

Brown, C. D., M. Higgins, et al. (2000). "Body mass index and the prevalence of hypertension and dyslipidemia." Obes Res 8(9): 605-619.

Buchwald, H., R. Estok, et al. (2009). "Weight and type 2 diabetes after bariatric surgery: systematic review and meta-analysis." Am J Med 122(3): 248-256 e245.

Caruana, J. A., M. N. McCabe, et al. (2005). "Incidence of symptomatic gallstones after gastric bypass: is prophylactic treatment really necessary?" Surg Obes Relat Dis 1(6): 564-567; discussion 567-568.

Casey, K. R., K. O. Cantillo, et al. (2007). "Sleep-related hypoventilation/hypoxemic syndromes." Chest 131(6): 1936-1948.

Chan, J. M., E. B. Rimm, et al. (1994). "Obesity, fat distribution, and weight gain as risk factors for clinical diabetes in men." Diabetes Care 17(9): 961-969.

Chiolero, A., D. Faeh, et al. (2008). "Consequences of smoking for body weight, body fat distribution, and insulin resistance." Am J Clin Nutr 87(4): 801-809.

Chobanian, A. V., G. L. Bakris, et al. (2003). "Seventh report of the Joint National Committee on Prevention, Detection, Evaluation, and Treatment of High Blood Pressure." Hypertension 42(6): 1206-1252.

Choices, N. (2011, 21/3/2011). "Food labels." Retrieved 26/8/2011, from http://www.nhs.uk/Livewell/Goodfood/Pages/food-labelling.aspx.

Clain, D. J. and J. H. Lefkowitch (1987). "Fatty liver disease in morbid obesity." Gastroenterol Clin North Am 16(2): 239-252.

Collop, N. A., W. M. Anderson, et al. (2007). "Clinical guidelines for the use of unattended portable monitors in the diagnosis of obstructive sleep apnea in adult patients.

Portable Monitoring Task Force of the American Academy of Sleep Medicine." J Clin Sleep Med 3(7): 737-747.
Corley, D. A. and A. Kubo (2006). "Body mass index and gastroesophageal reflux disease: a systematic review and meta-analysis." Am J Gastroenterol 101(11): 2619-2628.
Davtyan, C. and M. Ma (2008) "Drug-induced weight gain." Proceedings of UCLA Healthcare 12, 1-9.
de la Maza, M. P., A. Estevez, et al. (1994). "Ventricular mass in hypertensive and normotensive obese subjects." Int J Obes Relat Metab Disord 18(4): 193-197.
De Ridder, R. J., E. J. Schoon, et al. (2007). "Review article: Non-alcoholic fatty liver disease in morbidly obese patients and the effect of bariatric surgery." Aliment Pharmacol Ther 26 Suppl 2: 195-201.
Delgado-Aros, S., G. R. Locke, 3rd, et al. (2004). "Obesity is associated with increased risk of gastrointestinal symptoms: a population-based study." Am J Gastroenterol 99(9): 1801-1806.
Detitians in obesity management (2007). The dietetic weight management intervention for adults in the one to one setting. Is it time for radical rethink? , DOM UK.
Diaz, M. E. (2002). "Hypertension and obesity." J Hum Hypertens 16 Suppl 1: S18-22.
Dicker, D. (2011). "DPP-4 inhibitors: impact on glycemic control and cardiovascular risk factors." Diabetes Care 34 Suppl 2: S276-278.
Dixon, J. B., M. E. Dixon, et al. (2001). "Pre-operative predictors of weight loss at 1-year after Lap-Band surgery." Obes Surg 11(2): 200-207.
Eichinger, S., G. Hron, et al. (2008). "Overweight, obesity, and the risk of recurrent venous thromboembolism." Arch Intern Med 168(15): 1678-1683.
Eisenstein, I., J. Edelstein, et al. (1982). "The electrocardiogram in obesity." J Electrocardiol 15(2): 115-118.
El-Serag, H. B., D. Y. Graham, et al. (2005). "Obesity is an independent risk factor for GERD symptoms and erosive esophagitis." Am J Gastroenterol 100(6): 1243-1250.
Elfhag, K. and S. Rossner (2005). "Who succeeds in maintaining weight loss? A conceptual review of factors associated with weight loss maintenance and weight regain." Obes Rev 6(1): 67-85.
Epstein, L. J., D. Kristo, et al. (2009). "Clinical guideline for the evaluation, management and long-term care of obstructive sleep apnea in adults." J Clin Sleep Med 5(3): 263-276.
Farooqi, I. S. and S. O'Rahilly (2007). "Genetic factors in human obesity." Obes Rev 8 Suppl 1: 37-40.
Farquhar, C. (2007). Obesity and fertility. London, RCOG press.
Flegal, K. M., R. P. Troiano, et al. (1995). "The influence of smoking cessation on the prevalence of overweight in the United States." N Engl J Med 333(18): 1165-1170.
Flum, D. R., S. H. Belle, et al. (2009). "Perioperative safety in the longitudinal assessment of bariatric surgery." N Engl J Med 361(5): 445-454.
Foster, G. D., T. A. Wadden, et al. (2001). "Obese patients' perceptions of treatment outcomes and the factors that influence them." Arch Intern Med 161(17): 2133-2139.
Fox, C. S., S. Coady, et al. (2007). "Increasing cardiovascular disease burden due to diabetes mellitus: the Framingham Heart Study." Circulation 115(12): 1544-1550.
Frank, S., J. A. Colliver, et al. (1986). "The electrocardiogram in obesity: statistical analysis of 1,029 patients." J Am Coll Cardiol 7(2): 295-299.
Gardner, C. D., A. Kiazand, et al. (2007). "Comparison of the Atkins, Zone, Ornish, and LEARN diets for change in weight and related risk factors among overweight premenopausal women: the A TO Z Weight Loss Study: a randomized trial." JAMA 297(9): 969-977.

Gibbons, L. M., D. B. Sarwer, et al. (2006). "Previous weight loss experiences of bariatric surgery candidates: how much have patients dieted prior to surgery?" Obesity (Silver Spring) 14 Suppl 2: 70S-76S.

Gibson, G. J. (2000). "Obesity, respiratory function and breathlessness." Thorax 55 Suppl 1: S41-44.

Ginsberg, H. N. and P. R. Maccallum (2009). "The obesity, metabolic syndrome, and type 2 diabetes mellitus pandemic: II. Therapeutic management of atherogenic dyslipidemia." J Clin Hypertens (Greenwich) 11(9): 520-527.

Gluck, M. E., A. Geliebter, et al. (2001). "Night eating syndrome is associated with depression, low self-esteem, reduced daytime hunger, and less weight loss in obese outpatients." Obes Res 9(4): 264-267.

Goodpaster, B. H., J. P. Delany, et al. (2010). "Effects of diet and physical activity interventions on weight loss and cardiometabolic risk factors in severely obese adults: a randomized trial." JAMA 304(16): 1795-1802.

Greenman, Y., K. Tordjman, et al. (1998). "Increased body weight associated with prolactin secreting pituitary adenomas: weight loss with normalization of prolactin levels." Clin Endocrinol (Oxf) 48(5): 547-553.

Grief, S. N. and R. L. Miranda (2010). "Weight loss maintenance." Am Fam Physician 82(6): 630-634.

Guelinckx, I., R. Devlieger, et al. (2009). "Reproductive outcome after bariatric surgery: a critical review." Hum Reprod Update 15(2): 189-201.

Hammoud, A., M. Gibson, et al. (2009). "Effect of Roux-en-Y gastric bypass surgery on the sex steroids and quality of life in obese men." J Clin Endocrinol Metab 94(4): 1329-1332.

Heinberg, L. J., K. Keating, et al. (2010). "Discrepancy between ideal and realistic goal weights in three bariatric procedures: who is likely to be unrealistic?" Obes Surg 20(2): 148-153.

Heymsfield, S. B., C. A. van Mierlo, et al. (2003). "Weight management using a meal replacement strategy: meta and pooling analysis from six studies." Int J Obes Relat Metab Disord 27(5): 537-549.

Hezelgrave, N. L. and E. Oteng-Ntim (2011). "Pregnancy after bariatric surgery: a review." J Obes 2011: 501939.

Howell, M. J., C. H. Schenck, et al. (2009). "A review of nighttime eating disorders." Sleep Med Rev 13(1): 23-34.

Hubert, H. B., M. Feinleib, et al. (1983). "Obesity as an independent risk factor for cardiovascular disease: a 26-year follow-up of participants in the Framingham Heart Study." Circulation 67(5): 968-977.

Huerta, S., S. Dredar, et al. (2008). "Preoperative weight loss decreases the operative time of gastric bypass at a Veterans Administration hospital." Obes Surg 18(5): 508-512.

Jakicic, J. M. (2009). "The effect of physical activity on body weight." Obesity (Silver Spring) 17 Suppl 3: S34-38.

Johns, M. W. (1991). "A new method for measuring daytime sleepiness: the Epworth sleepiness scale." Sleep 14(6): 540-545.

Jones, L. R., C. I. Wilson, et al. (2007). "Lifestyle modification in the treatment of obesity: an educational challenge and opportunity." Clin Pharmacol Ther 81(5): 776-779.

Jones, R. L. and M. M. Nzekwu (2006). "The effects of body mass index on lung volumes." Chest 130(3): 827-833.

Jones, S., V. Srinivasan, et al. (2007). Treating menstrual disturbance including pelvic pain (excluding PCOS). London, RCOG press.

Jonsson, S., B. Hedblad, et al. (2002). "Influence of obesity on cardiovascular risk. Twenty-three-year follow-up of 22,025 men from an urban Swedish population." Int J Obes Relat Metab Disord 26(8): 1046-1053.

Kaila, B. and M. Raman (2008). "Obesity: a review of pathogenesis and management strategies." Can J Gastroenterol 22(1): 61-68.

Kannel, W. B. (1996). "Blood pressure as a cardiovascular risk factor: prevention and treatment." JAMA 275(20): 1571-1576.

Knowler, W. C., E. Barrett-Connor, et al. (2002). "Reduction in the incidence of type 2 diabetes with lifestyle intervention or metformin." N Engl J Med 346(6): 393-403.

Knudsen, N., P. Laurberg, et al. (2005). "Small differences in thyroid function may be important for body mass index and the occurrence of obesity in the population." J Clin Endocrinol Metab 90(7): 4019-4024.

Koh-Banerjee, P., Y. Wang, et al. (2004). "Changes in body weight and body fat distribution as risk factors for clinical diabetes in US men." Am J Epidemiol 159(12): 1150-1159.

Kok, P., F. Roelfsema, et al. (2004). "Prolactin release is enhanced in proportion to excess visceral fat in obese women." J Clin Endocrinol Metab 89(9): 4445-4449.

Kok, P., F. Roelfsema, et al. (2006). "Increased circadian prolactin release is blunted after body weight loss in obese premenopausal women." Am J Physiol Endocrinol Metab 290(2): E218-224.

Kopelman, P. G. (2000). "Physiopathology of prolactin secretion in obesity." Int J Obes Relat Metab Disord 24 Suppl 2: S104-108.

Kuchenbecker, W. K., H. Groen, et al. (2010). "The subcutaneous abdominal fat and not the intraabdominal fat compartment is associated with anovulation in women with obesity and infertility." J Clin Endocrinol Metab 95(5): 2107-2112.

Kulie, T., A. Slattengren, et al. (2011). "Obesity and women's health: an evidence-based review." J Am Board Fam Med 24(1): 75-85.

Kulkarni, S. K. and G. Kaur (2001). "Pharmacodynamics of drug-induced weight gain." Drugs Today (Barc) 37(8): 559-571.

Lagergren, J., R. Bergstrom, et al. (1999). "Symptomatic gastroesophageal reflux as a risk factor for esophageal adenocarcinoma." N Engl J Med 340(11): 825-831.

Lauer, M. S., K. M. Anderson, et al. (1991). "The impact of obesity on left ventricular mass and geometry. The Framingham Heart Study." JAMA 266(2): 231-236.

Lavie, C. J., R. V. Milani, et al. (2009). "Obesity and cardiovascular disease: risk factor, paradox, and impact of weight loss." J Am Coll Cardiol 53(21): 1925-1932.

Leslie, W. S., C. R. Hankey, et al. (2007). "Weight gain as an adverse effect of some commonly prescribed drugs: a systematic review." QJM 100(7): 395-404.

Liew, P. L., W. J. Lee, et al. (2006). "Hepatic histopathology of morbid obesity: concurrence of other forms of chronic liver disease." Obes Surg 16(12): 1584-1593.

Lim, E. L., K. G. Hollingsworth, et al. (2011). "Reversal of type 2 diabetes: normalisation of beta cell function in association with decreased pancreas and liver triacylglycerol." Diabetologia.

Liu, R. C., A. A. Sabnis, et al. (2005). "The effects of acute preoperative weight loss on laparoscopic Roux-en-Y gastric bypass." Obes Surg 15(10): 1396-1402.

Locke, G. R., 3rd, N. J. Talley, et al. (1997). "Prevalence and clinical spectrum of gastroesophageal reflux: a population-based study in Olmsted County, Minnesota." Gastroenterology 112(5): 1448-1456.

Lopez-Jimenez, F. and M. Cortes-Bergoderi (2011). "Update: systemic diseases and the cardiovascular system (i): obesity and the heart." Rev Esp Cardiol 64(2): 140-149.

Lupsor, M., R. Badea, et al. (2010). "Performance of unidimensional transient elastography in staging non-alcoholic steatohepatitis." J Gastrointestin Liver Dis 19(1): 53-60.
MacDonald, A. A., G. P. Herbison, et al. (2010). "The impact of body mass index on semen parameters and reproductive hormones in human males: a systematic review with meta-analysis." Hum Reprod Update 16(3): 293-311.
Maenhaut, N. and J. Van de Voorde (2011). "Regulation of vascular tone by adipocytes." BMC Med 9: 25.
Makimattila, S., K. Nikkila, et al. (1999). "Causes of weight gain during insulin therapy with and without metformin in patients with Type II diabetes mellitus." Diabetologia 42(4): 406-412.
McClean, K. M., F. Kee, et al. (2008). "Obesity and the lung: 1. Epidemiology." Thorax 63(7): 649-654.
McGill, H. C., Jr., C. A. McMahan, et al. (2002). "Obesity accelerates the progression of coronary atherosclerosis in young men." Circulation 105(23): 2712-2718.
Mechanick, J. I., R. F. Kushner, et al. (2009). "American Association of Clinical Endocrinologists, The Obesity Society, and American Society for Metabolic & Bariatric Surgery medical guidelines for clinical practice for the perioperative nutritional, metabolic, and nonsurgical support of the bariatric surgery patient." Obesity (Silver Spring) 17 Suppl 1: S1-70, v.
Miller, E. R., 3rd, T. P. Erlinger, et al. (2006). "The effects of macronutrients on blood pressure and lipids: an overview of the DASH and OmniHeart trials." Curr Atheroscler Rep 8(6): 460-465.
Mokhlesi, B. (2010). "Obesity hypoventilation syndrome: a state-of-the-art review." Respir Care 55(10): 1347-1362; discussion 1363-1345.
Mokhlesi, B., M. H. Kryger, et al. (2008). "Assessment and management of patients with obesity hypoventilation syndrome." Proc Am Thorac Soc 5(2): 218-225.
Mokhlesi, B. and A. Tulaimat (2007). "Recent advances in obesity hypoventilation syndrome." Chest 132(4): 1322-1336.
Movahed, M. R., A. Martinez, et al. (2009). "Left ventricular hypertrophy is associated with obesity, male gender, and symptoms in healthy adolescents." Obesity (Silver Spring) 17(3): 606-610.
Myers, R. P., G. Pomier-Layrargues, et al. (2011). "Feasibility and diagnostic performance of the fibroscan xl probe for liver stiffness measurement in overweight and obese patients." Hepatology.
Narkiewicz, K. (2006). "Obesity and hypertension--the issue is more complex than we thought." Nephrol Dial Transplant 21(2): 264-267.
Nathan, D. M., J. B. Buse, et al. (2009). "Medical management of hyperglycaemia in type 2 diabetes mellitus: a consensus algorithm for the initiation and adjustment of therapy: a consensus statement from the American Diabetes Association and the European Association for the Study of Diabetes." Diabetologia 52(1): 17-30.
National Heart, L., I. Blood, et al. (1998). Clinical guidelines on the identification, evaluation, and treatment of overweight and obesity in adults [electronic resource]: the evidence report. [Bethesda, Md.?], National Heart, Lung.
Ness-Abramof, R. and C. M. Apovian (2005). "Drug-induced weight gain." Drugs Today (Barc) 41(8): 547-555.
Netzer, N. C., R. A. Stoohs, et al. (1999). "Using the Berlin Questionnaire to identify patients at risk for the sleep apnea syndrome." Ann Intern Med 131(7): 485-491.
Nguyen, R. H., A. J. Wilcox, et al. (2007). "Men's body mass index and infertility." Hum Reprod 22(9): 2488-2493.

Nieman, L. K., B. M. Biller, et al. (2008). "The diagnosis of Cushing's syndrome: an Endocrine Society Clinical Practice Guideline." J Clin Endocrinol Metab 93(5): 1526-1540.

Nihalani, N., T. L. Schwartz, et al. (2011). "Weight gain, obesity, and psychotropic prescribing." J Obes 2011: 893629.

Nordmann, A. J., A. Nordmann, et al. (2006). "Effects of low-carbohydrate vs low-fat diets on weight loss and cardiovascular risk factors: a meta-analysis of randomized controlled trials." Arch Intern Med 166(3): 285-293.

Nyrnes, A., R. Jorde, et al. (2006). "Serum TSH is positively associated with BMI." Int J Obes (Lond) 30(1): 100-105.

O'Reardon, J. P., K. C. Allison, et al. (2006). "A randomized, placebo-controlled trial of sertraline in the treatment of night eating syndrome." Am J Psychiatry 163(5): 893-898.

Orth, D. N. (1995). "Cushing's syndrome." N Engl J Med 332(12): 791-803.

Pasquali, R., L. Patton, et al. (2007). "Obesity and infertility." Curr Opin Endocrinol Diabetes Obes 14(6): 482-487.

Pasquali, R., C. Pelusi, et al. (2003). "Obesity and reproductive disorders in women." Hum Reprod Update 9(4): 359-372.

Paulen, M. E., L. B. Zapata, et al. (2010). "Contraceptive use among women with a history of bariatric surgery: a systematic review." Contraception 82(1): 86-94.

Peeters, A., J. J. Barendregt, et al. (2003). "Obesity in adulthood and its consequences for life expectancy: a life-table analysis." Ann Intern Med 138(1): 24-32.

Poirier, P., T. D. Giles, et al. (2006). "Obesity and cardiovascular disease: pathophysiology, evaluation, and effect of weight loss: an update of the 1997 American Heart Association Scientific Statement on Obesity and Heart Disease from the Obesity Committee of the Council on Nutrition, Physical Activity, and Metabolism." Circulation 113(6): 898-918.

Pontiroli, A. E., P. Pizzocri, et al. (2004). "Left ventricular hypertrophy and QT interval in obesity and in hypertension: effects of weight loss and of normalisation of blood pressure." Int J Obes Relat Metab Disord 28(9): 1118-1123.

Priou, P., J. F. Hamel, et al. (2010). "Long-term outcome of noninvasive positive pressure ventilation for obesity hypoventilation syndrome." Chest 138(1): 84-90.

Pull, C. B. (2010). "Current psychological assessment practices in obesity surgery programs: what to assess and why." Curr Opin Psychiatry 23(1): 30-36.

Qatanani, M. and M. A. Lazar (2007). "Mechanisms of obesity-associated insulin resistance: many choices on the menu." Genes Dev 21(12): 1443-1455.

Quesada, B. M., G. Kohan, et al. (2010). "Management of gallstones and gallbladder disease in patients undergoing gastric bypass." World J Gastroenterol 16(17): 2075-2079.

Rabec, C., P. de Lucas Ramos, et al. (2011). "Respiratory complications of obesity." Arch Bronconeumol 47(5): 252-261.

Reinehr, T. (2010). "Obesity and thyroid function." Mol Cell Endocrinol 316(2): 165-171.

Ruhl, C. E. and J. E. Everhart (2005). "Joint effects of body weight and alcohol on elevated serum alanine aminotransferase in the United States population." Clin Gastroenterol Hepatol 3(12): 1260-1268.

Ruxton, C. H. and T. R. Kirk (1997). "Breakfast: a review of associations with measures of dietary intake, physiology and biochemistry." Br J Nutr 78(2): 199-213.

Ryden, A., J. Karlsson, et al. (2003). "Coping and distress: what happens after intervention? A 2-year follow-up from the Swedish Obese Subjects (SOS) study." Psychosom Med 65(3): 435-442.

Salgado Junior, W., J. S. Santos, et al. (2006). "Nonalcoholic fatty liver disease and obesity." Acta Cir Bras 21 Suppl 1: 72-78.

Scaglioni, F., S. Ciccia, et al. (2011). "ASH and NASH." Dig Dis 29(2): 202-210.
Scottish Intercollegiate Guidelines (2003). Management of obstructive sleep apnoea/hypopnoea syndrome in adults. Edinburgh, Scottish Intercollegiate Guidelines Network.
Scottish Intercollegiate Guidelines (2010). Management of obesity: a national clinical guideline. Edinburgh, Scottish Intercollegiate Guidelines Network.
Seyfeli, E., M. Duru, et al. (2006). "Effect of obesity on P-wave dispersion and QT dispersion in women." Int J Obes (Lond) 30(6): 957-961.
Shah, D. K. and E. S. Ginsburg (2010). "Bariatric surgery and fertility." Curr Opin Obstet Gynecol 22(3): 248-254.
Shai, I., D. Schwarzfuchs, et al. (2008). "Weight loss with a low-carbohydrate, Mediterranean, or low-fat diet." N Engl J Med 359(3): 229-241.
Sjostrom, L., A. K. Lindroos, et al. (2004). "Lifestyle, diabetes, and cardiovascular risk factors 10 years after bariatric surgery." N Engl J Med 351(26): 2683-2693.
Sjostrom, L., K. Narbro, et al. (2007). "Effects of bariatric surgery on mortality in Swedish obese subjects." N Engl J Med 357(8): 741-752.
Smith, D. E., C. E. Lewis, et al. (1994). "Longitudinal changes in adiposity associated with pregnancy. The CARDIA Study. Coronary Artery Risk Development in Young Adults Study." JAMA 271(22): 1747-1751.
Snyder, A. G. (2009). "Psychological assessment of the patient undergoing bariatric surgery." Ochsner J 9(3): 144-148.
Sood, A. (2009). "Altered resting and exercise respiratory physiology in obesity." Clin Chest Med 30(3): 445-454, vii.
Srivastava, S. and Z. M. Younossi (2005). "Morbid obesity, nonalcoholic fatty liver disease, and weight loss surgery." Hepatology 42(2): 490-492.
Stamler, R., J. Stamler, et al. (1978). "Weight and blood pressure. Findings in hypertension screening of 1 million Americans." JAMA 240(15): 1607-1610.
Stein, P. D., A. Beemath, et al. (2005). "Obesity as a risk factor in venous thromboembolism." Am J Med 118(9): 978-980.
Wilcox, I. (2010). Cardiovascular consequences of obesity. UK, Wiley-Blackwell.
Still, C. D., P. Benotti, et al. (2007). "Outcomes of preoperative weight loss in high-risk patients undergoing gastric bypass surgery." Arch Surg 142(10): 994-998; discussion 999.
Stunkard, A. J., K. C. Allison, et al. (2009). "Development of criteria for a diagnosis: lessons from the night eating syndrome." Compr Psychiatry 50(5): 391-399.
Susan F. Franks, a. K. A. K. (2008). "Predictive factors in bariatric surgery outcomes: what is the role of the preoperative psychological evaluation?" Primary psychiatry 15(8): 74-83.
Svetkey, L. P., D. Simons-Morton, et al. (1999). "Effects of dietary patterns on blood pressure: subgroup analysis of the Dietary Approaches to Stop Hypertension (DASH) randomized clinical trial." Arch Intern Med 159(3): 285-293.
Talley, N. J., S. Howell, et al. (2004). "Obesity and chronic gastrointestinal tract symptoms in young adults: a birth cohort study." Am J Gastroenterol 99(9): 1807-1814.
Thomas, D. E., E. J. Elliott, et al. (2007). "Low glycaemic index or low glycaemic load diets for overweight and obesity." Cochrane Database Syst Rev(3): CD005105.
Tsai, A. G. and T. A. Wadden (2006). "The evolution of very-low-calorie diets: an update and meta-analysis." Obesity (Silver Spring) 14(8): 1283-1293.
Tsigos, C., V. Hainer, et al. (2008). "Management of obesity in adults: European clinical practice guidelines." Obes Facts 1(2): 106-116.

Tuomilehto, J., J. Lindstrom, et al. (2001). "Prevention of type 2 diabetes mellitus by changes in lifestyle among subjects with impaired glucose tolerance." N Engl J Med 344(18): 1343-1350.

Dietitians in obesity management (2007). The dietetic weight management intervention for adults in the one to one setting. Is it time for radical rethink? , DOM UK.

Valencia-Flores, M., A. Orea, et al. (2000). "Prevalence of sleep apnea and electrocardiographic disturbances in morbidly obese patients." Obes Res 8(3): 262-269.

van Hout, G. and G. van Heck (2009). "Bariatric psychology, psychological aspects of weight loss surgery." Obes Facts 2(1): 10-15.

Vetter, M. L., L. F. Faulconbridge, et al. (2010). "Behavioral and pharmacologic therapies for obesity." Nat Rev Endocrinol 6(10): 578-588.

Vuppalanchi, R. and N. Chalasani (2009). "Nonalcoholic fatty liver disease and nonalcoholic steatohepatitis: Selected practical issues in their evaluation and management." Hepatology 49(1): 306-317.

Wadden, T. A., M. L. Butryn, et al. (2007). "Lifestyle modification for the management of obesity." Gastroenterology 132(6): 2226-2238.

Wannamethee, S. G. and A. G. Shaper (1999). "Weight change and duration of overweight and obesity in the incidence of type 2 diabetes." Diabetes Care 22(8): 1266-1272.

Wee, C. C., D. B. Jones, et al. (2006). "Understanding patients' value of weight loss and expectations for bariatric surgery." Obes Surg 16(4): 496-500.

Wei, S., M. D. Schmidt, et al. (2009). "Obesity and menstrual irregularity: associations with SHBG, testosterone, and insulin." Obesity (Silver Spring) 17(5): 1070-1076.

Williams, B., N. R. Poulter, et al. (2004). "Guidelines for management of hypertension: report of the fourth working party of the British Hypertension Society, 2004-BHS IV." J Hum Hypertens 18(3): 139-185.

Williamson, D. F., J. Madans, et al. (1991). "Smoking cessation and severity of weight gain in a national cohort." N Engl J Med 324(11): 739-745.

Wilson, P. W., R. B. D'Agostino, et al. (2002). "Overweight and obesity as determinants of cardiovascular risk: the Framingham experience." Arch Intern Med 162(16): 1867-1872.

Wing, R. R. (2010). "Long-term effects of a lifestyle intervention on weight and cardiovascular risk factors in individuals with type 2 diabetes mellitus: four-year results of the Look AHEAD trial." Arch Intern Med 170(17): 1566-1575.

Wing, R. R. and S. Phelan (2005). "Long-term weight loss maintenance." Am J Clin Nutr 82(1 Suppl): 222S-225S.

Wise, R. A., P. L. Enright, et al. (1998). "Effect of weight gain on pulmonary function after smoking cessation in the Lung Health Study." Am J Respir Crit Care Med 157(3 Pt 1): 866-872.

Wolfe, B. L. and M. L. Terry (2006). "Expectations and outcomes with gastric bypass surgery." Obes Surg 16(12): 1622-1629.

Wolk, R., P. Berger, et al. (2003). "Body mass index: a risk factor for unstable angina and myocardial infarction in patients with angiographically confirmed coronary artery disease." Circulation 108(18): 2206-2211.

Wyatt, H. R., G. K. Grunwald, et al. (2002). "Long-term weight loss and breakfast in subjects in the National Weight Control Registry." Obes Res 10(2): 78-82.

Zoungas, S., J. Chalmers, et al. (2010). "The efficacy of lowering glycated haemoglobin with a gliclazide modified release-based intensive glucose lowering regimen in the ADVANCE trial." Diabetes Res Clin Pract 89(2): 126-133.

5

Rethinking the Preoperative Psychological Evaluation – A New Paradigm for Improved Outcomes and Predictive Power

Susan F. Franks[1] and Kathryn A. Kaiser[2]
[1]*University of North Texas Health Science Center, Fort Worth, Texas,*
[2]*University of Alabama at Birmingham, Birmingham, Alabama*
Unites States of America

1. Introduction

Weight loss surgery (WLS) has become increasingly commonplace, as rates of morbid obesity and its serious medical consequences continue to rise in developed countries worldwide (Nguyen et al., 2005; Steinbrook, 2004). From 1998 to 2002, an increase in WLS of approximately 450% was observed in the United States alone, and from 2002 to 2004, it was estimated that more than 357,300 adults in the United States had undergone WLS (Wysoker, 2005). Most patients benefit from the procedure; however there remain at least 20% of patients who fail to lose the expected amount of weight or who regain a significant amount of lost weight (Christou, Look, & Maclean, 2006; Kalarchian et al., 2007; Kinzl et al., 2006). Some researchers have identified 7-10 year failure rates of up to 35% for gastric bypass patients and up to 57% for laparoscopic banding patients (Ayyad & Andersen, 2000; Fischer et al., 2007). A recent long-term follow-up of 200 gastric banded patients found that excess weight loss (EWL) was gradually regained, resulting in only 15.6% EWL after 14 years and a reoperation rate of 30.5% (Stroh, Hohmann, Schramm, Meyer, & Manger, 2011). While a minority of these failures or suboptimal outcomes may be due to technical surgical errors or complications, the majority of them are attributable to psychological and behavioral factors that interfere with patients' abilities to make or maintain lasting changes in lifestyle (Boeka, Prentice-Dunn, & Lokken, 2010; Buchwald et al., 2004; Pessina, Andreoli, & Vassallo, 2001). Long-term failure rates highlight the need to selectively identify patients at-risk for minimal weight loss or weight regain (O'Brien, McPhail, Chaston, & Dixon, 2006; Stroh et al., 2011).

It is widely accepted that obesity is multifactorial in nature, and that psychological and behavioral influences play an integral role in the development and maintenance of an obese state (Buchwald et al., 2004; Kinzl et al., 2006). The preoperative psychological evaluation for WLS candidates was uniformly put into practice following the 1991 National Institutes of Health Consensus Panel recommendations that officially recognized the key role of psychological and behavioral factors toward the ability of a patient to ultimately be successful with WLS (Buchwald, 2005; Buddeberg-Fischer, Klaghofer, Sigrist, & Buddeberg, 2004; Kinzl et al., 2006; NIH Consensus Panel, 1991). A majority of WLS programs and insurance carriers subsequently began requiring a presurgical psychological evaluation in order to clear the candidate for surgery (Bauchowitz et al., 2005; Kalarchian et al., 2007). At its outset, it was widely assumed that a preoperative psychological evaluation would be useful in identifying patients who would be at-risk for suboptimal or failed outcomes (Ashton, Favretti, & Segato, 2008; Bauchowitz et al., 2005; Kalarchian et al., 2007). This assumption was largely based on research that had been able to identify various psychological and behavioral patterns among obese patients that were associated with failure or suboptimal outcomes for conventional weight loss programs (Bauchowitz et al., 2005).

Research to date has found few consistently significant associations between independently studied traditional psychological risk factors that were assumed to be equally problematic for WLS patients (Franks & Kaiser, 2008; Greenberg, 2003; Greenberg, Sogg, & Perna, 2009; Grothe, Dubbert, & O'jile, 2006; Herpertz, Kielmann, Wolf, Hebebrand, & Senf, 2004; van Hout, Verschure, & van Heck, 2005). For example, our review of the literature found that Axis I pathology such as Mood Disorders, Anxiety Disorders, and Eating Disorders; while higher in the WLS candidates as compared to the normal population, have not uniformly predicted poorer weight loss or other health outcomes (Franks & Kaiser, 2008). In contrast, weight loss subsequent to WLS predicted improvement in depression and anxiety following the surgery and subsequent weight loss (Swan-Kremier, 2005). Other studies have suggested that it is the degree of psychopathology and the past history of psychiatric treatment that is relevant to WLS outcomes rather than the presence or absence of a diagnosable condition at the time of the presurgical evaluation (Ashton et al., 2008; van Hout et al., 2005).

The paucity of research findings for the utility of the preoperative evaluation in predicting outcomes has led to criticism of the field (Ashton et al., 2008; Greenberg et al., 2009). Some have demanded that the validity of the preoperative psychological evaluation be demonstrated for justification of its requirement for WLS (Ashton et al., 2008). It has become clear that the field of psychology must take a critical look at the current state of the science in this area, identify the problems, and revise its approach to meet the scientific rigor of evidence-based medicine. The lack of predictive power for any particular element of the psychological evaluation has been noted, and various reviews of the literature have been consistent in their observations about the problems with much of the research. Sogg and Mori (2004) point out that the research in this area generally has been hampered by the fact that the approach to the psychological evaluation for bariatric patients is non-standardized, resulting in heterogeneity of data, definitions, and measurements of constructs of interest. They further point out that many of the published studies suffer from methodological flaws. Others contend that because the psychological evaluation is not independent of clinical decision-making, patients get triaged out of WLS or get deferred into other treatments (both psychological and weight control-related) prior to the surgery (Greenberg et al., 2009; Kalarchian et al., 2007). Still others have pointed out that there is still no consensus of what constitutes WLS success (Franks & Kaiser, 2008). In addition to the aforementioned problems, we propose that there exists a more fundamental issue; the lack of a theory-based approach from which to systematically investigate and understand research findings.

In this chapter we will: 1) review and critique the current approach to the psychological evaluation for WLS candidates, 2) discuss attempts that have been made to improve the predictive utility of the evaluation, 3) highlight the specific areas of inquiry that have shown merit for predicting postoperative outcomes, 4) explore the reasons for the poor predictive power of the current medical model, and 5) propose a new paradigm from which to approach the evaluation with supportive evidence from the extant literature. A suggested theory-driven clinical intake and psychological assessment procedure will be outlined, with guidelines for clinical decision making. Finally, future considerations for research and clinical practice will be discussed.

2. State of the psychological science in bariatric evaluations

The initial medical model approach to the preoperative psychological evaluation of WLS candidates was based on the clinical convention of information gathering that is used to rule out or to formulate a mental health diagnosis. This involves gathering information relevant to a chief complaint and its associated symptoms and history, the past medical history, the psychosocial history, and the family history. The approach is contemporary in that it also incorporates a whole-person view that is supposed to integrate biological, psychosocial and environmental dimensions into formulating a diagnosis, as opposed to relying solely on the physical and biological aspects. Some psychologists also utilize psychological testing and may administer the mini-mental status exam or some other form of cognitive screen as well.

The intended purpose for gathering this information is to select a rational treatment approach by applying the information to diagnostic schema and their associated interventions. Optimally, these interventions should be based on a scientific evidence-base that links treatments with demonstrated outcomes. However, there are few interventions that are specifically tailored to the multiple determinants of a given psychological diagnosis. A similar issue exists for obesity, where the available treatments are not yet tailored to the complex and multiple determinants of the condition. Given that the goal for the preoperative psychological evaluation for WLS is to predict who will be successful and who is at risk for failure or suboptimal outcomes, the initial approach to the evaluation was not sufficiently designed with prediction in mind. In 2004, a behavioral health committee for the American Society of Metabolic and Bariatric Surgery (ASMBS) attempted to improve the utility of the presurgical evaluation by publishing which elements were thought to be important in conducting the assessment (LeMont, Moorehead, Parish, Reto, & Ritz, 2004). Due to the lack of empirical data in this area, however, no consensus or practice guidelines were able to be firmly established. Thus, little progress has been made in standardization of assessment and data collection from which to draw conclusions about relationships to postsurgical outcomes (Sogg & Mori, 2004).

2.1 What is known – paradoxical results

While there has been no agreed-upon defined outcome for WLS, a general professional consensus may be gleaned based on what is most consistently used in the research literature. Over the years, the field appears to have adopted a ">50% excess weight loss" (EWL) as a cut-point indicating "success." The use of EWL as the sole basis for defining success or failure is scientifically problematic, particularly when we are to set practice standards according to an evidence-base. The 50% EWL criterion is essentially an arbitrary standard, as it is calculated based on a statistical comparison to ideal weight standards, which are themselves arbitrarily defined (Franks & Kaiser, 2008). Additionally, the 50% EWL criterion is independent of associated health improvements and has not yet been shown to have any clinical superiority over lower amounts. Even less clear are what criteria should be used to discriminate "suboptimal" weight loss and "failure." Many patients will reduce their medication needs, resolve co-morbid medical conditions, and experience improved psychosocial function and quality of life (QOL) well before achieving the >50% EWL mark. Yet, few psychological studies rely on criteria other than EWL as their prediction standard. Thus, the research in psychological prediction of outcomes has been severely limited by a significant methodological flaw in the selection of prediction criteria.

Nonetheless, several reviews of the literature, including our own, have yielded consistent results about what appears to influence EWL, psychosocial function, and/or QOL (Ashton et al., 2008; Franks & Kaiser, 2008; Greenberg, 2003; Greenberg et al., 2009; Grothe et al., 2006; Herpertz et al., 2004; van Hout et al., 2005). These include a history of psychiatric inpatient admissions, outpatient psychiatric treatment or counseling, social support, body image, and depression. With regard to prior psychiatric admissions, it appears that inpatient admissions, irrespective of the quantity, are related to increased postsurgical medical and psychological complications and reduced patient satisfaction (Ashton et al., 2008; van Hout et al., 2005). However, a history of outpatient psychological treatment appears to be a positive predictor for postsurgical weight loss. It has been assumed that these findings related to a patient's ability to develop positive coping skills that carries over to the behavioral and psychological challenges faced during the postsurgical phase (Grothe et al., 2006). Presurgical body dissatisfaction, present in about 70% of patients, appears to be inversely related to postsurgical weight loss; however, a causal connection has not been established (Swan-Kremier, 2005). The presence of presurgical depression may result in less postsurgical weight loss than for non-depressed patients (van Hout et al., 2005). However, depression has not been a prognostic indicator of overall failure based on % EWL, psychosocial function, or quality of life (Kalarchian et al., 2005; Ma et al., 2006; Swan-Kremier, 2005). Some have reported that it may actually promote greater short-term weight loss (Averbukh et al., 2003; Ma et al., 2006).

Reviews of the literature have also been consistent in reporting findings that are not yet well-elucidated, but are nonetheless provocative. For example, marital relationship appears to be an important mediator of postsurgical results, although the nature of the association is unclear. Limited research suggests a possible U-shaped relationship, with marital satisfaction as well as dissatisfaction showing a positive association with postsurgical weight loss (Herpertz et al., 2004; van Hout et al., 2005). Also unclear is the effect of social support on complications and weight loss in the postsurgical phase (Grothe et al., 2006; Herpertz et al., 2004). Our own study of postsurgical support group attendance for laparoscopic banded patients demonstrated that increased attendance was associated with higher rates of weight loss one year after surgery (Kaiser, Franks, & Smith, 2011). This is consistent with a previous review of the literature that concluded that social support appeared to impact weight loss through the influence on adherence to postsurgical lifestyle modifications (Herpertz et al., 2004). Limited research has shown that the presence of anxiety in conjunction with presurgical obesity-related psychosocial stress may be positively associated with postsurgical weight loss (Herpertz et al., 2004; Ryden, Karlsson, Sullivan, Torgerson, & Taft, 2003; van Hout et al., 2005); however, the specific nature of the role of anxiety and a causal relationship to postsurgical outcomes have not been well-studied (Kalarchian et al., 2007; Rosik, 2005). Areas of research that continue to show conflicting results with regard to postsurgical outcomes include self-esteem (van Hout et al., 2005) and a presurgical diagnosis of binge eating disorder (Franks & Kaiser, 2008).

Finally, a consistent body of literature shows no strong relationship to postsurgical outcomes for specific personality traits, presurgical life stress, or a history of childhood abuse. Childhood sexual abuse and maltreatment, while more prevalent in the severely obese population (Grilo et al., 2005; Wildes, Kalarchian, Marcus, Levine, & Courcoulas, 2008), do not appear to have any relationship with postsurgical weight loss (Fujioka, Yan, Wang, & Li, 2008; Grilo, White, Masheb, Rothschild, & Burke-Martindale, 2006). Presurgical life stress, in and of itself, does not appear to have a negative impact on weight loss (Herpertz et al., 2004; van Hout et al., 2005). While poor postsurgical weight loss may be observed in personality disordered patients (Grothe et al., 2006; Herpertz et al., 2004), studies of personality traits have shown no consistent prognostic value with regard to weight loss or psychosocial outcomes (Herpertz et al., 2004). One study of gastric bypass patients, utilizing the Minnesota Multiphasic Personality Inventory - 2 (MMPI-2), found that patients with <50% EWL one year postsurgery had higher presurgical elevations of the Hypochondriasis and Hysteria scales. However, since the elevations were not above the clinical cut-off for these scales, the clinical significance of this finding is unclear. A recent study using both the MMPI-2 and the Millon Multiphasic Clinical Inventory (MCMI- III) found that the K-scale from the MMPI-2 and the Schizoid, Schizotypal, and Compulsive scales from the MCMI-III predicted weight loss, but differentially at various post-operative time points (Belanger, Wechsler, Nademin, & Virden, III, 2010). Additionally, the sample used in this study was inclusive of patients who had been approved without reservation and patients who had received psychological/psychiatric treatment presurgically or concurrent with the procedure, making it difficult to draw conclusions. In a cluster analytic approach to determine psychological profiles in 153 candidates for vertical banded gastroplasty, 3 distinct patterns were found that were comprised of combinations of high to low functioning, but these occurred across 7 domains (personality, coping, eating behavior, locus of control, body attitude, social functioning, and health-related quality of life) (van Hout, van Oudheusden, Krasuska, & van Heck, 2006). Generally, the research in the area of personality profiles has pointed to the heterogeneity of presurgical candidates and an inability to uniformly predict outcomes (Belanger 2010).

2.2 Second generation approaches to assessment

Given the disappointment of standard personality tests such as the Minnesota Multiphasic Personality Inventory (MMPI-2) in predicting WLS outcomes, more health- and behavior-specific assessment tools were investigated or newly developed. Based on its predictive utility with other health conditions, the Millon Behavioral Medicine Diagnostic (MBMD™) came into favor for use with bariatric patients (Fabricatore, Crerand, Wadden, Sarwer, & Krasucki, 2006; Walfish, Vance, & Fabricatore, 2007). Within two years of its introduction to the bariatric field, the authors of the test provided adjusted norms for the bariatric population (Millon, Antoni, Millon, Minor, & Grossman, 2007). Two problems very quickly came to light. First, there were no studies establishing that the instrument was valid or reliable for the bariatric population. Second, the method that was used to develop the adjusted norms was not reported. To date, the procedure for establishing the adjusted norms has not been published, making it difficult for consumers of the Bariatric version of the test to verify that it is a psychometrically sound instrument for the bariatric population. A recent study by Walfish, et al. urged caution for the use of the MBMD™ - Bariatric Norms with WLS patients due to the lack of adequate reliability for many of the scales (Walfish, Wise, & Streiner, 2008).

Behavior-specific tools (as opposed to personality measures) have been used to assess constructs related to various aspects of eating behavior. Using the Questionnaire on Eating and Weight Patterns (QWEP and QWEP-R), no differences were found in rates of postsurgical weight loss at one year follow-up between subjects who were preoperatively classified as binge-eaters or non-binge eaters (Fischer et al., 2007). However, pre-surgical grazing behavior was found to predict 19.5% of the variance in postsurgical % EWL (Colles, Dixon, & O'Brien, 2008). The Eating Disorder Inventory has also been utilized as a standardized assessment tool to characterize presurgical eating behavior. Regardless of which assessment tool is utilized, some studies find smaller % EWL for patients with presurgical binge eating, but still report significant weight loss. Patients with presurgical binge eating who have undergone laparoscopic banding surgery have been reported to undergo more frequent band adjustments and have more postsurgical complications than patients without disordered eating (Busetto et al., 2005).

The Three Factor Eating Questionnaire (TFEQ – Stunkard & Messick, 1985) and other similar surveys used to assess cognitive restraint, disinhibition, and hunger have been consistently useful in demonstrating postsurgical changes in eating behavior (Kaiser et al., 2004; Smith, Franks, Kaiser, & Carrol, 2008). In and of themselves, various presurgical eating behavior constructs do not appear to independently predict postsurgical outcomes such as weight loss. Less understood, however, has been how presurgical eating behaviors may interact with other psychological characteristics. For example, higher presurgical non-hungry eating, measured by TFEQ, when combined with symptoms of depression as measured by the Beck Depression Inventory (BDI), was associated with poorer % EWL in laparoscopic banding patients (Colles et al., 2008).

Another attempt to standardize the preoperative evaluation has been through the use of a semi-structured interview. For example, the Weight and Lifestyle Inventory (WALI - (Wadden & Foster, 2006) covers information relevant to weight history, weight loss history and goals, eating habits, food intake, eating patterns, physical activity, family and social support, self-perceptions, psychiatric history, stress, and medical history. Thus far, it appears that data from the WALI has been used to describe various preoperative characteristics of patients rather than for postoperative predication (Allison et al., 2006; Fabricatore et al., 2006; Gibbons et al., 2006). In addition to including the QEWP, the WALI incorporates a survey on Eating Habits. Factor analysis of the Eating Habits Survey demonstrated the presence of 5 factors: eating in response to negative affect, eating in response to positive affect and social cues, general overeating and impaired appetite regulation, overeating at early meals, and snacking (Fabricatore et al., 2006). Preliminary data using the survey show that it may hold promise in identifying patients at risk for non-hunger related eating (Fabricatore et al., 2006; Kaiser, Franks, Carrol, & Smith, 2009).

Just prior to the introduction of the WALI for use with bariatric patients, the Boston Interview for Gastric Bypass was introduced (Sogg & Mori, 2004). Its stated purpose was to address the variability in type of assessments that were being conducted between sites, and to provide a mechanism by which to gather consistent and comparable information for research in outcome prediction. Components of the semi-structured interview include: weight/diet/nutrition history, current eating behaviors, medical history, knowledge of surgical procedures/risks/postsurgical regimen, motivation and expectations of surgical outcome, relationships and support system, and past/current psychiatric functioning. It was revised to the Boston Interview for Bariatric Surgery in consideration of subsequent advances in knowledge (Sogg & Mori, 2004). The authors point out that the role of the psychological evaluation is evolving beyond that of a screening process and argue for its use as part of a presurgical program of education, intervention, and treatment planning (Sogg & Mori, 2004).

Recently, others have proposed the utilization and exploration of more newly developed instruments such as the Personality Assessment Inventory (PAI - Corsica, Azarbad, McGill, Wool, & Hood, 2010), the PsyBari (Mahony, 2010), and the Revised Master Questionnaire (Corsica, Hood, Azarbad, & Ivan, 2011). Corsica et al. demonstrated that the PAI has sound psychometric properties for use with the bariatric population (Corsica et al., 2010). Given the established psychometric strengths of the PAI and its proven applicability in medical settings, it appears to hold an advantage over other personality assessments. Furthermore, the PAI's ability to provide information descriptive of self-concept, interpersonal style and functioning, and perception of stress and social support may prove it to be useful in providing information under a model from which to predict postsurgical outcomes.

The PsyBari is a self-report survey comprised of questions designed to assess constructs that were thought by the author and "other bariatric surgery professionals" to be important to measure preoperatively (Mahony, 2010). These include surgical motivation, emotional eating, anger, binge eating, obesity-related depression, weight-related social impairment, knowledge of postsurgical dietary restrictions, substance/alcohol abuse, and surgical anxiety. As useful as the PsyBari may be in streamlining the evaluation process and providing a way to standardize data collection, it is lacking in a clearly delineated rationale for construct selection or a theoretical framework from which to operationalize the various constructs. The PsyBari is still under development and needs further refinement and demonstration of validity and reliability.

The Revised Master Questionnaire (MQR) was recently evaluated for its potential use for WLS candidates (Corsica et al., 2011). It was originally developed in 1984 as a self-report survey to assess constructs thought to be important to success in conventional weight loss programs (Straw et al., 1984). Factors assessed by the MQR include stimulus control, motivation for weight loss and weight loss behaviors, hopefulness about weight loss and the future, unchangeable versus changeable attributions for weight, and understanding the caloric value of specific foods and activities. These 5 factors were reported to have been empirically supported as valid constructs for obese individuals seeking conventional treatment and to have demonstrated usefulness in prediction of weight loss. Based on these findings and the need for tools to assess weight control-related constructs, Corsica et al.

sought to determine its applicability for WLS candidates (Corsica et al., 2011). They administered the MQR to 790 candidates for gastric banding surgery and gastric bypass surgery. Results indicated acceptable reliability, confirmation of the factor structure, and convergent validity between factors and relevant psychological tests. Corsica, et al. (2011) also presented preliminary norms for use with WLS candidates. The usefulness of the MQR in determining postsurgical outcomes remains to be empirically tested.

These various second generation approaches to the preoperative evaluation of the bariatric patient hold promise for identifying different factors that may be relevant to postsurgical outcomes. However, they are likely to be of limited value in and of themselves. If a principal goal is indeed to establish predictive utility, adjustments will need to be made to the preoperative psychological evaluation to gather construct-specific data that have a basis for their use in the prediction of outcomes. In order to make such adjustments, we will need to decide what outcomes are important to predict. These defined outcomes should be linked to measurable prediction (mediating) variables, i.e. those that have the potential to directly influence the outcome. In order to accomplish this, we first need to establish a systematized way of selecting information related to these prediction variables. While several practitioners have published standardized clinical assessments (Mahony, 2010; Sogg & Mori, 2004; Wadden & Foster, 2006), the information determined important continues to be based largely on clinical convention and not systematically tied to an empirical basis. Empirical evidence without an overarching framework prohibits a broader understanding of relationships among complex determinants and the outcome(s) of interest, and thus does little to guide clinical practice (Green, 2000). In order to effectively discriminate which assessments will be useful, we need to operate under a theoretical framework that can serve as to guide our selection of constructs. We suggest using a theory-driven approach to formulating the presurgical evaluation as a way to understand the nature of what we are trying to predict, and as a framework to (a) select variables for which interventions may be approached, (b) to organize the information, and (c) to systematically test the relationships between variables and outcomes through the course of treatment and follow-up.

3. Empirical support for theoretical models in weight loss studies

According to a recent review (Painter, Borba, Hynes, Mays, & Glanz, 2008), the most common health behavior theories referenced in a random sample of studies published in high profile journals in 2004 - 2007 were: 1) the *Health Belief Model,* which has undergone several revisions and versions since the original work (Hochbaum, 1958); 2) the *Transtheoretical Model (Prochaska, Diclemente, & Norcross, 1992)* and 3) *Social Cognitive Theory* (Bandura, 1986). Another recent review was undertaken to evaluate several health behavior change models in relation to their utility in obesity prevention (Baranowski, Cullen, Nicklas, Thompson, & Baranowski, 2003). Of the various motivational models reviewed, the *Theory of Planned Behavior* was judged to be the most promising for applicability to weight management based on empirical evidence. Less frequently applied theories/explanatory models include the *Theory of Self-determination* (Deci & Ryan, 1985b) and the *Health Behavior Internalization Model* (Bellg, 2003), which both seek to understand motivation and change processes pertinent to long-term behavior maintenance. An *Integrated Model* recently proposed (Hagger, Chatzisarantis, & Biddle, 2002) has been tested for predictive ability in weight loss behaviors and maintenance (Hagger, Chatzisarantis, & Harris, 2006; Jacobs, Hagger, Streukens, De, I, & Claes, 2011). This model combines aspects of the Theory of Planned Behavior and Self-determination Theory. We discuss each theory or model in terms of the advantages and disadvantages one may hold over another relative to the bariatric population and the goal of long-term maintenance of lifestyle behavior changes.

3.1 Health belief model

The core concept of the *Health Belief Model*, as put forth by Hochbaum in 1958, is that health behavior depends on personal beliefs about a disease and the resources or strategies available to the individual that will decrease the likelihood of contracting the disease. The version of the *Health Belief Model* (Becker & Rosenstock, 1984) includes four beliefs or components that work individually and in concert to predict health behaviors. These components include 1) perceived threats, 2) perceived seriousness, 3) perceived benefits, and 4) perceived barriers. In reviewing contemporary models of health behavior change, Baranowski et al. found little support for the Health Belief Model as applied to weight management (Baranowski et al., 2003). Few studies were able to demonstrate that there exists an interaction between perceived susceptibility and perceived seriousness, and that these in turn determine motivation to change or relate to actual behavior change. Cues to action have not been well studied, possibly because they are not stable or predictable. Studies of cues to action suggested that people are not able to accurately rate personal salience. There was only modest support for the effectiveness of using fear-based communication to affect perceived susceptibility and seriousness in effecting behavior change (Baranowski et al., 2003).

3.2 Transtheoretical model

The Transtheoretical Model (TTM - Prochaska et al., 1992) draws on several different theories to incorporate a number of change processes and concepts such as decisional balance and self-efficacy, that are purported to determine movement between stages of behavior change (Prochaska & Velicer, 1997). It assumes that individuals go through five progressive stages of behavior change: *precontemplation, contemplation, preparation, action,* and *maintenance.* The theory assumes that individuals do not move from one stage to another in a linear fashion. Rather, individuals may sustain multiple relapses in their effort to change their behavior, moving back and forth between the stages in a recursive fashion until the behavior change is permanent. The model proposes that there are four *dimensions* to change: the aforementioned stages of change, processes of change, decisional balance, and self-efficacy. Appropriate interventions for behavior change vary according to each stage of change and/or dimension of change in the TTM.

Our review of 14 studies focusing on weight loss and the Transtheoretical Model found that only four were specifically obesity intervention trials and none were performed on bariatric samples. Only two of the four had follow-up periods of longer than six months, the duration which the TTM model specifies is necessary to progress to the stage of maintenance of the new behavior. Furthermore, there has been little to no empirical work done to support the segregation of the stages and the dimensions of the TTM. Various reviews have not found strong support for the TTM as an explanatory or predictive basis for health behavior change, including dietary interventions (Salmela, Poskiparta, Kasila, Vahasarja, & Vanhala, 2009) and exercise (Hutchison, Breckon, & Johnston, 2009). It has been pointed out, however, that many of the interventions studied were built around limited constructs (stages of change) rather than incorporating concepts from the broader TTM model itself (Armitage, 2009; Prochaska, 2006). Particularly understudied have been the specific processes of change. While there appears to be some general support for several of the independent TTM constructs, much work remains to be done in the application of this theory *in toto* to weight loss, especially for the bariatric population.

3.3 Social cognitive theory

Put forth by Bandura in 1986, *Social Cognitive Theory* (SCT) posits a "triadic interaction model" between personal factors, behavior, and the environment that is central to adaptation and change. Reciprocal interactions between each element determine thoughts, actions, beliefs, cognitive competencies, and behavior. For Bandura, cognition plays a central role in a person's construction of reality and thus the ability to self-regulate. Individuals are seen as proactive and as holding beliefs about themselves that affect their sense of personal agency and in turn, influence their behaviors. A core cognition affecting the belief system is self-efficacy, which is seen as providing the foundation for motivation. Efficacy belief is believed to be the major impetus of action, and can be modified through mastery experiences, vicarious experiences, modeling, and social persuasion. A person's outcome expectancies form the primary motivation for action, while self-efficacy and capabilities provide resources for action. Several primary capabilities are thought to be fundamental, including the capacity to symbolize and extract meaning; the ability for forethought and planning; the ability to learn vicariously; and the ability to self-regulate through self-observation, self-monitoring, and self-reflection.

These latter constructs have not been as well-studied as have the concepts of self-efficacy and outcome expectancies (Baranowski et al., 2003). Baranowski et al.'s review of SCT found support for many of its constructs with regard to behavior change, particularly self-efficacy and outcome expectancies. However, they also describe a great deal of variability that is not yet well-understood between genders and across different age groups in relation to the role of outcome expectancies and self-efficacy for diet or physical activity (Baranowski et al., 2003).

3.4 Theory of reasoned action, theory of planned behavior

As an elaboration of social learning theory (Miller & Dollard, 1941) and Bandura's *Social Cognitive Theory*, the *Theory of Reasoned Action* was an extension to socially learned attitudes and norms (Fishbein & Ajzen, 1975). Later, this was expanded to the *Theory of Planned Behavior* (TPB) (Ajzen, 1985), which asserts that individuals form intentions to behaviors based on beliefs, norms and attitudes (Figure 1). Behavior is largely determined by *the intention* to act or not act, although significant perceived barriers may moderate this relationship. Intention is thought to be the closest measurable construct proximal to the behavioral act, therefore the model attempted to identify variables that determine intention.

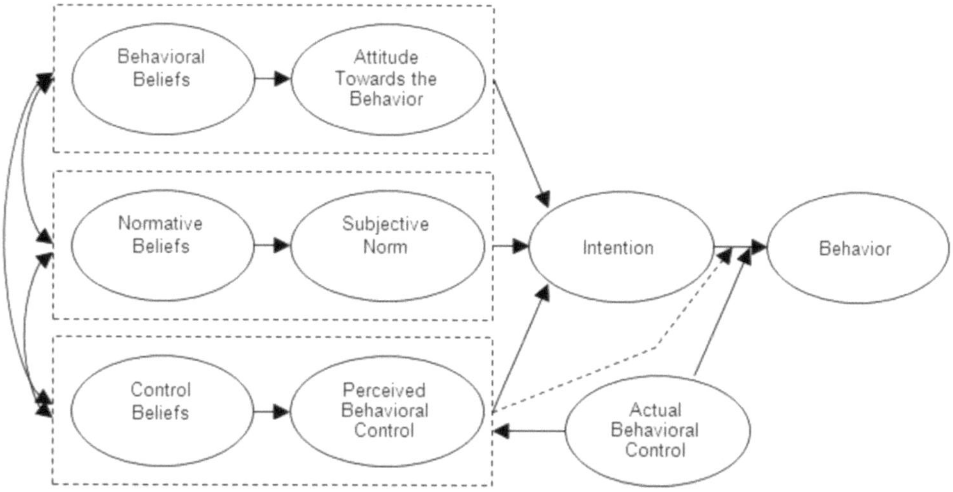

Fig. 1. Model diagram of the Theory of Planned Behavior (Ajzen, 1991)

In the original theory (Theory of Reasoned Action), intentions are moderated by two factors: 1) *attitude toward the behavior* (i.e., personal evaluation of the behavior), and 2) *subjective norm* (i.e., perception of social pressure to engage or not engage in the behavior). *Attitude toward the behavior* is based on the individual's belief that the behavior will lead to a desired outcome or away from an undesired outcome. One's *subjective norm* is created by the perception of the evaluation (either positive or negative) of a particular individual (or group of individuals) placed on the behavior and one's motivation to comply with norms set by others with whom one identifies or is influential. Thus, personal attitudes toward the behavior are weighed against subjective norms or opinions of presumably important others. The *Theory of Planned Behavior* (Ajzen, 1991) added the concept of "perceived behavioral control". That is, one's perception of how much control one has over a particular behavior or action greatly predicts whether or not an action or behavior will be undertaken. The more resources and opportunities an individual believes are personally available, the stronger the belief in the ability to control the target behavior. In essence, the easier the behavior appears to be, the more likely the behavior will be performed. For example, behaviors that are almost automatic will be the most predictable behaviors as these are the behaviors that individuals are more likely to *intend* to perform. Thus, predictions of behavior can be made from knowledge of an individual's attitude toward the behavior, one's subjective norm, and the perceived behavioral control. These three factors are thought to work in concert to shape an individual's intention to behave. Later research suggested that the relationship between actual and perceived behavioral control is a determinant of whether or not intention resulted in actual performance of the behavior (Ajzen, 2001).

In a review of behavior change models relative to weight control, the component of attitude from the TPB appears to be the strongest determinant of dietary behavior, with perceived behavioral control and subjective norms demonstrating less predictive power (Baranowski et al., 2003). A review of studies comparing perceived controllability and self-efficacy found that only perceived difficulty in performance of the behavior (self-efficacy) was significant in the prediction of change in dietary behavior (Ajzen, 2001). With regard to multiple behaviors but primarily physical activity, a meta-analysis (Hagger & Chatzisarantis, 2009) determined that prior behavior accounted for much of the variance predicted by the constructs of the TBP. A recent study specifically applied the TBP to the prediction of exercise in 212 bariatric patients during the preoperative stage through the postsurgical stage for more than one year (Hunt & Gross, 2009). Results were reportedly consistent with other reports in the literature that found moderate to large correlations among the various constructs of the model as well as strong associations between perceived behavioral control, exercise intention and behavior. Only a weak association between subjective norms and intention to exercise was found, which appears to be consistent across many studies. One limitation was the use of subjective self-report surveys of physical activity rather than objective measures. The review by Baranowski et al. concluded that the constructs of TPB, while moderately predictive of *subjective* estimates of health behaviors, are poorly predictive when objective measurements of health behaviors are utilized (Baranowski et al., 2003). Another common criticism of TPB has been that, while it may provide information that is useful for prediction of behavior, it has not provided a useful foundation for developing interventions because there are no constructs included to help understand behavior change processes (Baranowski et al., 2003; Hobbis & Sutton, 2005). However, the TPB has undergone modifications to incorporate such concepts as belief salience and accessibility, past behavior and experience, moral norms, values, self-identity, goal desirability, mood, cognition, and affect on the formation and modification of attitudes, as well as the role of temporal stability and cognition on the relationship between intention and actual behavior (Ajzen, 2001). Baranowski and colleagues' review of health behavioral change models concluded that the TBP, with its more recent modifications, held the most promise for application to diet and physical activity changes in the treatment of obesity (Baranowski et al., 2003).

3.5 Self-determination theory (Deci and Ryan, 1985)

Much research reflects the challenge of maintaining weight loss, no matter the means by which it was initially lost (Sarwer, von Sydow, Vetter, & Wadden, 2009). According to self-determination theory, the level of motivation must be internally regulated and have an orientation of autonomy for long-term behavior maintenance to occur (Deci & Ryan, 1985b). Phases across the internalization continuum reflect the developmental process and styles of regulation going from non-regulation to fully integrated regulation (Figure 2).

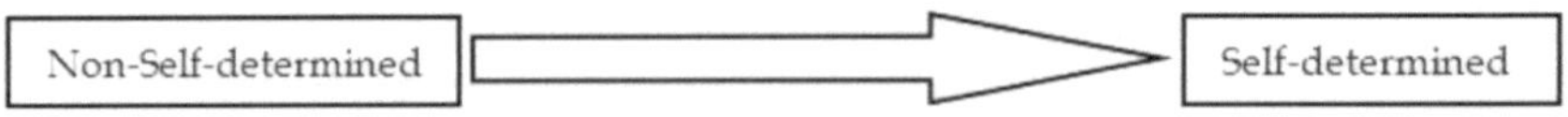

Motivation	Amotivation	Extrinsic Motivation				Intrinsic Motivation
Regulatory Styles	Non-Regulation	External Regulation	Introjected Regulation	Identified Regulation	Integrated Regulation	Intrinsic Regulation
Source of Motivation	Impersonal	External	Somewhat external	Somewhat internal	Internal	Internal
What regulates the motivation?	Non-intentional, non-valuing, Incompetence, Lack of control	Compliance, External rewards and punishments	Self-control, Ego-involvement, Internal rewards and punishments	Personal Importance, Conscious Valuing	Congruence, Awareness, Synthesis with Self	Interest, Enjoyment, Inherent Satisfaction
Causality orientation	Impersonal	Control				Autonomy

Fig. 2. The self-determination continuum (Based on Deci & Ryan, 1985b; Ryan & Deci, 2000)

For long term behavioral regulation to become fully integrated and therefore maintained, the person must develop: 1) an integrated identity and 2) a locus of causality that is *internal* (deCharms, 1968; Deci & Ryan, 1985b). This locus of causality is distinguished from locus of control (Rotter, 1966) in that the perceived source and initiation of the motivated behaviors are inside the self (autonomous) or outside the self (therefore, controlled, e.g. by directives of others or external rewards and contingencies) (Deci & Ryan, 1985b; Williams, Grow, Freedman, Ryan, & Deci, 1996). The goal state of integrated regulation results from the adoption of the behavior into one's core set of values.

An important aspect of self-determination is that of seeking ideal challenge and competency. Individuals tend to approach activities that are at an optimal level of psychological incongruity, i.e. interesting and enjoyable challenges that are optimal for one's abilities (Bandura, 1986; Deci & Ryan, 1985b). Three important factors relating to perceived competence are: 1) the task must be optimally challenging, 2) the task must be associated with immediate, spontaneous feedback or interpersonal feedback from a significant other, and 3) the action and feedback must be experienced as informational rather than controlling. The third characteristic is essential for integrated internalization. The factors increasing perceived competence highlight the importance of setting and generating focus on intermediate, realistic goals. Successive approximations use tasks and goals that are hierarchically structured to provide a person with increased perceptions of competence and lowered levels of anxiety (Bellg, 2003). Research has demonstrated that efficacy expectations are key to successful behavior change (Ajzen, 2001). Increasing perceived competence through treatment gains is a result of enhanced perception of internal causality.

Self Determination Theory (Deci & Ryan, 1985, pp. 153-159) also described three causality orientations: 1) autonomy, 2) control, and 3) impersonal. *Autonomy orientation* is the tendency for behavior to be initiated and regulated by events internal to one's sense of self as well as events in the environment that are interpreted as *informational*. In both, the locus of causality is internal. *Control orientation* is the tendency for behavior to be initiated by events that are external to one's integrated sense of self (i.e., introjected values or internally conflicting events) and by events in the environment that are interpreted as controlling. In both, perceived locus of causality is external. *Impersonal orientation* is based on a sense of one's being incompetent to deal with challenges. It is erratic and non-intentional, for the person lacks the necessary psychological structures for coping with internal and external forces. Impersonal orientation involves the beliefs that behavior and outcomes are independent and that the associated forces are uncontrollable, resulting in the perception of incompetence leading to amotivation.

The role of autonomy has been shown to be an important determinant for behavioral change in obesity intervention programs. For example, patients with a greater sense of autonomy in selecting a weight loss program were shown to have greater attendance in the program, to lose more weight, to adopt a better exercise regimen, and to maintain greater weight loss (Williams et al., 1996). Other studies have consistently demonstrated a strong relationship between positive health behaviors in patients who report a high sense of autonomy, and a greater sense of autonomy and perceived competence when health care environments were perceived as autonomy supportive (Shigaki et al., 2010; Williams et al., 2002).

3.6 A Needs-focused model of self-determination theory – the health behavior internalization model (HBIM - Bellg, 2003)

The HBIM focuses on four self-needs (identity, self-determination, security and support) as well as four behavior-related needs (preference, context, competence and coping) as components of the development of internalized regulation of health behaviors (Figure 3). Internalization of self-regulation is characterized by low conflict/high acceptance, high autonomy, high security, high perceived support, high satisfaction with behavior choices/context, high perceived competence, and adequate coping without undesired behavior co-occurring. This HBIM builds on Self-determination theory by adding it into a context of needs that interact in order to resolve into internalization and self-regulation. The security component refers to perceived threats associated with an adverse medical situation. Fear of declining health may be perceived as a threat that initially promotes treatment-seeking and/or behavioral adherence, but it is not likely to lead to long-term behavioral change as people tend not to maintain levels of fear, anxiety and guilt (conflict states) (Bellg, 2003). This model shows promise, but has not yet been tested.

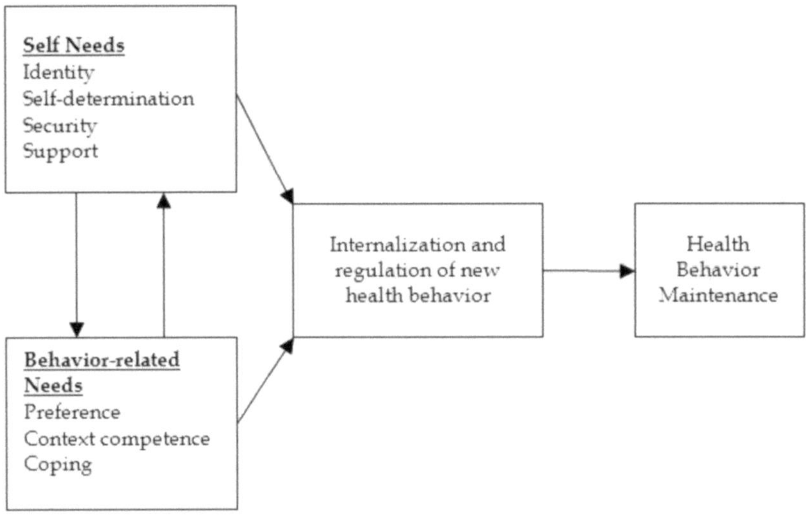

Fig. 3. Health behavior internalization model (Bellg, 2003).

Bellg (2003) describes the transition to internalization as being a product of the need to reduce conflict. In externally controlled behaviors, conflict occurs between the values of self-related needs and behavior-related needs of the individual. Bellg states that the process of transforming the external ideas and regulations of the social environment (when these are perceived as a desirable goal to obtain) to becoming personally held values is a fundamental human need. The new, integrated state is stable and free of conflict or a feeling of external control.

3.7 The integrated model (Hagger, 2006)

Hagger and colleagues performed a structural modeling study on an integrated model that linked Self-determination Theory and the Theory of Planned Behavior (SDT/TPB), testing effects of change in antecedents on exercise and dieting (Hagger et al., 2006). Later, Jacobs and colleagues reported further testing and refinement of this integrated model on dieting and physical activity behaviors in undergraduates at baseline and at a one-year follow-up (Jacobs et al., 2011). In this integrated model, changes in autonomous and controlled motivation were assessed for effects on changes in attitudes and self-efficacy. All four of these constructs were tested for relationships to change in behavioral intentions and the subsequent change in diet/exercise behavior. While for both diet and exercise behaviors, increased autonomous motivation was associated with increased self-efficacy and behavioral intentions, the intensity of the exercise intervention moderated the relationship between self-efficacy and intentions (Jacobs et al., 2011). Both studies used assessments designed to measure constructs specific to Self-determination Theory.

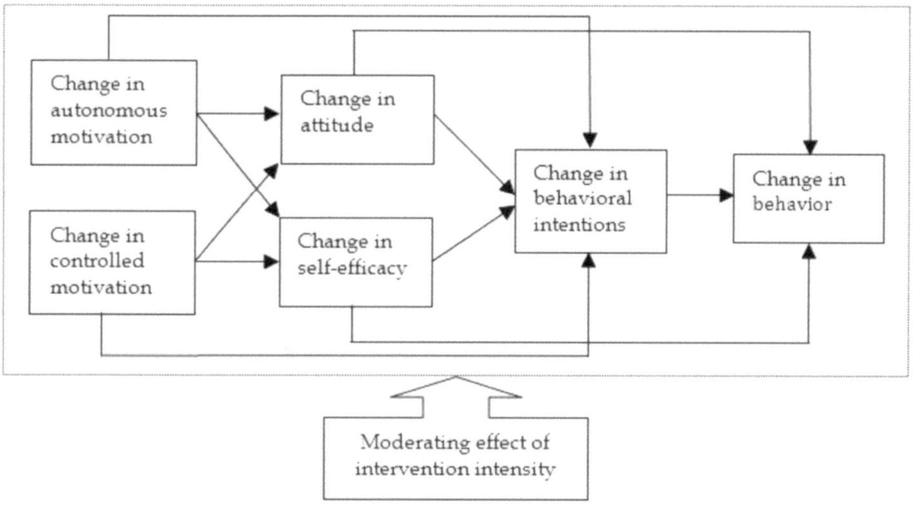

Fig. 4. Integrated model of the Theory of Planned Behavior and Self-determination theory (Jacobs et al., 2011).

3.8 Summary of theories and relevance in bariatric psychological evaluation

In examination of the application of these most popular or relevant theories to weight loss treatment-seeking or bariatric populations, we found few thorough and long-term studies of the mechanisms and processes of lifestyle behavior change maintenance. Also, we found that many of these theories or models are modestly descriptive but not explanatory. Further, we found little support in the predictive power of measuring some of these constructs for maintenance of postsurgical weight loss. Since the evolution of the presurgical psychological evaluation has origins in the medical diagnostic model rather than a prognostic model, we believe that a more systematic approach to the evaluation is needed to advance our understanding of the constructs and processes of long-term postsurgical behavioral change. Based on our limited review, it appears that aspects of both Self-determination Theory and the Theory of Planned Behavior have the most demonstrated empirical support thus far, such that the integrated SDT/TPB model has the greatest potential application for this purpose. Additionally, the Health Belief Internalization Model appears to hold promise in providing constructs relevant to the specific needs-satisfaction processes required for internalization to occur. More empirical work is needed, including the development and validation of assessments of its constructs before it can be applied in the clinical setting.

4. Proposal for applying a new, theoretically-based model to presurgical assessment

We propose that a paradigm shift is needed in order to address the apparent deficiencies of the current approach to the presurgical psychological evaluation of WLS candidates. Specifically, we propose that the presurgical psychological evaluation undergo a reformulation with a theory-based, integrated stage and motivational basis to inform the selection of pertinent areas of inquiry and assessment tools. Ideally, the theory would be one that is applicable to understanding health behavior changes that are relevant to positive postoperative outcomes. Based on the current body of literature, it appears that following a bariatric diet, following an exercise program, and attending a bariatric support group comprise targeted activities that support the goals of long-term maintenance in improved health and optimum weight loss. We propose basing the presurgical psychological evaluation on an integrated theoretical model (SDT/TPB), so that clinicians can begin to assess constructs pertinent to long-term maintenance of these relevant health behaviors (Figure 4). In order to effectively assess the constructs relevant to the integrated theoretical model, the presurgical psychological evaluation must be coordinated to occur subsequent to patient interactions with the surgeon and the dietician so that the patient has a reference point and exposure to postsurgical expectations from which to answer questions.

Based on this new paradigm and empirical evidence to date, the recommended presurgical psychological evaluation would ideally evaluate the constructs and areas listed below. Assessments should be utilized that have demonstrated validity and reliability for use with the bariatric population. This list is not intended to be exhaustive, but is based on our review of the current literature related to WLS outcomes and to a plausible theoretical framework.

1. **Psychological functioning, including personality disorders, psychopathology, self-esteem, and coping**. The Personality Assessment Inventory (PAI) (Morey, 2007) has recently been shown to be a valid and reliable instrument that offers data relevant to clinical decision making for these constructs. Other personality tests, such as the Millon Behavioral Medicine Diagnostic™ - Bariatric (Millon et al., 2007) and the Millon Clinical Multiaxial Inventory – III™ (Millon, Millon, Davis, & Grossman, 2009) need further research to demonstrate their use with the bariatric population.
2. **Eating disorders and body dissatisfaction**. The Eating Disorder Inventory – 2 offers a valid assessment of these constructs. The Body Shape Questionnaire (BSQ- Cooper, Taylor, Cooper, & Fairburn, 1987) has also been utilized as an effective measurement of body dissatisfaction with bariatric patients. Additionally, semi-structured interviews such as the Weight and Lifestyle Inventory (WALI – Wadden & Foster, 2006) or the Boston Interview for Bariatric Surgery (Sogg & Mori, 2004) utilize questions designed to evaluate these constructs.
3. **Autonomous motivation for bariatric lifestyle changes**. The Treatment Self-Regulation Questionnaire (TSRQ - Levesque et al., 2007; Ryan & Connell, 1989;

Williams et al., 1996) assesses four factors (autonomous regulation, introjection, external regulation and amotivation) that could be used to evaluate the degree to which the patient has adopted autonomous motivation for the bariatric diet, an exercise program, and support group attendance. The TSRQ is a 15-item self-report survey that takes less than 5 minutes to complete for each behavioral topic. Items could be responses to the following suggested stems: "The reason I would follow a bariatric diet/an exercise program/attend support group is because…". Item responses represent various autonomous, controlled, and amotivational statements. Responses are according to a seven-point, Likert-type scale ranging from 1 (not at all true) to 7 (very true). Internal consistencies across several health behaviors ranged for the four factors from .73 - .93 with the exception of one dataset where amotivation was .41, but three other datasets ranged from .73 - .79 for this factor (Levesque et al., 2007).

4. **Self-efficacy**. Perceived Competence Scale (PCS - Williams & Deci, 1998; Williams, Freedman, & Deci, 1998). The PCS is a 4-item self-report survey that can be adapted and used to determine a patient's perceived competence, or self-efficacy, for maintaining a bariatric diet, an exercise program, and attendance in support group. Responses are according to a seven-point, Likert-type scale ranging from 1 (not at all true) to 7 (very true). It takes approximately one minute to complete for each behavior domain. In two studies, internal consistencies were above .80 (Williams & Deci, 1998; Williams et al., 1998).
5. **Clinical support resources**. Health Care Climate Questionnaire (HCCQ - Williams et al., 1996). The HCCQ is a 15-item self-report survey (or a 5 item short version) used to assess the level of autonomy support that a patient perceives is provided by the bariatric surgeon and staff. It takes approximately 5 minutes to complete. Ratings are on a 7-point scale which indicates the degree to which health care providers are perceived to be autonomy supportive. Higher scores indicate greater perceived autonomy support. Across domains, the alpha coefficient of internal consistency is above .90.
6. **Control orientation**. General Causality Orientations Scale (GCOS - Deci & Ryan, 1985a). The GCOS is a 36-item self-report survey of various vignettes used to determine the degree to which a patient is oriented toward autonomy as a general tendency. It takes approximately 20 minutes to complete. The GCOS is available in two forms. The original scale consists of 12 vignettes and 36 items. Each vignette describes a typical social or achievement oriented situation with three types of possible responses: an autonomous, a controlled, or an impersonal type. Respondents indicate (on 7-point, Likert-type scales) the extent to which each response is typical for them. Higher scores indicate higher amounts of the particular orientation. Subscale scores are generated by summing the 12 responses on items corresponding to each subscale. This scale has been shown to be reliable, with Cronbach alpha values of about .75 and a test-retest coefficient of .74 over two months (Deci & Ryan, 1985a).
7. **Attitudes Toward Behaviors** (Ajzen, 2001; Ajzen & Fishbein, 1980). Cognitive and affective attitude toward the bariatric diet, exercise, and support group attendance can be assessed using two sets of three bipolar items on a 7 point scale. Cognitive attitude is

comprised of the following scales: useful to useless, wise to foolish, beneficial to harmful. Affective attitude is comprised of the following poles: pleasant to unpleasant, interesting to boring, and enjoyable to unenjoyable.

8. **Perceived Behavior Control** (Ajzen, 2001). The measurement of PBC occurs on a 7-point, Likert-type scale (-3 not at all, +3 extremely) that measures confidence, ease-difficulty, and control ability for following a bariatric diet, maintaining an exercise program, and regularly attending support group. The extent to which this scale may overlap with the Perceived Competence scale (#4 above) is not known.

The use of an assessment battery that is based on current empirical evidence and a theoretical model for prediction of long-term behavior change, as we are proposing, should generate information that will inform prognostic statements and guide recommendations needed to improve prognosis that are based on specific processes under the model. Using this battery, it would be anticipated that patients who were autonomy oriented; high in autonomous motivation, confidence, and perceived control for the expected postsurgical lifestyle behavior changes; and who perceive the health care climate as supportive would receive a favorable prognosis for maintenance of behavioral changes. Ideally, these would support postsurgical success, as defined by maintenance of EWL corresponding to improved health and quality of life. Patients found to have an impersonal orientation; who were amotivated, who lack confidence or perceive themselves to have little control for lifestyle modifications; and who perceive the health care climate as non-supportive would receive the poorest prognosis. Furthermore, patients with a personality disorder diagnosis or who have a high degree of psychopathology (including disturbed eating) or body dissatisfaction would also be considered at risk for poor postsurgical behavioral adherence. Low self-esteem or poor coping skills would warrant caution. It is unclear to what extent these non-theoretically based psychological constructs are related to and may be picked up by constructs under the integrated model, such as causality orientation, autonomous motivation, self-efficacy/competence, and perceived behavioral control.

By evaluating the current status as well as the attitudes and perceptions of the bariatric patient using the integrated principles of SD/TPB, clinicians can identify key issues that may need to be addressed to assist a patient in achieving intrinsically motivated health behavior maintenance to achieve sustained behavior changes that support the long-term goals of the surgery. We are in agreement with Sogg and Mori's (2004) assertion that the role of the presurgical psychological evaluation should be used for treatment planning, but propose that treatment recommendations and components are based on a theoretically sound, motivational model for systematic testing.

Based on our view of the SDT/TPB integrated model, key targets for increasing intentions (and therefore behaviors) are: 1) facilitating development of an autonomous orientation within the patient, 2) maximizing a perception of internal regulation of behavioral goals, 3) increasing positive attitudes associated with desired behaviors, and 4) optimizing self-efficacy surrounding skills needed to easily maintain lifestyle patterns. Theoretically-based guidelines for promoting these areas in relation to behavioral targets such as dietary change, physical activity, and regular attendance in a supportive group intervention have been described throughout the literature and can help guide the development of interventions specific to the bariatric population.

5. Conclusions

In conclusion, it is our contention that bariatric clinical practice and outcomes research would benefit from the application of theories and models that describe and model behavior change processes, and that psychological evaluation and assessments should be framed in theory and based on empirical evidence. Our proposal to use the SDT/TPB integrated model to guide the presurgical psychological evaluation for bariatric surgery represents the first attempt to establish an empirically-justified approach. As a framework for understanding the processes that determine the long-term behavior changes needed for postsurgical success, clinicians are in a better position to provide prognostic statements and treatment recommendations that have a scientifically-based rationale.

Future studies should seek to validate and establish the psychometric properties of psychological tests or questionnaires for the bariatric population. Studies should also determine their validity across age, gender, and cultural groups. Assessments that are designed to measure the various constructs of a theoretical model should be validated. This will allow for sound systematic investigations of the relationships of the validated measures with defined behavioral targets. In this way, we will begin to amass empirical evidence of the predictive utility of our instruments. However, selected behavioral targets should also be evaluated for their relationship to various parameters thought to represent postsurgical success. Furthermore, if a specific % EWL cut-off is to be used as a criterion of success, its clinical utility needs to be firmly established.

The role of the presurgical psychological evaluation should be expanded to incorporate treatment planning. Often, abrupt lifestyle prescriptions are directed at patients who are very far from a level of mastery at attempting, much less maintaining a new pattern of behavior. In the case of the postsurgical phase, patients are often unlikely to have ever encountered an eating plan similar to a bariatric diet. They are also not likely to be able to perform 30 minutes of moderate physical activity several times per week. Thus, it is likely that the process involved in change is recursive and prone to derailing without a supportive, patient-centered plan. Future studies should seek to characterize postsurgical phases and develop treatment plans to address their corresponding challenges. According to SDT/TPB, plans that are too rigid (not strongly identifiable to the patient) or directive (not autonomy supporting) will not likely aid the patient in making the needed internalization transition required for long-term maintenance of change.

With the advent of evidence-based medicine and the increasing need to justify evaluative and other clinical psychological services for bariatric patients, the presurgical psychological evaluation has been in need of a critical review. Our review suggests that a paradigm shift is in order to broaden our knowledge and advance the field. By suggesting a theory-based approach and presenting an example of a theory-based assessment battery, we hope to generate dialogue and stimulate further discussion and research on this topic in order to improve bariatric care.

6. Acknowledgements

We thank Susan Frensley, Ph.D. for providing a review and summary of various health behavior theories used to inform our investigation of the literature.

7. References

Ajzen, I. (1985). From intentions to actions: A theory of planned behavior. In J.Kuhl & J. Beckman (Eds.), *Action-control: From cognition to behavior* (pp. 11-39). Heidelberg: Springer.

Ajzen, I. (1991). The theory of planned behavior. *Organizational behavior and human decision processes, 50,* 179-211.

Ajzen, I. (2001). Nature and operation of attitudes. *Annual Review of Psychology, 52,* 27-58.

Ajzen, I. & Fishbein, M. (1980). *Understanding attitudes and predicting social behavior.* Englewood Cliffs, NJ: Prentice-Hall.

Allison, K. C., Wadden, T. A., Sarwer, D. B., Fabricatore, A. N., Crerand, C. E., Gibbons, L. M. et al. (2006). Night eating syndrome and binge eating disorder among persons seeking bariatric surgery: Prevalence and related features. *Surgery for Obesity & Related Disorders, 2,* 153-158.

Armitage, C. J. (2009). Is there utility in the transtheoretical model? *British Journal of Health Psychology, 14,* 195-210.

Ashton, D., Favretti, F., & Segato, G. (2008). Preoperative psychological testing--another form of prejudice. *Obesity Surgery, 18,* 1330-1337.

Averbukh, Y., Heshka, S., El-Shoreya, H., Flancbaum, L., Geliebter, A., Kamel, S. et al. (2003). Depression score predicts weight loss following Roux-en-Y gastric bypass. *Obesity Surgery, 13,* 833-836.

Ayyad, C. & Andersen, T. (2000). Long-term efficacy of dietary treatment of obesity: A systematic review of studies published between 1931 and 1999. *Obesity Reviews, 1,* 113-119.

Bandura, A. (1986). *Social foundations of thought and action: A social cognitive theory.* Englewood Cliffs, NJ: Prentice-Hall.

Baranowski, T., Cullen, K. W., Nicklas, T., Thompson, D., & Baranowski, J. (2003). Are current health behavioral change models helpful in guiding prevention of weight gain efforts? *Obesity Research, 11 Suppl,* 23S-43S.

Bauchowitz, A. U., Gonder-Frederick, L. A., Olbrisch, M. E., Azarbad, L., Ryee, M. Y., Woodson, M. et al. (2005). Psychosocial evaluation of bariatric surgery candidates: a survey of present practices. *Psychosomatic Medicine, 67,* 825-832.

Becker, M. H. & Rosenstock, I. M. (1984). Compliance with medical advice. In A.Steptoe & A. M. Matthews (Eds.), *Health care and human behavior* (London: Academic Press.

Belanger, S. B., Wechsler, F. S., Nademin, M. E., & Virden, T. B., III (2010). Predicting outcome of gastric bypass surgery utilizing personality scale elevations, psychosocial factors, and diagnostic group membership. *Obesity Surgery, 20,* 1361-1371.

Bellg, A. J. (2003). Maintenance of health behavior change in preventive cardiology. Internalization and self-regulation of new behaviors. *Behavior Modification, 27,* 103-131.

Boeka, A. G., Prentice-Dunn, S., & Lokken, K. L. (2010). Psychosocial predictors of intentions to comply with bariatric surgery guidelines. *Psychology, Health & Medicine, 15,* 188-197.

Buchwald, H. (2005). Consensus conference statement bariatric surgery for morbid obesity: health implications for patients, health professionals, and third-party payers. *Surgery for Obesity & Related Disorders, 1,* 371-381.

Buchwald, H., Avidor, Y., Braunwald, E., Jensen, M. D., Pories, W., Fahrbach, K. et al. (2004). Bariatric surgery: a systematic review and meta-analysis. *JAMA, 292,* 1724-1737.

Buddeberg-Fischer, B., Klaghofer, R., Sigrist, S., & Buddeberg, C. (2004). Impact of psychosocial stress and symptoms on indication for bariatric surgery and outcome in morbidly obese patients. *Obesity Surgery, 14,* 361-369.

Busetto, L., Segato, G., De, L. M., De, M. F., Foletto, M., Vianello, M. et al. (2005). Weight loss and postoperative complications in morbidly obese patients with binge eating disorder treated by laparoscopic adjustable gastric banding. *Obesity Surgery, 15,* 195-201.

Christou, N. V., Look, D., & Maclean, L. D. (2006). Weight gain after short- and long-limb gastric bypass in patients followed for longer than 10 years. *Annals of Surgery, 244,* 734-740.

Colles, S. L., Dixon, J. B., & O'Brien, P. E. (2008). Grazing and loss of control related to eating: two high-risk factors following bariatric surgery. *Obesity, 16,* 615-622.

Cooper, P. J., Taylor, M. J., Cooper, M., & Fairburn, C. G. (1987). The development and validation of the Body Shape Questionnaire. *International Journal of Eating Disorders, 6,* 485-494.

Corsica, J. A., Azarbad, L., McGill, K., Wool, L., & Hood, M. (2010). The Personality Assessment Inventory: clinical utility, psychometric properties, and normative data for bariatric surgery candidates. *Obesity Surgery, 20,* 722-731.

Corsica, J. A., Hood, M. M., Azarbad, L., & Ivan, I. (2011). Revisiting the Revised Master Questionnaire for the Psychological Evaluation of Bariatric Surgery Candidates. *Obesity Surgery.* 2011 May 13. [Epub ahead of print].

deCharms, R. (1968). *Personal causation.* New York: Academic.

Deci, E. L. & Ryan, R. M. (1985a). The general causality orientations scale: Self-determination in personality. *Journal of Research in Personality, 19,* 109-134.

Deci, E. & Ryan, R. (1985b). *Intrinsic Motivation and Self-Determination in Human Behavior.* New York: Plenum Press.

Fabricatore, A. N., Crerand, C. E., Wadden, T. A., Sarwer, D. B., & Krasucki, J. L. (2006). How do mental health professionals evaluate candidates for bariatric surgery? Survey results. *Obesity Surgery, 16,* 567-573.

Fabricatore, A. N., Wadden, T. A., Sarwer, D. B., Crerand, C. E., Kuehnel, R. H., Lipschutz, P. E. et al. (2006). Self-reported eating behaviors of extremely obese persons seeking bariatric surgery: A factor analytic approach. *Surgery for Obesity & Related Disorders, 2,* 146-152.

Fischer, S., Chen, E., Katterman, S., Roerhig, M., Bochierri-Ricciardi, L., Munoz, D. et al. (2007). Emotional eating in a morbidly obese bariatric surgery-seeking population. *Obesity Surgery, 17,* 778-784.

Fishbein, M. & Ajzen, I. (1975). *Belief, attitude, intention, and behavior: An introduction to theory and research.* Reading, MA: Addison-Wesley.

Franks, S. F. & Kaiser, K. A. (2008). Predictive factors in bariatric surgery outcomes: What is the role of the preoperative psychological evaluation? *Primary Psychiatry, 15,* 74-83.

Fujioka, K., Yan, E., Wang, H. J., & Li, Z. (2008). Evaluating preoperative weight loss, binge eating disorder, and sexual abuse history on Roux-en-Y gastric bypass outcome. *Surgery for Obesity & Related Disorders, 4,* 137-143.

Gibbons, L. M., Sarwer, D. B., Crerand, C. E., Fabricatore, A. N., Kuehnel, R. H., Lipschutz, P. E. et al. (2006). Previous weight loss experiences of bariatric surgery candidates: how much have patients dieted prior to surgery? *Surgery for Obesity & Related Disorders, 2,* 159-164.

Green, J. (2000). The role of theory in evidence-based health promotion practice. *Health Education Research, 15,* 125-129.

Greenberg, I. (2003). Psychological aspects of bariatric surgery. *Nutrition in Clinical Practice, 18,* 124-130.

Greenberg, I., Sogg, S., & Perna, M. (2009). Behavioral and psychological care in weight loss surgery: best practice update. *Obesity, 17,* 880-884.

Grilo, C. M., Masheb, R. M., Brody, M., Toth, C., Burke-Martindale, C. H., & Rothschild, B. S. (2005). Childhood maltreatment in extremely obese male and female bariatric surgery candidates. *Obesity Research, 13,* 123-130.

Grilo, C. M., White, M. A., Masheb, R. M., Rothschild, B. S., & Burke-Martindale, C. H. (2006). Relation of childhood sexual abuse and other forms of maltreatment to 12-month postoperative outcomes in extremely obese gastric bypass patients. *Obesity Surgery, 16,* 454-460.

Grothe, K. B., Dubbert, P. M., & O'jile, J. R. (2006). Psychological assessment and management of the weight loss surgery patient. *American Journal of the Medical Sciences, 331,* 201-206.

Hagger, M. S. & Chatzisarantis, N. L. (2009). Integrating the theory of planned behaviour and self-determination theory in health behaviour: A meta-analysis. *British Journal of Health Psychology, 14,* 275-302.

Hagger, M. S., Chatzisarantis, N. L., & Biddle, S. J. (2002). The influence of autonomous and controlling motives on physical activity intentions within the Theory of Planned Behaviour. *British Journal of Health Psychology, 7,* 283-297.

Hagger, M. S., Chatzisarantis, N. L., & Harris, J. (2006). From psychological need satisfaction to intentional behavior: testing a motivational sequence in two behavioral contexts. *Personality & Social Psychology Bulletin, 32,* 131-148.

Herpertz, S., Kielmann, R., Wolf, A. M., Hebebrand, J., & Senf, W. (2004). Do psychosocial variables predict weight loss or mental health after obesity surgery? A systematic review. *Obesity Research, 12,* 1554-1569.

Hobbis, I. C. & Sutton, S. (2005). Are techniques used in cognitive behaviour therapy applicable to behaviour change interventions based on the theory of planned behaviour? *Journal of Health Psychology, 10,* 7-18.

Hochbaum, G. M. (1958). Public participation in medical screening programs: A socio-psychological study. Washington, D.C., Government Printing Office.

Hunt, H. R. & Gross, A. M. (2009). Prediction of exercise in patients across various stages of bariatric surgery: A comparison of the merits of the theory of reasoned action versus the theory of planned behavior. *Behavior Modification, 33,* 795-817.

Hutchison, A. J., Breckon, J. D., & Johnston, L. H. (2009). Physical activity behavior change interventions based on the transtheoretical model: A systematic review. *Health Education & Behavior, 36,* 829-845.

Jacobs, N., Hagger, M. S., Streukens, S., De, B., I, & Claes, N. (2011). Testing an integrated model of the theory of planned behaviour and self-determination theory for different energy balance-related behaviours and intervention intensities. *British Journal of Health Psychology, 16,* 113-134.

Kaiser, K. A., Franks, S. F., Carrol, J. F., & Smith, A. B. (2009). Disinhibitory eating and the bariatric patient. *Surgery for Obesity & Related Disorders, 5,* 3, S75.

Kaiser, K. A., Franks, S. F., Hall, J., McGill, J., Berbel, G., & Smith, A. (2004). Changes in psychological dimensions of eating behavior after laparoscopic banding: A preliminary analysis. *Obesity Research,* 12, A91.

Kaiser, K. A., Franks, S. F., & Smith, A. B. (2011). Positive relationship between support group attendance and one-year postoperative weight loss in gastric banding patients. *Surgery for Obesity & Related Disorders, 7,* 89-93.

Kalarchian, M. A., Marcus, M. D., Levine, M. D., Courcoulas, A. P., Pilkonis, P. A., Ringham, R. M. et al. (2007). Psychiatric disorders among bariatric surgery candidates: relationship to obesity and functional health status. *American Journal of Psychiatry, 164,* 328-334.

Kalarchian, M. A., Marcus, M. D., Levine, M. D., Haas, G. L., Greeno, C. G., Weissfeld, L. A. et al. (2005). Behavioral treatment of obesity in patients taking antipsychotic medications. *Journal of Clinical Psychiatry, 66,* 1058-1063.

Kinzl, J. F., Schrattenecker, M., Traweger, C., Mattesich, M., Fiala, M., & Biebl, W. (2006). Psychosocial predictors of weight loss after bariatric surgery. *Obesity Surgery, 16,* 1609-1614.

LeMont, D., Moorehead, M. K., Parish, M. S., Reto, C. S., & Ritz, S. J. (2004). Suggestions for the pre-surgical psychological assessment of bariatric surgery candidates. Available at: http://s3.amazonaws.com/publicASMBS/GuidelinesStatements/Guidelines/PsychPreSurgicalAssessment.pdf. Accessed 7-Aug-2011.

Levesque, C. S., Williams, G. C., Elliot, D., Pickering, M. A., Bodenhamer, B., & Finley, P. J. (2007). Validating the theoretical structure of the Treatment Self-Regulation Questionnaire (TSRQ) across three different health behaviors. *Health Education Research, 22,* 691-702.

Ma, Y., Pagoto, S. L., Olendzki, B. C., Hafner, A. R., Perugini, R. A., Mason, R. et al. (2006). Predictors of weight status following laparoscopic gastric bypass. *Obesity Surgery, 16,* 1227-1231.

Mahony, D. (2010). Assessing sexual abuse/attack histories with bariatric surgery patients. *Journal of Childhood Sexual Abuse, 19,* 469-484.

Miller, N. E. & Dollard, J. (1941). *Social learning and imitation.* New Haven, CT: Yale University Press.

Millon, T., Antoni, M. H., Millon, C., Minor, S., & Grossman, S. (2007). *MBMD manual supplement: Bariatric report.* Minneapolis, MN: Pearson Assessments.

Millon, T., Millon, C., Davis, R., & Grossman, S. (2009). *Millon Clinical Multiaxial Inventory-III.* Minneapolis, MN: Pearson Assessments.

Morey, L. C. (2007). *The Personality Assessment Inventory professional manual.* Lutz, FL: Psychological Assessment Resources.

Nguyen, N. T., Root, J., Zainabadi, K., Sabio, A., Chalifoux, S., Stevens, C. M. et al. (2005). Accelerated growth of bariatric surgery with the introduction of minimally invasive surgery. *Archives of Surgery, 140,* 1198-1202.

NIH Consensus Panel (1991). Gastrointestinal Surgery for Severe Obesity. In *Consensus Development Conference* (pp. 1-20).

O'Brien, P. E., McPhail, T., Chaston, T. B., & Dixon, J. B. (2006). Systematic review of medium-term weight loss after bariatric operations. *Obesity Surgery, 16,* 1032-1040.

Painter, J. E., Borba, C. P., Hynes, M., Mays, D., & Glanz, K. (2008). The use of theory in health behavior research from 2000 to 2005: A systematic review. *Annals of Behavioral Medicine, 35,* 358-362.

Pessina, A., Andreoli, M., & Vassallo, C. (2001). Adaptability and compliance of the obese patient to restrictive gastric surgery in the short term. *Obesity Surgery, 11,* 459-463.

Prochaska, J. O. (2006). Moving beyond the transtheoretical model. *Addiction, 101,* 768-774.

Prochaska, J. O., Diclemente, C. C., & Norcross, J. C. (1992). In search of how people change: Applications to addictive behaviors. *American Psychologist, 47,* 1102-1114.

Prochaska, J. O. & Velicer, W. F. (1997). The transtheoretical model of health behavior change. *American Journal of Health Promotion, 12,* 38-48.

Rosik, C. H. (2005). Psychiatric symptoms among prospective bariatric surgery patients: Rates of prevalence and their relation to social desirability, pursuit of surgery, and follow-up attendance. *Obesity Surgery, 15,* 677-683.

Rotter, J. B. (1966). Generalized expectancies for internal versus external control of reinforcement. *Psychological Monographs, 80,* 1-28.

Ryan, R. M. & Connell, J. P. (1989). Perceived locus of causality and internalization: Examining reasons for acting in two domains. *Journal of Personality & Social Psychology, 57,* 749-761.

Ryan, R. M. & Deci, E. L. (2000). Self-determination theory and the facilitation of intrinsic motivation, social development, and well-being. *American Psychologist, 55,* 68-78.

Ryden, A., Karlsson, J., Sullivan, M., Torgerson, J. S., & Taft, C. (2003). Coping and distress: what happens after intervention? A 2-year follow-up from the Swedish Obese Subjects (SOS) study. *Psychosomatic Medicine, 65,* 435-442.

Salmela, S., Poskiparta, M., Kasila, K., Vahasarja, K., & Vanhala, M. (2009). Transtheoretical model-based dietary interventions in primary care: a review of the evidence in diabetes. *Health Education Research, 24,* 237-252.

Sarwer, D. B., von Sydow, G. A., Vetter, M. L., & Wadden, T. A. (2009). Behavior therapy for obesity: Where are we now? *Current Opinion in Endocrinology, Diabetes & Obesity, 16,* 347-352.

Shigaki, C., Kruse, R. L., Mehr, D., Sheldon, K. M., Bin, G., Moore, C. et al. (2010). Motivation and diabetes self-management. *Chronic Illness, 6,* 202-214.

Smith, A. B., Franks, S. F., Kaiser, K. A., & Carrol, J. F. (2008). Eating behavior patterns and weight loss one year after laparoscopic banding surgery. *Surgery for Obesity & Related Disorders, 4,* 3, 331-332.

Sogg, S. & Mori, D. L. (2004). The Boston interview for gastric bypass: Determining the psychological suitability of surgical candidates. *Obesity Surgery, 14,* 370-380.

Steinbrook, R. (2004). Surgery for severe obesity. *New England Journal of Medicine, 350,* 1075-1079.

Straw, M. K., Straw, R. B., Mahoney, M. J., Rogers, T., Mahoney, B. K., Craighead, L. W. et al. (1984). The Master Questionnaire: Preliminary report on an obesity assessment device. *Addictive Behaviors, 9,* 1-10.

Stroh, C., Hohmann, U., Schramm, H., Meyer, F., & Manger, T. (2011). Fourteen-year long-term results after gastric banding. *Journal of Obesity, 2011,* doi:10.1155/2011/128451.

Stunkard, A. J. & Messick, S. (1985). The three-factor eating questionnaire to measure dietary restraint, disinhibition and hunger. *Journal of Psychosomatic Research, 29,* 71-83.

Swan-Kremier, L. A. (2005). Psychosocial outcomes of bariatric surgery. In J.E.Mitchell & M. de Zwann (Eds.), *Bariatric surgery: A guide for mental health professionals* (pp. 101-118). New York: Taylor & Francis Group.

van Hout, G. C., van Oudheusden, I., Krasuska, A. T., & van Heck, G. L. (2006). Psychological profile of candidates for vertical banded gastroplasty. *Obesity Surgery, 16,* 67-74.

van Hout, G. C., Verschure, S. K., & van Heck, G. L. (2005). Psychosocial predictors of success following bariatric surgery. *Obesity Surgery, 15,* 552-560.

Wadden, T. A. & Foster, G. D. (2006). Weight and Lifestyle Inventory (WALI). *Surgery for Obesity & Related Disorders, 2,* 180-199.

Walfish, S., Vance, D., & Fabricatore, A. N. (2007). Psychological evaluation of bariatric surgery applicants: Procedures and reasons for delay or denial of surgery. *Obesity Surgery, 17,* 1578-1583.

Walfish, S., Wise, E. A., & Streiner, D. L. (2008). Limitations of the Millon Behavioral Medicine Diagnostic (MBMD) with bariatric surgical candidates. *Obesity Surgery, 18,* 1318-1322.

Wildes, J. E., Kalarchian, M. A., Marcus, M. D., Levine, M. D., & Courcoulas, A. P. (2008). Childhood maltreatment and psychiatric morbidity in bariatric surgery candidates. *Obesity Surgery, 18,* 306-313.

Williams, G. C. & Deci, E. L. (1998). The importance of supporting autonomy in medical education. *Annals of Internal Medicine, 129,* 303-308.

Williams, G. C., Freedman, Z. R., & Deci, E. L. (1998). Supporting autonomy to motivate patients with diabetes for glucose control. *Diabetes Care, 21,* 1644-1651.

Williams, G. C., Grow, V. M., Freedman, Z. R., Ryan, R. M., & Deci, E. L. (1996). Motivational predictors of weight loss and weight-loss maintenance. *Journal of Personality & Social Psychology, 70,* 115-126.

Williams, G. C., Minicucci, D. S., Kouides, R. W., Levesque, C. S., Chirkov, V. I., Ryan, R. M. et al. (2002). Self-determination, smoking, diet and health. *Health Education Research, 17,* 512-521.

Wysoker, A. (2005). The lived experience of choosing bariatric surgery to lose weight. *Journal of the American Psychiatric Nurses Association, 11,* 26.

6

Bariatric Surgery – Anesthesiologic Concerns

Johan Raeder
University of Oslo,
Oslo University Hospital,
Oslo,
Norway

1. Introduction

Both in developed and under developed countries the total number of obese people and their fraction of the population are increasing, and they live longer. The need for bariatric surgery is rapidly increasing (Buchwald, 2009) and the concept of fast-track surgery and laparoscopy (Kehlet, 2008) has made bariatric surgery a cost-effective and efficient way of treating the morbididly obese when other non-surgical options have been unsuccessful. Whereas ambulatory care is evolving for medium invasive bariatric procedures (i.e. gastric banding or minor laparoscopic procedures) in some places, most bariatric patients are still in-patients, although a short stay and accelerated recovery should be feasible and encouraged (Raeder, 2007). There is a general trend, especially in the obese, to supply anesthetic care with loco-regional techniques whenever possible (Raeder 2010a). This has to do with less physiologic and especially respiratory physiologic, derangement, when loco-regional techniques are used instead of general anesthesia. Also, as ultrasound technology has emerged as a valuable tool in locating regional anesthesia bone-marks in the obese, the use of brachial plexus techniques and spinal/epidural techniques has grown in the obese. Still, the bariatric procedures usually imply an upper abdomen surgical procedure and a predominantly laparoscopic approach. This kind of surgery is hard to do with success and patient satisfaction in the awake, even if they have a perfect spinal or epidural anesthesia. Similarly local anesthesia is not possible to apply sufficiently for laparoscopy, both due to the complexity of anatomical structures involved and the risk of toxicity from high total doses of local anesthetic agents. Still, local anesthesia is a very valuable, many will say mandatory, supplement to general anesthesia in these patients for improved postoperative pain management, together with other measures (see later). There are hardly any reports on bariatric surgery in epidural or spinal anesthesia, but there are a very few scattered reports on use of epidural pain relief for the postoperative period (Kira, 2007; Nishiyama 2011). Considered the technical challenge with these techniques in the obese and the modest pain problems in these patients when a proper multimodal approach is used, almost all anesthesiologist will abstain from using regional techniques in these procedures.

2. Preoperative concerns

Obese patients may present for any kind of surgery throughout their life; minor or major, emergency or elective, well prepared or with severe concomitant problems. Many general precautions and warnings linked to anesthesia in these patients are based on worst case scenario in an unstable and poorly prepared patient. The bariatric patient, although quite huge per definition, is still in many ways less problematic. They are highly motivated, well prepared - often through weeks, they are usually young or middle aged, and they usually understand that their cooperation and own efforts are very important during the recovery phase.

Although the obese has reduced physiologic reserves, both cardiovascular and respiratory; the obesity per se is usually not a major risk factor or reason for not accepting these patients for general anesthesia and bariatric surgery (Dindo, 2003). The rare non-acceptance of these patients has to do with the total picture of obesity, co-morbidity, preparation, co-operation and potential for improvements by postponing the procedure and spend some efforts in medical optimization.

The list of co-morbidity which are more frequent in the obese population include: diabetes, hypertonia, gastro-oesophageal reflux, artrosis and musculo-sceletal pain, sleep apnoea syndrome and in more severe cases pulmonary hypoventilation and atelectasis or heart failure (Chung 1999). It is beyond the scope of this chapter to go in depth with these concomitant diseases; the reader is advised to look in general anesthesia textbooks (Raeder 2010a).

Useful tests are ECG, spirometri, resting bloodgas while breathing room-air, pulmonary x-ray and a functional test, such as walking a flight of stairs.

Baseline blood pressure is important to obtain. Also, a 12-lead routine ECG should be taken in these patients upon age above 40 yrs or any suspicion of cardiovascular disease. Still, many important aspects of the ECG will be displayed anyway on the one-lead routine monitoring peri-operatively. The one-lead ECG is displayed before any drugs are given and will tell you about arrhythmia, P-Q prolongation or heart block and any ST segment changes in the pre-cordial area. What you will miss by a one-lead ECG are signs of heartfailure, hypertrophia and previous infarction.

Body mass index is the most common way of classifying obesity, and this figure is also useful for the anaesthesiologist for classification, risk-stratifying and need of extra consults and measures. However, for dosing of anesthetic drugs, different weight concepts are more useful. Some definitions of weight is listed in the frame below:

Different types of weight:

- Actual weight : = Total weight
- Ideal weight: Height ÷ 100 (105 in women)
- Lean weight: = fat-free body mass
- Corrected ideal weight:
  = ideal weight + 20-40% (?) of difference to actual weight
- Body mass index: weight / height x height

2.1 Concomitant pulmonary disease

Breathing disorders may be classified into problems of airways and lungs, problems with respiratory control and problems of muscular function for breathing. In patients with respiratory problems, especially chronic obstructive disease, it may be useful to refer the patient to a physiotherapist in advance in order to clean up and get instructions on how to cough, breathe and mobilize lungs after surgery.

Patients with an episode of airway infection should generally be postponed until 1-2 weeks after the infection is fully resolved. Postoperative sore-throat or coughing may be a problem being no good for the healing after a bariatric surgical procedure, thus also mild viral symptoms should call for postponing the case.

As with all patients; stop of smoking at least 4-5 weeks before scheduled surgery will improve the respiratory function, and this is especially valuable in the obese because they are more prone to airway problems than others. Also, smoking may impair wound healing. Offering the patients this kind of elective, planned surgery may also be a good opportunity to try to convince patients to stop smoking, and some clinics even put this token of patient cooperation as a condition for being accepted for surgery. Stopping 1-3 weeks before surgery, if the patient is a daily smoker, is not advised; as airway reactivity and secretions may be temporarily increased for some weeks after stop of smoking. If stop of smoking is not possible, they should at least not smoke on day of surgery, as even a single cigarette will result in some carboxy haemoglobin formation which will reduce the oxygen binding capacity of blood for some hours afterwards.

For patients with severe airway or pulmonary disease or infections, a more thorough approach should be undertaken for preoperative evaluation. Patient history with ability to walk one flight of stairs, the amount of coughing and secretion, as well as episodic changes versus stability in condition should be taken. Preoperative lung x-ray, arterial blood gas and spirometry with vital capacity and forced expiratory volume (FEV1), with and without bronchodilator are further options. Generally, a vital capacity of less than 1.5-2 litres in an adult or a FEV1 Less than 1-1.5 liter should indicate increased likelihood of severe problems and need of ventilatory support post-operatively.

2.1.1 Sleep apnoea syndrome (SAS)

Sleep apnoea syndrome is under diagnosed, but probably occurs in 4% of adult male population and 2% of females. It is associated with obesity and also with large tonsils or adenoids, especially in small children, but could be present without any of these (Young, 1993). Although these patients manage someway at home preoperatively the chance of respiratory arrest will be increased especially first night after surgery in general anesthesia or any use of post-operative opioids. Although fatalities are very rare, 8 cases were reported in a big US survey (Lofsky, 2002), one case is one too much and could be avoided by overnight continuous monitoring of respiration, either by pulse-oxymetri or better with respiratory rate monitoring of some kind (see below).

The symptoms of SAS almost always include snoring but should be accompanied with more problems to make the diagnosis: respiratory arrest (> 10 sec), frequent change in position during sleep, tired in spite of normal "length of sleep", morning headache and family history of SAS (Chung, 2008). A more specific and detailed diagnosis could be made with polysomnography done well in advance, and then eventually fit and become familiar with using a CPAP device. Patients with a CPAP device should be urged to bring this with them on day of surgery, in order to have ready for use in the PACU if needed and mandatory use the first nights.

During polysomnograpy the patient is monitored continuously during full overnight sleep with pulse oxymeter, ECG, number and lengths of apnea episodes etc. More than 30 episodes of hypopnoea or apnea per hour signal a serious condition, whereas less than 15 is mild. A fairly precise prediction of a serious condition could be made clinically if the patient tests positively on these four anamnestic items: load snoring (heard through wall or door), observed apnea during sleep, tired in spite of normal length of sleep in bed, hypertension (Chung, 2008).

A rational approach to these patients may be (table):

Known SAS:

- If treated with CPAP → OK *
- If minor surgery with no opioids postop → OK
- If seriously affected SAS and use of opioids → Continuous respiratory monitor!

Suspected SAS:

- If serious symptoms → polysomnography (or →continous monitor)
- Mild symptoms (not tired, no major apnoea or distress)
  - → OK if not opioid effects after discharge to ward
  - Otherwise: monitor

No SAS mentioned:

- Ask for symptoms, partner/comparent information
- If in doubt → = suspected and plan with monitoring

*It has been shown that SAS patient who use a CPAP will not have increased risk of apnoea, even during first night after surgery.

Importantly, when these patients are considered to be extra risk, ordinary stay at the ward will not be good enough; they have to be monitored continuously during the night. A pulse oxymeter may do, although signs of hypoxia are somewhat delayed, even better is a respiratory rate monitor with alarm of apnoea. Such respiratory rate monitoring may be: end-tidal CO2, breast cage movements or respiratory sound monitor on neck.

2.2 Patients with cardio-vascular disease

Generally; a patient who is unable to climb 1 flight of stairs in normal speed without cardiovascular symptoms (angina or heart failure, dyspnoea), have a recent cardiac event (infarction, revascularisation) within last 3 months or have a serious unstable condition or serious limitation in activity; should be postponed and go to cardiology consult and be optimized before elective surgery.

2.3 General advices and measures in advance

Especially when these intra-abdominal bariatric procedures (laparoscopy, laparotomy) is planned, it is a good safety advice to make the patient reduce even a minor bit in weight during the weeks ahead of surgery, by using a high protein-low carbohydrate diet. The reason is that most obese have an enlarged and fragile fatty liver. By diet and weight reduction for some weeks, the liver will shrink and become less fragile. This may be important in order to facilitate surgical access in the abdomen and reduce the risk of liver tear or bleeding.

In the obese patients gastro-oesophageal reflux disease (GERD) occur in about 20-30% of cases, and these patients may be at risk for peri-operative regurgitation of acid stomach juice into the airways. A good way of reducing both amount and acidity of the gastric content is to use a proton pump inhibitor (e.g. omeprazole or other). The first dose should be at least some hours ahead of surgery, but best if already given the evening before and then repeated on morning of surgery. If this had not been accomplished, some sips of non-pulmonary toxic fluid antacid (sodium-citrate) in front of anesthetic induction may be an alternative solution, although not so effective as a proton pump inhibitor.

As to fasting rules, the gastric emptying speed in obese patients is similar as to lean patients (Soreide, 2005). Thus, if no physiologic cause of gastrointestinal obstruction or slowing is evident, they should have nothing to eat (including milk and milk products) for the last six hours in front of surgery and no clear fluids for the last 2 hours. Still, some preoperative tablets may be allowed in a few sips of water up to 1 hour ahead of anesthetic induction.

2.3.1 Premedication

Due to the increased incidence and risk of airway obstruction in the obese patients, one should generally be restrictive with anxiolytic or opioid premedication. If there is a strong indication, an oral benzodiazepine may be used, either the short acting midazolam (5-7.5 mg orally) or more longacting diazepam, 5-15 mg. The patients should then not be left alone, but have attendance or pulse-oximetry applied. Establishing an IV line in the ward for premedication will enable a more precise targeting of effect, both because midazolam or diazepam may be carefully titrated and also because rapid injection of the benzodiazepine antagonist, flumazenil, is an option if needed for overdosing or respiratory problems. Establishment of an IV line on the preoperative ward is also a good measure in terms of avoiding stress and time consuming search for a vein in the busy operating room (OR) just before start of anesthesia. Whereas the usual veins on the dorsum of the hand may be difficult to find in the obese, the thin volar veins are usually accessible without covering fat pads. It may also be a case for ultrasound location of veins in these patients, either in the elbow or the medial upper arm (basilica vein) or the central veins (internal jugular or subclavian) in the more difficult cases. Opioid premedication should only be used when needed for pre-operative pain, and then in titrated iv doses with subsequent monitoring.

The time for potential premedication, 1-2 hours ahead of surgery, may be a time for giving other drugs of benefit for the patient such as oral analgesics (paracetamol and NSAIDs or cox-II inhibitor) or prophylactic antibiotics or thrombosis prophylaxis. As the obese are more prone to both thrombosis, pulmonary embolism and wound infections in general, and even more so with intra-abdominal surgery, appropriate antibiotic (e,g. Cefuroxim 1.5g) and antitrombotic (e.g. low molecular heparine 5000IU sc, day before and every day for one week) is usually indicated.

3. Anesthetic technique

3.1 Surgeons contribution

Even though general anesthesia is needed, it is very important that the surgeon use an optimal protocol of local anaesthesia extensive infiltrated in wound areas and surrounding structures (LIA-technique) in order to reduce postoperative opioid consume. The surgeon should typically use a total of 40 mls of either bupivacaine 2.5 mg/ml or ropivacain 2.0 mg/ml for superficial and deep wound infiltration. If more than 40 ml is needed, ropivacaine should be the drug of choice, as the toxicity from general absorption is less than with bupivacaine. Whether the injection should be done at the start of surgery or at the end is disputed. Injection at the start will potentially contribute to preoperative analgesia, but the resultant effect on general anesthetic dose reduction has been none or negligible in most studies. With injection by the end, the effect will last longer than if the injection is done 1-2 hours previously. Some surgeons may even prefer to do both; before and at the end. The injection initially may then be with a rapid and shortacting agent such as 5-10 mg/ml lidocaine, eventually with a vaso-constructive agent (i.e. epinephrine added) in order to reduce wound bleeding.

There are also some studies in the literature advocating installation of local anesthesia in the peritoneal cavity (Kahokehr, 2011). This seems to be more effective for dedicated upper abdominal surgery, such a liver or gallbladder surgery, whereas the effect in general laparoscopy, such as bariatric, is more doubtful. Whatever local anesthesia techniques are used, the surgeon should take care to obey the rules of maximal doses for general toxicity of the drugs, and these considerations should be based on mg local anesthesia per kg ideal weight, not actual weight.

The obese patient will generally benefit from spending as short time as possible on the operating table, thus, a rapid and technical accurate surgeon is very highly appreciated in these patients.

3.2 For the anesthetist

Tthe goal will be to have proper anesthesia when needed, but a rapid emergence and resumption of adequate respiration and physiology very shortly after the end of the procedure (Bergland, 2008). Anything done to minimize the need of postoperative opioids and minimize the risk of postoperative nausea and vomiting is very valuable.

3.2.1 Issues for general anesthesia induction (see also recipe)

Usually it will be possible to find an IV access in these patients, for instance at the inside of the lower underarm there are some thin veins not covered by fat. However, occasionally there may be an indication for ultrasound guided access to a central vein if nothing else is possible (see above). The patients should be with 20-30 degrees elevated trunk (half-sitting) during induction, preferably be a special pillow or by adjusting the operation table. This position has three functions: it will prevent regurgitation, improve lung function (compared to supine) and also facilitate mask ventilation and laryngoscopy for intubation. A potential drawback may be increased risk of hypotention after induction with this position, thus titrated dosing is advisable and a ready availability of vasopressors, such as ephedrine or fenylefrine. Also a rapid running infusion of crystalloid or colloid is useful. Rapid sequence induction is not needed in these patients if they otherwise fulfil fasting criteria. In case of rapid sequence induction there may be a case for high dose rocuronium (i.e. 0.8-1.2 mg/kg ideal weight) instead of suxamethonium, as the latter is associated with an increased risk of anaphylactoid reactions compared with the non-depolarising agents.

Proper pre-oxygenation with a tight fitting mask and PEEP of 10 cm H2O is very useful, and shown to result in an extra 1-2 minutes before de-saturation occurs, if some airway problems arise later on. An end-tidal oxygen concentration of 80-90% on mask is a good sign of successful pre-oxygenation. Laryngeal mask airway (LMA) and spontaneous ventilation is basically beneficial for minimizing airway reactivity and optimizing lung physiology, especially in the obese. However, in the obese there is a need for high inspiratory pressure in order to overcome the resistance of the fat-coat surrounding the rib cage. With an LMA this higher pressure may result in inspiratory leakage, and frequently transition to endotracheal tube is needed. With laparoscopy and bariatric surgery even more so, because there is a considerable intrabdominal pressure adding to the resistance during inspiration. In conclusion, endotracheal intubation is recommended as routine airway management in these patients (Raeder, 2010a). Intubation may be achieved with propopfol + remifentanil only, but the high dose need and subsequent risk of hemodynamic instability makes the use of non-depolarising neuromuscular blocking agent a better choice. The intubation conditions will be more reliable and the anesthetic agents may be kept lower in dosing. After intubation, a recruitment manoeuvre is beneficial to blow up the lungs, and then maintain a PEEP of 10 cm H2O throughout the case, with a new recruitment before extubation. Whereas pressure control ventilation mode is better for lung physiology, the volume mode is safer in terms of delivering a proper and fixed tidal-volume, which again should be adjusted to ideal weight, 6-8 ml/kg. Especially during laparoscopy the high and variable peritoneal pressure may result in very low or variable tidal volumes with the pressure control mode, unless the settings are frequently adjusted.

Recommended drugs for induction will be propofol + remifentanil (see recepe below)

3.2.2 Issues during maintenance

All the fat soluble agents are problematic to dose in the obese, because they distribute according to slightly more than ideal weight at start (i.e. corrected ideal body weight) and then more and more to total weight as the fat gets slowly loaded with drug (Servin, 2006; Raeder 2010a). An exception is remifentanil which is degraded before diffusing into the fat, and thus is very suitable for continued use in the obese. Propofol may be used for induction according to corrected ideal weight, but maintenance beyond 30-60 min calls for increase in dose, which is best titrated by using a brain function monitor, such as the BIS or similar device. Among inhalational agents, desflurane is the best in terms of less tissue binding and more rapid emergence compared with the other potent inhalational agents. Still, sevoflurane or even isoflurane may be used in these patients, but then more care is needed to taper down the concentration during the last part of the operation in order to ensure reasonable fast emergence (Baerdemaeker, 2003). Nitrous oxide is very rapidly acting and rapidly eliminated, but the potency is low and this agent may only be used as an adjunct to either propofol or a potent inhalational agent for anesthetic maintenance.

3.2.3 Issues for ending the case and postoperative issues

With dedicated use of maintenance drugs, it should be possible to have a rapid emergence, and extubation, also in the obese bariatric cases. It is very important to be generous with anti-emetic prophylaxis in these patients as well as providing an optimal non-opioid analgesia (see below). The patients should be awake within 5 min to an extent enabling them to help in transfer from the operating table to the bed. During transport to the postoperative care unit, the patients should be laying on the side, with the head lightly elevated, 2-3 litres of oxygen per min by nose catheter. A pulse-oxymeter should be connected during the transport to recovery, as well as during the recovery stay. In the PACU, half sitting position should be rapidly encouraged and the patients should be tested for breathing room air when they are reasonable awake. A pulse-oxymeter saturation on room air of 92% or more is satisfactory. With such a value or higher the patient should not have oxygen supply. It has been shown that oxygen supply when not needed, may increase the risk of micro-atelectasis in the lung. Further monitoring in the PACU will include regular non-invasive blood-pressure measurements and continuous ECG registration. When the patient is fully awake, monitoring may be limited to pulse-oxymeter only. Slow intravenous fluid from the period of surgery may be continued until the patients drinks, typically an amount of 1-2 litres of krystalloid iv solution is sufficient for the total peri-operative period, unless there has been significant blood-loss.

Within 2-4 hours the patients should be able to mobilize on the floor, and be ready for discharge to the ward.

3.2.4 Prophylaxis and treatment of pain, nausea and vomiting

These are the most common and bothersome complications in the first period after surgery, and every measure should be taken to avoid and minimize the occurrence. The two important common principles for avoiding these complications will be to think prophylactic and multimodal. Multimodal means to address the problem with different drugs of different but additive analgesic action mechanisms and different potential and type of side-effects (Raeder, 2010a).

3.2.4.1 Postoperative pain

For pain the idea is to use as many different non-opioid additive acting analgesics as possible in order to minimize the need for opioids (Raeder, 2010a). As opioids should be used and given on top when necessary, they carry some dose-dependent side-effects which are non-beneficial in the postoperative period. These include: somnolescense, nausea, constipation, disrupted sleep pattern, and the more rare and serious respiratory depression and sleep apnea syndrome. While opioids usually are needed in small, titrated doses in bariatric patients, the potential of non-opioid pain prophylaxis and treatment should be addressed first.

The concept of starting analgesic treatment before start of surgery in order to reduce nociceptive input to central pain mechanisms is disputed, while everyone agrees upon the use of having proper pain prophylaxis established when the patients awake from general anesthesia shortly after end of the procedure is well established.

Drugs useful in this context include (Raeder, 2010):

a. Local wound anesthesia: This should be given by the surgeon either at the start or at the end of the procedure (see above). If a particular wound is especially painful after surgery, the infiltration may be repeated (bupivacaine 2.5 mg/ml, 5-10 ml per wound) every 5-10 hrs, but this is rarely indicated.
b. Paracetamol: Although a fairly week analgesic the incidence and type of side-effects are low, as long as high total doses with potential liver toxixcity is avoided. Paracetamol may be used in virtually all patients. It is very well and completely absorbed after oral administration and may be started 1-2 hours before surgery, while the alternative may be to start with an IV infusion at the start of surgery. The initial dose should be 2 g (1-2 g if IV), while the continued dosing should be 1 g bid 4, either orally or IV as long as the patient have some pain, that is for 4-7 days usually.
c. Non-steroidal analgesic drugs (NSAIDs): These are very useful analgesic drugs which may be used in most patients unless clearly contra-indicated. All NSAIDs carry a risk of renal failure upon hypoveolemia, and gastrointestinal ulceration and bleeding. In the bariatric setting the new subtype of cox-II selective NSAIDs (i.e. coxibs: celecoxib, etoricoxib, lumiraccoxib, parecoxib) have some beneficial characteristics and should therefore be preferred. They have less risk of allergy and asthma, they have no influence on trombocyte adhesion and no risk of bleeding, and the chance of developing gastric ulceration is less than with traditional NSADs (i.e. naproxen, ibuprofen, ketprofen, diclofenac). While an overt gastric ulcer or recent story of such is an absolute contraindication to these drugs, the coxibs may be used in patients with a cured gastric ulcer. Gastric regurgitation is no definite contraindication, unless there are overt wounds in the oesophagus. The combination of proton-pump inhibitor and a coxib is usually well tolerated, also as gastric regurgitation is mostly a defect in gastro-oesophageal sphincter and not a change in gastric juice or gastric mucosa constitution. The potential negative impact from NSAIDs on gastric anastomoses healing has not been proved; on the contrary the opioid sparing effect on gastric motility from using NSAIDs may be beneficial in this context. The much disputed risk of cardiovascular complications with these drugs is usually not relevant as these are long-term use effects. Still, all these drugs may cause some initial fluid retention and slight increase in blood-pressure, which should be monitored in high risk-patients.
d. Glucocorticoids: Although a lot of potential side-effects may occur with long term treatment, the beneficial analgesic and anti-emetic effect of a single dose perioperatively lasting up to 2-3 days is very useful. As the onset of action is slow (2-3 hours) a glucocorticoid is best given at start of surgery. Dexamethasone is most popular, because it is a pure glucocorticoid with minor effect on electrolyte and mineral balance, and because duration of a single IV dose is long. It may be wise to give dexamethasone after

the patient is asleep as there is a preservative in most dexamethasone solutions which may give strong perineal itching when given rapidly in the awake. While the dose of 8 mg IV has been proven efficacious in general laparoscopy, it may be wise to increase the dose to 16 mg in the obese bariatric patient. Alternatives to IV dexamethasone may be metylprednisolone (50-125 mg) or oral prednisolone given in advance (20-50 mg) or oral dexamethasone, 15-25 mg. As these drugs cause a slight increase in blood-sugar level, care should be taken to monitor blood-sugar levels if these drugs are used in the diabetic.

e. Opioids: These may surely be needed on top of the non-opioid multimodal regimen. Any opioid may do, but care should be taken to use small and titrated dosing. For that reason opioids with rapid onset and short duration, such as alfentanil or fentanyl, are most easy to adjust. Initially the IV route is best, for instance using fentanyl, oxycodone or morphine. Then, after the PACU period the oral alternative should be preferred. The newer opioid subclass of oral opioid agonist with norepinephric effects, such as tramadol and tapentadol, has less risk of respiratory depression, but the incidence of nausea and vomiting is quite high, especially with tramadol, whereas tapentadol so far seems promising. Buprenorphine is a weaker opioid agonist, but well absorbed orally and with long duration of effect and low risk of respiratory depression. Other oral alternatives include codeine and oxycodone. Codeine is an inactive prodrug of morphine and 5-10% of the population do not have the converting enzyme and then they have no effect of the drug. Oxycodone is a potent, well absorbed opioid which may be given in rapid acting 5 mg tablets or slow-release formulations of 10-20 mg. Some studies show less sedation or somnolescense with oxycodone when compared to equipotent doses of morphine (Lenz, 2009). As this opioid also seems to work very well on visceral pain, it may be the preferred oral opioid for the bariatric patients.
f. Other analgesics: There are quite some other non-opioid drugs which have a beneficial postoperative analgesic action: ketamine, iv lidocaine, gabapentin, pre-gabalin, cannabinoids (Raeder, 2010a).

The gabapentinoids (gabapentin, pre-gabalin) are well established for postoperative pain indication, but they may result in somnolescense, dizziness and fainting initially, when dosed to high. In bariatric patients with more than usual pain, these drugs may still be an alternative; then a modest starting dose of for instance 75-150 mg pre-gabalin may be tried, and then repeated twice a day, eventually increased carefully until 300 mg.

In the immediate postoperative period a low dose infusion (i.e. 1-2 microg/kg ideal weight/min) of ketamin may also be an option in patients with strong pain.

3.2.4.2 Postoperative nausea and vomiting (PONV)

This is a troublesome complication in the postoperative, obese bariatric patient and an aggressive approach as to multimodal prophylaxis should be applied. The reason for multimodality in this context is that no single drug is more than effective in 50% of the patients, but with different acting drug combination this incidence may be up in the 80-90% range (Raeder, 2010a). The known risk factors of postoperative nausea and vomiting include: more than average tendency of travel sickness, more than average nausea after general anesthesia, opioid use, non-smoking status, female gender. Also type of surgery, such as laparoscopy, has been associated with higher incidence of PONV, and the use of inhalational anesthetic agents as opposed to propofol which is anti-emetic (Apfel, 2004).

A first measure to reduce the incidence of PONV is to minimize opioid effects and use in the postoperative care unit. This is achieved by using optimal non-opioid analgesic prophylaxis and treatment, and by using shortacting opioid (i.e. remifentanil) with minimal residual effect after general anesthesia.

Then, secondly, a mixture of anti-emetic prophylaxis should be used in these patients.

The basis will be a 5-HT3 blocker (e.g. ondansetron 4 mg) given by end of anesthesia and glucocorticoid given by start (see above, glucocorticoid for pain) in all bariatric patients. In patients with more than average risk it may be useful to add droperidol 1.25 mg into the prophylaxis, and consider ending the anesthesia with a period of propofol infusion instead of desflurane all way through.

If the patient develops nausea in the postoperative unit, it is important to rule out and treat some non-pharmacologic reasons for PONV: dehydration, hypotention, hypoxia or sudden movement. If anti-emetic drug treatment is needed it is wise to supplement with a drug the patient not already has received; that may be either metoclopramid (10 mg iv, eventually repeated) or ephedrine 5-10 mg IV. Ephedrine is especially efficient in those patients who experience nausea when moving or mobilizing, and if this is a consistent problem a sc injection of 25-40 mg ephedrine may be of help.

In more resistant cases the new class of NK-1 antogonisk anti-emetics may be tried.

4. Anesthetic recepe

There are many successfyl ways to run general anesthesia in bariatric surgical patients, but this is a well tested recepe, now being applied to more than 2000 consecutive patients in a dedicated clinic for these procedures (Bergland, 2008). These patients should have standard monitoring with ECG, noninvasive blood pressure measurement, pulse oximetry, nerve stimulation test of neuromuscular block (i.e., TOF guard®), end-tidal CO_2 measurement, and anesthetic gas analysis. An arterial line for invasive blood pressure measurement is only inserted if specifically indicated, e.g., patients with known cardiovascular problems.

It may be useful to monitor the depth of anesthesia in these patients, but this may be skipped during inhalational-based anesthesia if end-tidal MAC values are above 1 MAC all the time.

Our recipe for obese patients undergoing laparoscopy is as follows:

An iv infusion of 500 ml starch, colloid solution is running rapidly, followed by a slow infusion of crystalloid (0.5-1.0 liter during the procedure).

When preoxygenation is fulfilled, anesthesia is induced with fentanyl 100 micog, propofol and remifentanil plasma target controlled infusions (TCI) with targets of 6 microg/ml and 8 ng/ml, respectively. Both infusions are based on corrected ideal weight (height in centimeters minus 100, plus 20% of the difference between the real weight and ideal weight), propofol with the Marsh effect site model and remifentanil with the Minto effect site model.

Then, vecuronium 0.08 mg/kg corrected ideal weight is given.

Tracheal intubation is performed with the patient in the semi-sitting position with their torso flexed and the head extended in the neck ("sniffing the morning air" position). A standard laryngoscope with a short handle and an endotracheal tube with a stylet are used.

After the tracheal tube is secured, the propofol infusion is stopped and inhalation of desflurane at 3–6 % (i.e., 0.5 - 1 MAC) is started. Inspiratory oxygen is reduced to 40% and PEEP to 5 cmH_2O.

A gastric tube is inserted and the gastric content (if any) is aspirated.

Anesthesia is continued throughout the operation with remifentanil and desflurane. The doses are adjusted according to clinical observation, arterial blood pressure, and bispectral index (BIS). Typically, remifentanil TCI is adjusted within a wide range to keep systolic blood pressure within acceptable limits (i.e., 85–120 mmHg) and desflurane is adjusted to keep the BIS within the range of 45–55. If no BIS is available an endtidal concentration of 0.7-1.0 MAC desflurane should be used.

Droperidol 1.25 mg, ondansetron 4 mg, and dexamethasone 16 mg are given as routine iv antiemetic prophylaxis.

Parecoxib 40 mg and paracetamol 1g are given iv, and bupivacaine 2.5 mg/ml is infiltrated around the incisions, in a total volume of 30–40 ml, to prevent postoperative pain. Furthermore, fentanyl 100 microg is given before the end of surgery.

Desflurane and remifentanil are stopped upon removal of the laparoscope at the end of surgery, and a small dose of propofol (30–50 mg total) is then given. The neuromuscular block is reversed with neostigmine 2.5 mg and glycopyrrolate 1 mg and the patients are ventilated with 100% oxygen. The patients are extubated on the table when they are emerging, breathing, and showing the first signs of irritation from the tracheal tube. Then patients move themselves, with some assistance, into the bed.

Analgesia (present at emergence):

- bupivacaine/ropivacaine wound infiltration
- paracetamol 1.0 g iv
- parecoxib 40 mg iv (or ketorolac 30 mg iv)
- dexamethasone 16 mg iv
- fentanyl 1–2 microg/kg at the end of surgery

Anti-emesis:

- droperidol 1.25 mg iv
- (dexamethasone, also given for pain)
- ondansetron 4 mg iv
- propofol anesthesia + remifentanil anesthesia, no nitrous oxide, low opioid hangover

5. References

Apfel CC, Korttila K, Abdalla M, et al. A factorial trial of six interventions for the prevention of postoperative nausea and vomiting. N Engl J Med 2004;350:2441-51.

Bergland A, Gislason H, Raeder J. Fast-track surgery for bariatric laparoscopic gastric bypass with focus on anaesthesia and peri-operative care. Experience with 500 cases. Acta Anaesthesiol Scand 2008;52:1394-9.

Buchwald H, Oien DM. Metabolic/bariatric surgery Worldwide 2008. Obes Surg 2009;19:1605-11.

Chung F, Mezei G, Tong D. Pre-existing medical conditions as predictors of adverse events in day-case surgery. Br J Anaesth 1999;83:262-70.

Chung SA, Yuan H, Chung F. A systemic review of obstructive sleep apnea and its implications for anesthesiologists. Anesth Analg 2008;107:1543-63.

Chung SA, Yuan H, Chung F. A systemic review of obstructive sleep apnea and its implications for anesthesiologists. Anesth Analg 2008;107:1543-63.

De Baerdemaeker LE, Struys MM, Jacobs S, et al. Optimization of desflurane administration in morbidly obese patients: a comparison with sevoflurane using an 'inhalation bolus' technique. Br J Anaesth 2003;91:638-50.

De Baerdemaeker LE, Struys MM, Jacobs S, et al. Optimization of desflurane administration in morbidly obese patients: a comparison with sevoflurane using an 'inhalation bolus' technique. Br J Anaesth 2003;91:638-50.

Dindo D, Muller MK, Weber M, Clavien PA. Obesity in general elective surgery. Lancet 2003;361:2032-5.

Kahokehr A, Sammour T, Srinivasa S, Hill AG. Systematic review and meta-analysis of intraperitoneal local anaesthetic for pain reduction after laparoscopic gastric procedures. Br J Surg 2011;98:29-36.

Kehlet H, Wilmore DW. Evidence-based surgical care and the evolution of fast-track surgery. Ann Surg 2008;248:189-98.

Kira S, Koga H, Yamamoto S, et al. Anesthetic management of laparoscopic adjustable gastric banding in Japanese patients with morbid obesity. J Anesth 2007;21:424-8.

Leifsson BG, Gislason HG. Laparoscopic Roux-en-Y gastric bypass with 2-metre long biliopancreatic limb for morbid obesity: technique and experience with the first 150 patients. Obes Surg 2005;15:35-42.

Lenz H, Sandvik L, Qvigstad E, et al. A comparison of intravenous oxycodone and intravenous morphine in patient-controlled postoperative analgesia after laparoscopic hysterectomy. Anesth Analg 2009;109:1279-83.

Lofsky A. A Lofsky, Anesthesia Pt Safety Foundation Newsletter 2002; 17:24-5. Anesthesia Pt Safety Foundation Newsletter 2002;17:24-5.

Nishyiama, T, Kohno, Y, and Koishi, K. Anesthesia for Bariatric Surgery. Obes Surg . 2011. 2011. Ref Type: Online Source

Raeder J. Clinical ambulatory anaesthesia. Cambridge University Press, 2011.

Raeder J. Bariatric procedures as day/short stay surgery: is it possible and reasonable? Curr Opin Anaesthesiol 2007;20:508-12.

Servin F. Ambulatory anesthesia for the obese patient. Curr Opin Anaesthesiol 2006;19:597-9.

Soreide E, Eriksson LI, Hirlekar G, et al. Pre-operative fasting guidelines: an update. Acta Anaesthesiol Scand 2005;49:1041-7.

Young T, Palta M, Dempsey J, et al. The occurrence of sleep-disordered breathing among middle-aged adults. N Engl J Med 1993;328:1230-5.

7

Gastric Banding and Bypass for Morbid Obesity – Preoperative Assessment, Operative Techniques and Postoperative Monitoring

Brane Breznikar, Dejan Dinevski and Milan Zorman
Department of General and Abdominal Surgery, Slovenj Gradec General Hospital,
Faculty of Medicine & Faculty of Electrical Engineering
and Computer Science, University of Maribor,
Slovenia

1. Introduction

Morbid obesity is a chronic, lifelong, multifactorial, congenital disorder characterised by excessive fat deposits and associated medical, psychological, physical, social, and economic problems. It is also a significant health threat. The extra weight puts unusual stress on all parts of the body. It raises your risk of diabetes, stroke, heart disease, kidney disease, and gallbladder disease. Conditions such as high blood pressure and high cholesterol, which were once thought to mainly affect adults, are often seen in children who are obese. Obesity may also increase the risk for some types of cancer. Persons who are obese are more likely to develop osteoarthritis and sleep apnea. Obesity is the second leading cause of preventable death after smoking. A combination of genetics, environmental issues, and behavioral factors may contribute to the condition (Breznikar & Dinevski, 2009).

Nonsurgical treatment has relapse rates of up to 90%, irrespective of the choice of conservative treatment (Council of Scientific Affairs, 1988). As early as 1991, the U.S. National Institute of Health issued a statement recognizing the known lack of success with conservative forms of treatment, nothing that operations to constrict or bypass the stomach were justified for fully informed and consenting patients and constituted an acceptable risk (National Institute of Health, 1985, Oppert & Rolland-Cachera, 1998).

In 1954, Kremen and Linner introduced jejunoileal bypass. Modifications in the original procedures and the development of new techniques have led to 3 basic concepts for bariatric surgery, as follows: (1) gastric restriction by gastric banding (vertical-banded gastroplasty and adjustable banding), (2) gastric restriction with mild malabsorption (Roux-en-Y gastric bypass), and (3) a combination of mild gastric restriction and malabsorption (duodenal switch) (Masson et al., 1997, Belachew et al., 1997, Gravante et al. 2007).

Bariatric surgery can be undertaken by open and laparoscopic techniques. The latter has become the more popular approach because of its proven (and now well-known) advantages. GBP is currently the most popular procedure. More than 80% of bariatric procedures in the USA are GBP. It has earned the reputation of being the criterion standard against which other procedures are compared. The procedure has restrictive and malabsorptive components. GBP provides a substantial amount of dietary restriction. The restrictive element of the surgery consists of the creation of a small gastric pouch with a small outlet that, on distention by food, causes the sensation of satiety. In addition, GBP provides a small-to-moderate degree of intentional malabsorption due to the separation of food, which passes through the Roux alimentary limb of the Y, from the biliopancreatic secretions, which pass through the biliopancreatic limb of the Y. The degree of malabsorption can be adjusted by modifying the length of the alimentary and biliopancreatic limbs.

The diversity of clinical- and occult obesity-related comorbidities necessitates a multidisciplinary-team approach in the preoperative evaluation of a morbidly obese the patient: this evaluation enhances outcome. Preoperative cardiac, pulmonary, psychiatric, and endocrine evaluations may be necessary. These evaluations help to exclude patients who may not benefit from surgery. They simultaneously optimize those considered to be good candidates for this type of surgery. Patients should meet all necessary criteria for general surgery.

The contraindications specific to bariatric surgery are:

1. Absence of periods of identifiable medical management
2. A patient who cannot participate in prolonged follow-up
3. Non-stabilized psychotic disorders, severe depression and personality disorders (unless specifically advised by a psychiatrist experienced in obesity)
4. Alcohol abuse and/or drug dependencies
5. Diseases threatening life in the short-term
6. Patients who cannot care for themselves and have no long-term support from their family or social service that warrant such care.

The indications for bariatric surgery are: patients aged 18–60 years with a body mass index (BMI) >40 kg/m2 or with a BMI 35–40 kg/m2 with a comorbidity in which surgically induced weight loss is expected to improve the disorder (e.g., metabolic disorders, cardio-respiratory disease, severe joint disease, obesity-related severe psychological problems). The BMI criterion may be the current BMI or a documented previous BMI of identical severity. Bariatric surgery is indicated in patients who exhibit substantial weight loss in a conservative treatment program but who started to regain weight. To be considered for surgery, patients must have failed to lose weight or to maintain long-term weight loss despite appropriate medical care. Patients must have shown compliance with medical appointments. The indication for bariatric surgery for age >60 years or <18 years should be considered on an individual basis.

Preoperative consultation helps in obtaining a detailed diet history and in explaining preoperative and postoperative diet protocol. At our facility, patient preparation for surgery consisted of a detailed explanation (in written and oral form) of the developmental aspect of laparoscopic GBP and its benefits and risks. These included short- and long-term complications, side effects, nutritional sequelae, and the possibility of conversion to an open procedure. Antibiotics were administered perioperatively. Prophylaxis against venous thrombosis and pulmonary emboli consisted of perioperative pneumatic compression devices and low-dose heparin (s.c.).

After GBP, patients must remain on a high-protein, low-fat diet supplemented with multivitamins, iron, and calcium. Patients must modify their eating habits by avoiding "chewy" meats and other foods that may inhibit normal emptying of their stomach pouch. Nutritional and metabolic blood tests need to be carried out frequently (at 6 months after surgery, 12 months after surgery, and annually thereafter).

Outcomes related to changes in comorbidities, quality of life, and patient satisfaction are assessed for patients with 1 year or more of follow-up. The Bariatric Analysis and Reporting Outcome System (BAROS) was introduced to evaluate bariatric procedures and to compare them worldwide. It consists of a Moorehead Quality of Life (QoL) questionnaire, and documentation of excess weight loss (EWL), medical conditions, complications, and reoperations.

2. Bariatric procedures, gastric bypass (GBP)

GBP is currently the most popular procedure. It has earned the reputation of being the criterion standard, against which other procedures are compared. The procedure has both a restrictive component and a malabsorptive component. GBP provides a substantial amount of dietary restriction. The restrictive element of the operation consists of the creation of a small gastric pouch (approximately 20 mL in volume) with a small outlet that, on distention by food, causes the sensation of satiety. In addition, gastric bypass provides a small-to-moderate degree of intentional malabsorption due to the separation of food, which passes through the alimentary limb of the Y, from the biliopancreatic secretions, which pass through the biliopancreatic limb of the Y. The degree of malabsorption can be adjusted by modifying the length of the alimentary and biliopancreatic limbs.

For all bariatric procedures, pure reversal without conversion to another bariatric procedure is almost certainly followed by a return to morbid obesity. Gastric bypass can be reversed, though this is rarely required. Laparoscopic Roux-en Y gastric bypass results in substantial weight loss and resolves more than 80% of cases of type 2 diabetes. The investigators suggest that this bariatric operation should be considered the standard of care for morbidly obese type 2 diabetics5.

Vitamin D deficiency and elevated PTH are common following GBP and progress over time. There is a significant incidence of secondary hyperparathyroidism in short-limb GBP patients, even those with vitamin D levels ≥30 ng/mL, suggesting selective Ca2+ malabsorption. Thus, calcium malabsorption is inherent to gastric bypass. Careful calcium and vitamin D supplementation and long-term screening are necessary to prevent deficiencies and the sequelae of secondary hyperparathyroidism.

Laparoscopic Roux-en-Y gastric bypass is a major elective surgical procedure. The risks are as follows: mortality (1-2% of patients), mainly due to pulmonary embolism or gastrointestinal leak, wound infections, gastrojejunal stomal stricture, marginal ulcers, internal hernia, roux limb ischemia, blow-out of the stomach remnant, long-term nutrient deficiencies (eg, vitamin B12, folate, iron).

2.1 Preoperative details

The diversity of clinical and occult obesity-related comorbidities necessitates a multidisciplinary team approach in the preoperative evaluation of the patient who is morbidly obese. This evaluation enhances the postoperative outcome. Preoperative cardiac, pulmonary, psychiatric, and endocrine evaluations may be necessary. These evaluations help to exclude patients who may not benefit from surgery; at the same time, they optimize those considered being potential good candidates. Preoperative nutritional consultation helps in obtaining a detailed diet history and in explaining preoperative and postoperative diet protocol. At our facility, patient preparation for surgery consisted of a detailed explanation in written and oral form of the developmental aspect of laparoscopic GBP and its benefits and risks, including short- and long-term complications, side effects, nutritional sequelae, and the possibility of conversion to an open procedure. Perioperative antibiotics were administered. Prophylaxis against venous thrombosis and pulmonary embolus consisted of perioperative pneumatic compression devices and low-dose subcutaneous heparin.

2.2 Postoperative details

After surgery, patients must remain on a high-protein, low-fat diet supplemented with multivitamins, iron, and calcium. Patients must modify their eating habits by avoiding chewy meats and other foods that may inhibit normal emptying of their stomach pouch. Nutritional and metabolic blood tests need to be performed frequently (at 6 months after surgery, 12 months after surgery, and annually thereafter).

We have a monthly support group meeting, where the evaluation of the results is monitored. To evaluate the bariatric procedures and to compare them worldwide, Bariatric Analysis and Reporting Outcome System (BAROS) was introduced (Oria & Moorehead, 1998). It consists of Moorehead Quality of Life questionnaire (QoL), EWL, medical condition, complications, and reoperations (Table 1). Total score is between 1 and 9 in the group with comorbidities and between 0 and 6 in the group with no comorbidities (Table 2), each divided in 5 classes: bad, acceptable, good, very good, and excellent.

Outcomes related to changes in comorbidities, quality of life, and patient satisfaction were assessed for patients with 1 year or more of follow-up. The Moorehead-Ardelt Quality of Life Questionnaire specific for bariatric surgery was administered according to the protocol to assess quality of life changes.

2.3 Material and methods

Surgical procedures were performed at Slovenj Gradec General Hospital and Celje General Hospital, Slovenia. An extensive preoperative evaluation consisting of a history and physical examination, nutritional and psychiatric evaluation, and indicated specialty consultations was performed on all patients. Laboratory evaluation included complete blood count, serum chemistries, and thyroid function testing.

The surgical technique was a modification of the technique described by Wittgrove et al. (1994). The patient was placed in a supine position with the surgeon in between the legs, and two monitors above the patient's shoulders. After creation of carbon dioxide pneumoperitoneum (15 mmHg) using the Veress needle technique or entering the abdomen without gas, just with the optic trocar, ports were placed at the level of mesogastrium; the first one for the camera approximately 12 cm from the xyphoid. The operating table was placed in a steep reverse Trendelenburg position. To expose the esophagus and stomach, the liver retractor was placed through the inferior right subcostal port, and the left lateral segment of the liver was elevated. A 30 ml gastric pouch was created. The endo-linear stapler, 45-mm in length with 3.8-mm staples, was inserted and applied three or four times to staple and cut the gastric pouch with three rows of staples on each side. A gastroenteroanastomosis was than created 40 - 60 cm from the ligament of Treitz using either a circular end-to-end anastomosis stapled technique (first 20 cases) or a linear stapled technique (last 80 cases). The Roux limb was then measured 100 cm distally, or 150 cm distally for the superobese patients. A stapled side-to-side anastomosis was created with the proximal jejunal limb using the endo-linear stapler, 45-mm in length with 2.5-mm, white staples. The enterotomy sites were closed with running suture. All the anastomoses were tested with methylene blue. Lastly, the afferent loop close to the gastroenteroanastomosis was divided with a white cartridge of the linear stapler.

From February 2007 until March 2010, we performed 100 laparoscopic GBP surgeries. Patients were 42.2 years old on average (range 18.9 to 63.3). 87 females were 42.3 years old on average (range 18.9 to 63.3) and 13 males were 41.5 years old on average (range 26.4 to 53.0). Their BMI was 42.6 on average (range 33.4 to 72.3); females 42.7 (range 33.7 to 72.3), males 42.1 (range 33.4 to 49.6).

2.4 Results

The mean follow-up was 9.1 months (range 2 - 39 months); 53 patients had 1 or more, 17 patients had 2 or more and 3 patients had 3 or more years of follow up. We had one conversion because of adhesions and one because of bleeding from injured mesentery.

One year after the surgery, 53 patients (47 females and 5 males) lost 32.8 kg on average (range 7.0 to 53.0). Female patients lost 31.8 kg on average (range 7.0 to 53.0); male patients lost 43.0 kg (37.0 to 47.5), 17 patients lost 35.7 kg (11.0 to 57.0) after 2 years, and 3 patients lost 47.3 kg (43.0 to 55.0) after 3 years (Figure 1).

Excess Weight Loss (EWL) was 69.6 % (range 12.2 to 133.4) after 1 year, 76.5% (range 21.0% to 108.4%) after 2, and 86.0% after 3 years (range 71.8 to 104.9) (Figure 2).

EWL(t) = (max. weight - weight(t)) / (max. weight - weight (BMI25)), while "t" is the time of the interest and weight (BMI25) is the weight of the person at BMI=25 kg/m2

Body mass index (BMI) was reduced by 11.6 kg/m2; from an average of 42.6 before the operation to 31.0 at one year post-operatively (range 21.4 to 59.5). BMI was further reduced to 29.4 (range 23.5 to 43.5) at 2 years post-operatively, and to 27.4 at 3 years post-operatively (range 24.1 to 31.2) (Figure 3, Table 3). BMI= mass (kg)/(height, m)2

A total of 137 comorbidities were identified in our 100 patients. The most common comorbidities included hypertension (34 %), degenerative joint disease (22%), type II diabetes (16%), hypercholesterolemia (7%), and asthma (7%). The comorbidities and their resolution are presented in Table 4. The resolution of diabetes with respect to therapy prior to GBP surgery is presented in Table 5.

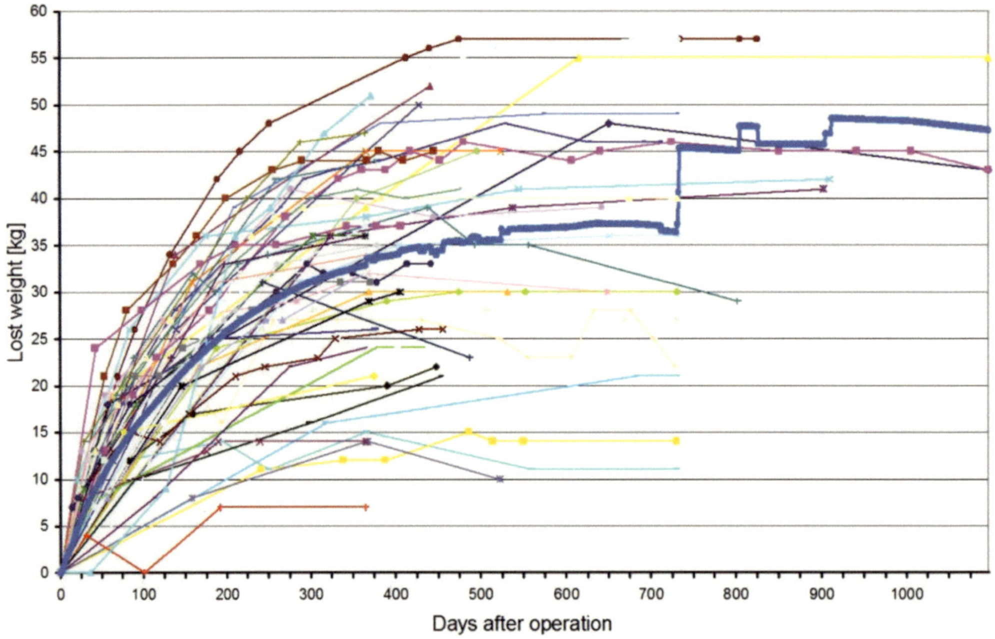

Fig. 1. Weight loss
(every line presents a patient, a dot in the line is the monitoring point, thick line is mean value)

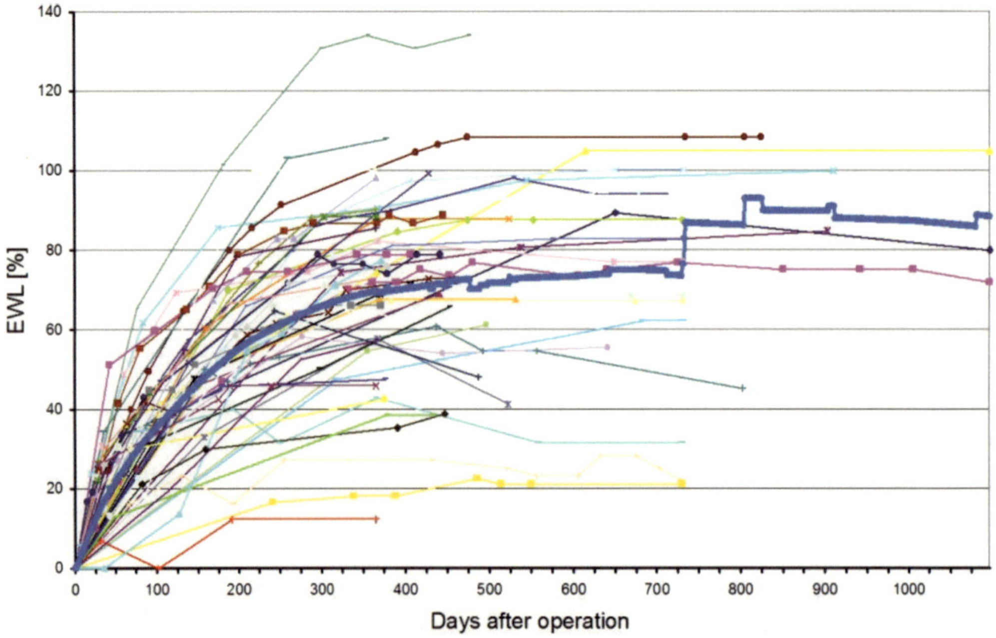

Fig. 2. Excess Weight Loss - EWL
(every line presents a patient, a dot in the line is the monitoring point, thick line is mean value)

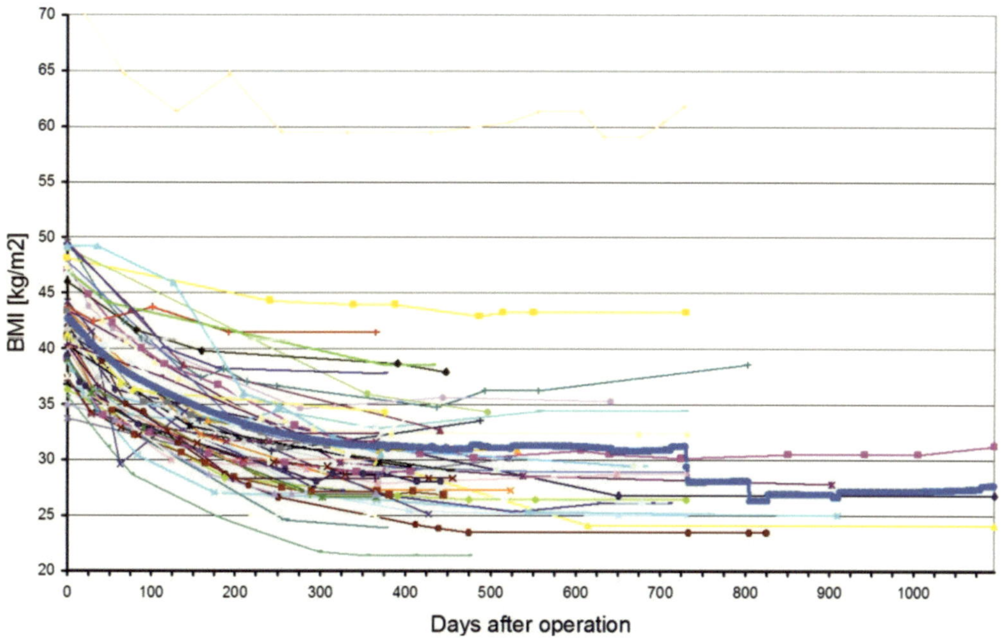

Fig. 3. BMI reduction
(every line presents a patient, a dot in the line is the monitoring point, thick line is mean value)

		points
Moorehead questionnaire of QoL		-3 to +3
EWL: weight gain	0 - 24% 25 - 49% 50 - 74% 75 - 100%	-1 0 +1 +2 +3
Medical condition:	worsened unchanged improved resolve a major comorbidity and improve others resolve all major comorbidities and improve others	-1 0 +1 +2 +3
Complications:	major minor	-1 -0.2
reoperation		-1

Table 1. BAROS

The overall mean operating time for the last 50 patients was 90.6 minutes (range 55 to 195). Four patients had early (<30 days) major complications: leakage, ileus, stenosis of entero-entero anastomosis, and small bowel injury. All complications were treated with an additional procedure. Among minor complications were two bleedings from the mesentery due to a mesentery suturing, and one bleed from the staple line intraluminally. Blood transfusions were sufficient. A port site abscess occurred in one patient. One instance of Peterson's hernia, a late complication, occurred two years after the first operation when Peterson's space wasn't closed. The problem was solved by repositioning the small bowel and closing the defect.

	Patients with comorbidities (total score)	Patients without comorbidities (total score)
bad	<1	<0
acceptable	1 - 3	0 -1.5
good	3 - 5	1.5 -3
very good	5 -7	3 – 4.5
excellent	7 - 9	4.5 - 6

Table 2. BAROS scoring

	1 year-53 pts	2 years-17 pts	3 years-3 pts
Lost weight (kg) (range)	32.8 (7.0-53.0)	35.7 (11.0-57.0)	47.3 (43.0-55.0)
EWL (%) (range)	69.6 (12.2-133.4)	76.5 (21.0-108.4)	86.0 (71.8-104.9
BMI (kg/m^2) (range)	31.0 (21.4-59.5)	29.4 (23.5-43.5)	27.4 (24.1-31.2)

Table 3. Results at 1, 2, and 3 years post-operatively

	all	improved	resolved	no change	no data
Orthopedic symptoms	22	9 (40.9%)	11 (50.0%)	1 (4.5%)	1
Hypertension	34	10 (29,4%)	23 (67,6%)		1
Diabetes	16	6 (37,5%)	9 (56.2%)		1
Hyperlipidemia	7	3 (42.9%)	4 (57.1%)		0
Asthma	7	2 (28.6%)	4 (57.1%)		1

Table 4. Comorbidities

	all	improved	resolved	months to resolution
DM - diet	4	0	4 (100%)	< 1
DM – oral medication	7	3 (42.9%)	4 (57.1%)	10.2 (1-29)
DM - insulin	4	3 (75.0%)	1 (25.0%)	< 1

Table 5. Resolution of diabetes with respect to therapy prior to surgery

Three patients had a gastric bypass performed after insufficient weight loss after sleeve gastrectomy, and four patients had GBP surgery after gastric banding. One bypass was performed because of migration of the band. Two out of four major complications (ileus and small bowel injury) occurred in redo procedures - after failed bandings. 50 out of 53 patients who were monitored for more than one year answered the Moorehead QoL questionnaire. The total average BAROS score was 6.5 for the group with comorbidities (range 2.8 to 9.0), and 3.2 for the group without comorbidities (range 0.3 to 5.0) - which is "very good" in both groups.

3. Bariatric procedures, Adjustable Gastric Banding (AGB)

The device consists of an adjustable inflatable band placed around the proximal part of the stomach. This creates a small gastric pouch (approximately 15 ml in volume) and a small stoma. Band restriction is adjustable by adding or removing saline from the inflatable band by a reservoir system of saline attached to the band and accessible through a port, which is attached by a catheter to the band. The port is placed subcutaneously in the anterior abdominal wall after the band is secured around the stomach. Adjustment of the band through the access port is an essential part of laparoscopic adjustable gastric banding therapy. Appropriate adjustments, performed up to 6 times annually, are critical for successful outcomes. Patients must chew food thoroughly to allow food to pass through the band. Adjusting the inflation of the cuff changes the size of the opening through which food passes but does not change the size of the gastric pouch; deflation of the cuff is useful when the outlet is obstructed.

Weight loss after laparoscopic adjustable gastric banding is about 50-60% of excess body weight in approximately 2 years. AGB can be completely reversed with removal of the band, tubing, and port.

Laparoscopic adjustable gastric banding was a safe and feasible technique with specific indications in moderately obese patients and, secondarily, in highly obese patients who are unfit for more invasive techniques. In patients with mild-to-moderate obesity, laparoscopic adjustable gastric banding appears to be significantly more effective than nonsurgical therapies in producing weight loss, resolving the metabolic syndrome, and improving quality-of-life outcomes, new study findings suggest.[8,9,11]

3.1 Material & methods

A clinical study was conducted at Slovenj Gradec General Hospital, Slovenia. We performed 264 gastric bandings (66.5% of all bariatric procedures) between May 2005 and May 2010. On average, patients were 41.0 years old (range 17.2 - 68.8) and had a BMI of 42.4 kg/m^2 (range 34.5 - 59.0). There were 224 female patients (84.8%) with an average age of 41.0 (range 19.5 - 68.8) and a BMI 42.0 kg/m^2 (range 34.5 - 59.0) - table 6. Out of 264 patients, 15 had to have the band removed because of either insufficient weight loss (6 patients, 2.3%), slippage (4 patients, 1.5%), migration (1 patient, 0.4%), band leakage (1 patient, 0.4%), intra abdominal abscess (1 patient, 0.4%), outlet obstruction (1 patient, 0.4%), and personal reasons (1 patient, 0.4%). 4 patients (1.5%) were lost to follow up - table 7 and 8. We followed 192 patients for more than one year. 155 patients (80.7%) were evaluated with BAROS - Bariatric Analysis and Reporting Outcome System, which is a questionnaire assessing the quality of life (QoL), excessive weight loss (EWL), medical conditions, and complications. Scoring is divided into 5 grades ranging from bad to excellent. There are 2 different scoring groups: a group with comorbidities (1 - 9 points) and a group without comorbidities (0 – 6 points). 155 of our patients (80.7%) responded and answered the BAROS questions; 101 with comorbidities and 54 without.

We excluded patients with hormonal disorders and other pathologies preoperatively. Because gastric banding is not appropriate for every patient, we performed a thorough psychological evaluation of all the patients. When needed, we offered preoperative and postoperative psychological and dietary support.

We performed the operation using a pars flaccida technique and secured the band with 1-3 stitches (fundus to the left crus and pouch).

To determine if there is a correlation between EWL and participation in the support group, we performed a statistical analysis on the 192 patients who were monitored for more than 1 year. Background data statistics included frequency and percentage distributions for categorical variables, along with mean values and standard deviations for continuous variables. Pearson correlation coefficient was calculated to conduct univariate strength association between EWL and the number of visits in the support group. We used the linear regression method for calculation of the EWL value (dependent variable) in relation to the number of visits, adjusted by age and gender (Figure7, Table 13). Statistical analysis was performed with the SPSS 15.0 software (SPSS Inc., Chicago, Il). P value < 0.05 was marked as statistically significant.

3.2 Results

192 out of 264 patients were monitored for more than one year after the procedure (172 females and 20 males).

Weight loss; In the first year, patients lost 23.4 kg on average (-1.1 - 52.9); (female 23.3 kg, range -1.1 - 52.9; male 24.6 kg, range 8.4 - 47.7).

Two years after the operation, 118 patients (106 females and 12 males) lost 31.4 kg on average, range -6.3 to 63.8 (female 31.4 kg, range -6.3 – 63.8; male 29.9, range 11.0 – 51.9).

Three years after the operation, 72 patients (67 females and 5 males) lost 33.7 kg on average, range 6.2 to 69.0. Fig. 4.

EWL; One year after the operation, EWL was 50.3% on average, range -2.0 -145.3% (female 51.7%, range -2.0 - 145.3%; male 38.3%, range 12.2 - 51.2%).

Two years after the operation, EWL was 65.6% on average (-11.2 to 135.9%); (female 68.0%, range -11.2 – 135.9%; male 43.9%, range 19.0 - 62.5%).

Three years after the operation, EWL was 69.8% on average, range 17.0 to 134.9. Fig 5

BMI; The average BMI of all patients before the operation was 42.4 kg/m^2 (range 34.5 – 59.0), 42.0 kg/m^2 for females (range 34.5 – 59.0),and 44.0 kg/m^2 for males (range 34.8 – 55.7).

One year after the procedure, the average BMI was 34.0 kg/m^2 for all patients (range 21.9 – 51.2), 33.6 kg/m^2 for females (range 21.9 – 51.2), and 37.4 kg/m^2 for males (range 29.0 – 45.5).

Two years after the procedure, the average BMI was 31.4 kg/m^2 (range 20.2 – 47.9), 31.0 kg/m^2 for females (range 20.2 – 47.9), and 36.4 kg/m^2 for males (range 31.8 – 43.0).

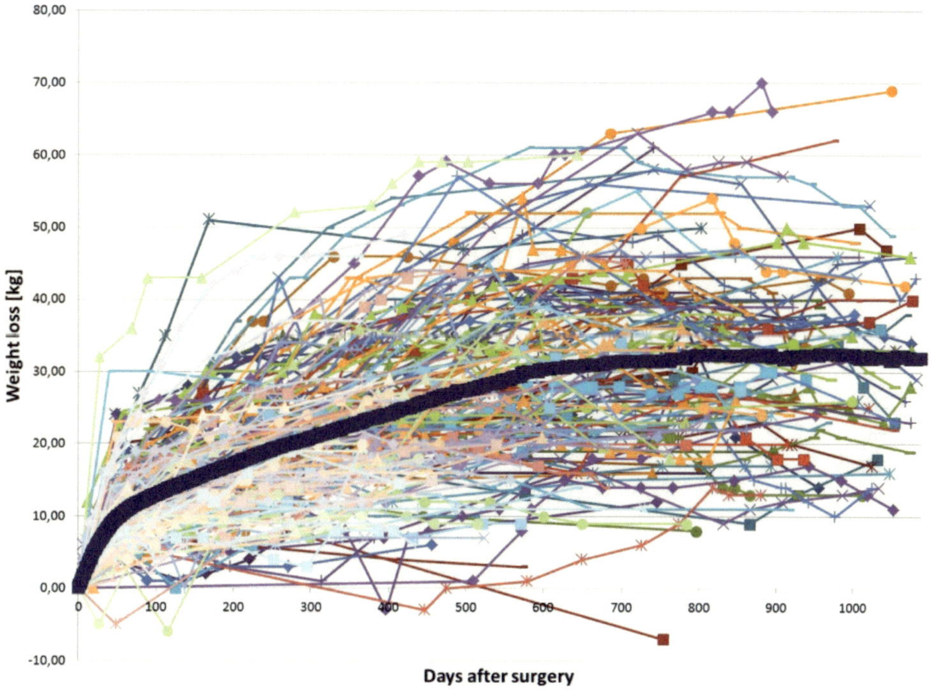

Fig. 4. Weight loss

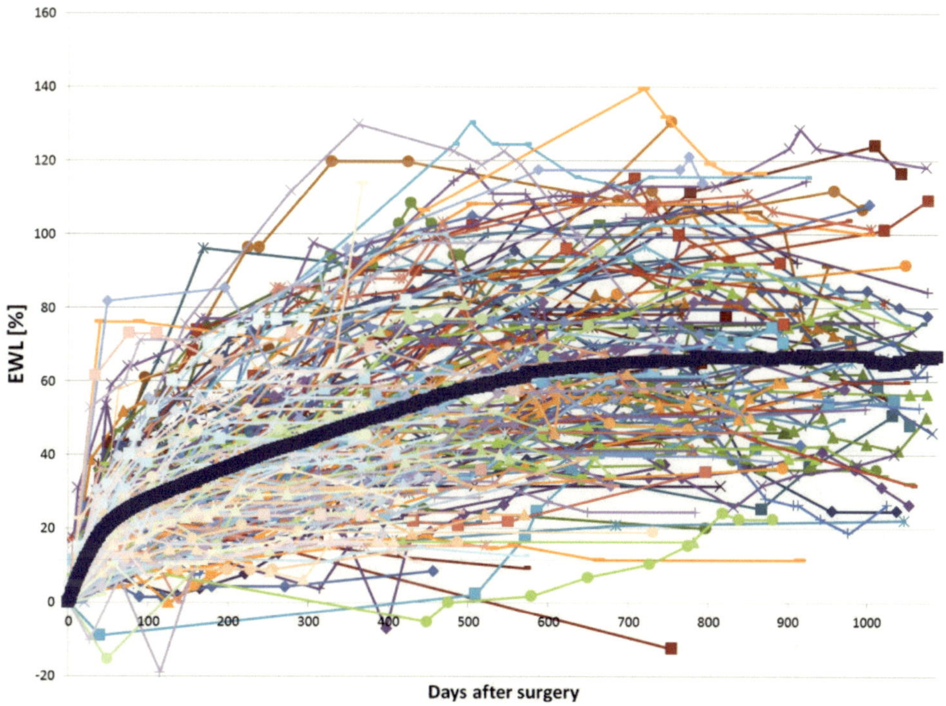

Fig. 5. EWL

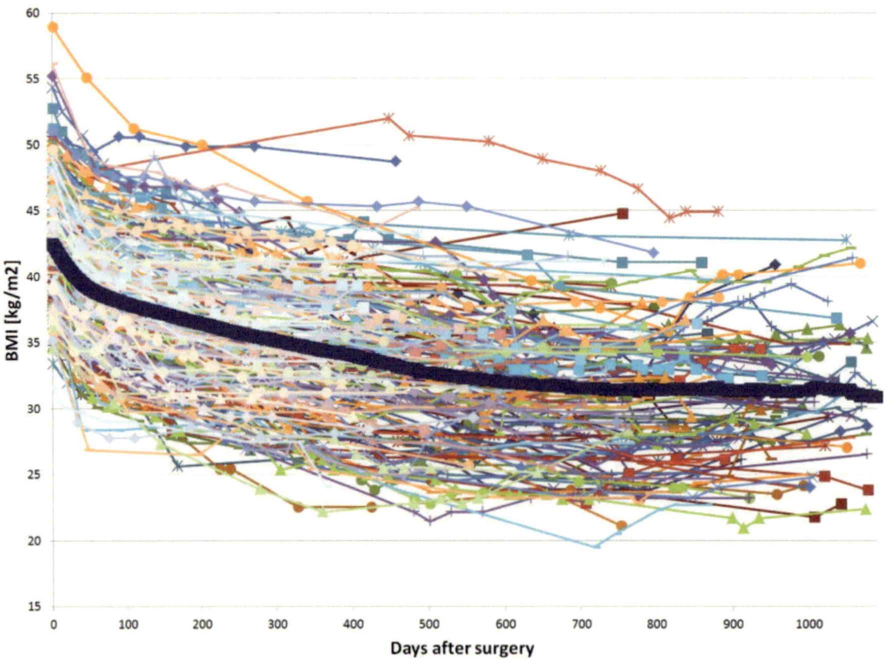

Fig. 6. BMI reduction:

	ALL	FEMALE	MALE
No	264	224	40
AGE	41.0(17.2-68.8)	41.0(19.5-68.8)	41.2(17.2-61.9)
BMI	42.4(34.5-59.0)	42.0(34.5-59.0)	44.0(34.8-55.7)

Table 6. Patients

YEAR OF THE SURGERY	PTS	WITH BAND	WITHOUT BAND	LOST
1st	11	4(36.4%)	6(54.5%)	1(9.1%)
2nd	76	68(89.5%)	8(10.5%)	0
3rd	49	46(94%)	1(2%)	2(4%)
4th	75	74(99%)	0	1
5th	53	53(100%)	0	0
ALL	264	245(92.8%)	15(5.7%)	4(1.5%)

Table 7. Monitoring

Three years after the procedure, the average BMI of all patients was 30.8 kg/m^2 (range 22.4 - 44.0) Fig. 6, Table 10a-c

Reoperations; We performed 15 re-operations: 4 (1.5%) bands were removed due to dilatation of the pouch and slippage, 6 (2.3%) due to insufficient reduction of the body weight, and one each (0.4%) due to migration, outlet obstruction, band leakage, intra abdominal abscess, and personal reasons.

Resolution of comorbidities; The main obesity-related comorbidities resolved as shown in table 6. We had 31 patients with diabetes. 13 of them (41.9%) improved, 17 (54.8%) had complete resolution of the disease, and one patient (3.2%) was lost to follow up. Out of 51 patients with hypertension, 21 (41.2%) improved, 28 (54.9%) had complete resolution of the disease, one patient (2.0%) showed no change, and one patient (2.0%) was lost to follow up. Out of 17 patients with hyperlipidemia, 6 (35.3%) improved, 9 (52.9%) had complete resolution of the disease, one patient (5.9%) showed no change, and one patient (5.9%) was lost to follow up.

Complications; There was no perioperative mortality, no pulmonary embolism, no stomach wall lesions, and no hemorrhage.

Early complications (within 1 month after the procedure): 1 (0.4%) intra abdominal abscess and 1 (0.4%) outlet obstruction.

Late complications (more than 1 month after the procedure): 1 (0.4%) band migration, 4 (1.5%) slippages/dilatations, and 1 (0.4%) band leakage.

Statistical analysis of support group visits and EWL; With the Pearson coefficient of $r=0.58$ ($p<0.001$), we are able to conclude that there is a "moderate to strong" correlation ($r>0.5$ is usually interpreted as a strong correlation) between the number of visits in the support group and EWL. The distribution between EWL and the number of visits is shown by a scattered plot in Table 12.

Table 12 shows that the number of visits has a statistically significant impact on EWL, while age and gender do not significantly correlate with the EWL.

Quality of life evaluation; The average BAROS score was a grade of "good" in both groups: 4.85 in the group with comorbidities and 2.64 in the group without comorbidities. 155 out of 193 patients (80.7%) answered the QoL questionnaire. In the group of 54 patients with comorbidities, the average score for QoL was 1.83 (range -0.4 - 3.0), 1.53 for EWL (range 0 - 3), and 1.66 for medical condition (range 0 - 3). In the group of 101 patients without comorbidities, the average score for quality of life (QoL) was 1.72 (range -2.5 - 3.0), and 1.48 for EWL (range 0 - 3), Table 13.

Year of the surgery	1st	2nd	3rd	4th	5th	TOTAL
migration		1				1(0.4%)
Slippage/dilatation	1	2	1			4(1.5%)
Insuficient weight loss	3	3				6(2.3%)
Outlet obstruction	1					1(0.4%)
Band leakage	1					1(0.4%)
Personal reasons		1				1(0.4%)
Intra abdominal abscess		1				1(0.4%)

Table 8. Reasons for removing of the band

Characteristics	Patient group (N=192)
EWL	50.3±24.2
Gender (%)	
male	12.4
female	87.6
Age in years	41.7±12.2
Number of visits	2.8±2.0

Table 9. Background data of the patients participating the support group

Monitored years/ No of patients	Weight loss(kg)	EWL(%)	BMI(kg/m^2)
>1/192	23.4(-1.1-52.9)	50.3(-2.0-145.3)	34.0(21.9-51.2)
>2/118	31.4(-6.3-63.8)	65.6(-11.2-135.9)	31.4(20.2-47.9)
>3/72	33.7(6.2-69.0)	69.8(17.0-134.9)	30.8(22.4-44.0)
>4/4	35.1(25.1-51.7)	82.2(69.0-97.3)	27.6(25.4-29.7)

Table 10.a) Results all

Monitored years/ No of patients	Weight loss(kg)	EWL(%)	BMI(kg/m^2)
>1/172	23.3(-1.1-52.9)	51.7(-2.0-145.3)	33.6(21.9-51.2)
>2/106	31.4(-6.3-63.8)	68.0(-11.2-135.9)	31.0(20.2-47.9)
>3/67	33.7(6.2-69.0)	71.6(19.5-134.9)	30.3(22.4-41.6)
>4/4	35.1(25.1-51.7)	82.2(69.0-97.3)	27.6(25.4-29.7)

Table 10.b) Results - female

Monitored years/ No of patients	Weight loss(kg)	EWL(%)	BMI(kg/m^2)
>1/20	24.6(8.4-47.7)	38.3(12.4-79.7)	37.4(29.0-45.5)
>2/12	29.9(11.0-51.9)	43.9(19.0-62.5)	36.4(31.8-43.0)
>3/5	33.5(12.2-51.2)	45.0(17.0-60.6)	36.2(30.9-44.0)
>4/4			

Table 10.c) Results - male

	all	improved	resolved	No change	No data
Diabetes	31	13(41.9%)	17(54.8%)		1(3.2%)
Hypertension	51	21(41.2%)	28(54.9%)	1(2.0%)	1(2.0%)
Hyperlipidemia	17	6(35.3%)	9(52.9%)	1(5.9%)	1(5.9%)

Table 11. Resolution of comorbidities

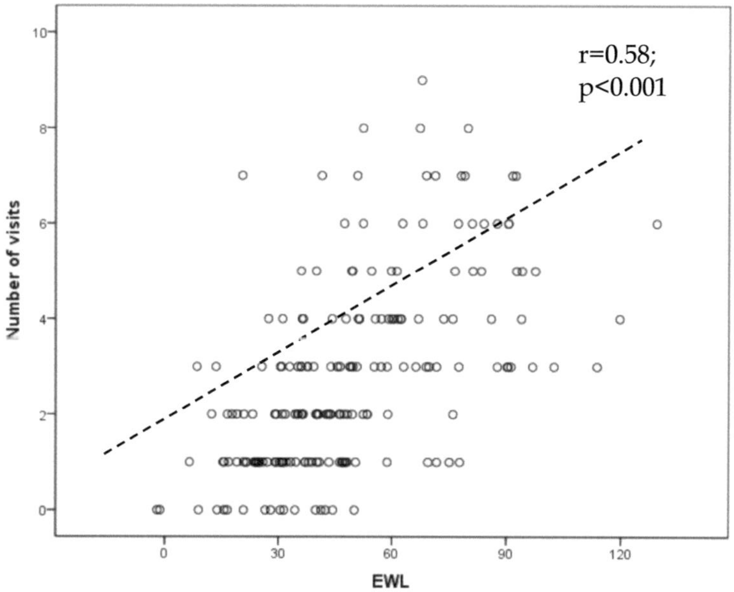

Fig. 7. Relation between number of visits and EWL

	Beta	t	p
Number of visits	0.56	9.32	<0.001
Age	-0.03	-0.57	0.571
Female gender	0.09	1.45	0.148

R^2=0.341

Table 12. Linear model to calculate EWL

	QoL	EWL	Medical condition	Total score
Comorbidity group	1.83(-0.4-3.0)	1.53(0-3)	1.66(0-3)	4.85(0.2-8.4)
Without comorbidity	1.72(-2.5-3.0)	1.48(0-3)		2.64(-2.5-5.9)

Table 13. BAROS

4. Bariatric procedures, laparoscopic sleeve gastrectomy (LSG)

LSG is a resection of the stomach along the greater curvature. For high-risk obese patients seeking gastric bypass, it may be safer and more effective to first conduct a laparoscopic sleeve gastrectomy, and then perform a Roux-en-Y procedure later, researchers reported at the Society of American Gastrointestinal Endoscopic Surgeons8. Laparoscopic sleeve gastrectomy has been advocated as the first of a 2-stage procedure for the high-risk, super-obese patient. More recently, LSG has been studied as a single-stage procedure for weight loss in the morbidly obese. LSG has been shown in initial studies to produce excellent excess weight loss comparable with laparoscopic Roux-en-Y gastric bypass in many series with a very low incidence of major complications and death10.LSG will cause many patients to lose weight, which could make them better candidates for the higher morbidity, higher mortality

Roux-en-Y gastric bypass. The data appear to show that LSG only causes short-term weight loss, so in most cases, the Roux-en-Y procedure will likely be required.

5. Discussion

Our results are comparable to the ones published in the literature (Schirmer, 2004, Wise et al., 2001, Lippincott & Wilkins, 2003, Gravante et al., 2007). In our case, there is a noticeable difference of the early results when we did not have such a strict interdisciplinary approach. Several of our first 20 cases were not really successful because of insufficient psychological and dietary treatment before the operation: our first patient had psychological problems we failed to recognize. She was willing to cooperate, but she did not tell us about her son who used drugs and husband who was an alcoholic. After two years we performed LSG on her. At the beginning, we did not have a psychologist of our own. Our second patient could not change his eating habits, which resulted in slippage of the band. We would be able to predict this deviation today. Next patient from the beginning ate too much and too fast- 5 weeks after the operation an outlet obstruction ocured and we had to remove the band. Among the first ten patients, failiures could be prevented with good psychological evaluation. AGB is a method where patients should be very motivated and willing to cooperate. If one has many of the obsessive-compulsive elements in his character, we cannot expect good results. Frequent monitoring after the operation in a support group is very important as well as immediate emptying of the band if necessary. The diference between those patients who participated in the support group and those who did not is significant- EWL of the group who did not participate in the support group was significantly lower than that of the group where patients were present at least 5 times during the first year (30.7% vs 75.7%).

AGB has indeed been shown in a randomized study to be superior to its open counterpart regarding hospital stay and readmissions (O'Brien et al., 2002). AGB is usually reported to be associated with a low perioperative complication rate and a very low mortality. The mean excess weight loss after 2 or more years is between 45% and 65% (Belachew et al., 2002, Zinzindohoue et al., 2003, Ceelen et al., 2003) ours is 66.9%. Commonly reported long-term complications are band slippage with or without pouch dilatation, band erosion (migration of the band into the stomach), band or port infection, and leaks from the band, port, or connecting tube. Overall, late morbidity affects between 6% and 25% of the patients in series including more than 100 patients. The frequency of each of these complications varies among series. For instance, band slippage occurs at rates between 0.6% and 20%, band erosion at rates between 0% and 11%, and leaks at rates between 1.4% and 26%. We have had two slippages among 120 patients in 2 years, no migrations and no leaks. These late complications lead to reoperations in up to 20% of the patients. Our reoperation rate is 7,5%. We are satisfied of not having fatalities, stomach wall lesions, pneumothorax, haemorrhages, port system complications wound ifections…(literature : fatalities up to 2,1%, somach wall lesions up to 3,5%,haemorrhage up to 2,0%, port or band system complications up to 10,4%...) (Miller, 2005).

The GBP procedure has generally been considered the gold standard based on the availability of long-term results that achieve an approximate 70% excess body weight loss over 7 to 10 years. The correction of comorbid conditions has been reported for diabetes mellitus (83%), hypertension (69%), gastric reflux (100%), urinary stress incontinence, and degenerative joint disease (Schauer et al., 2003, Sugerman et al., 2003, Perry et al., 2004, Lara et al., 2005). Flum and others have shown a significant improvement in survival for a group of patients treated with surgery compared with conventional treatment (Flum & Delinger, 2004). The cost analysis shows that the recovery of procedure cost is achieved in 12 months (Gallagher et al., 2003). When one considers the improvements in life expectancy, resolution of severe chronic disease, improvement in quality of life, and reduction in risk of cancer, there is hardly a procedure or medication in the history of medicine that can equal the GBP procedure.

Compared to published results our program in laparoscopic bariatric surgery is successful. Significant complications occurred in a few patients as a result of anastomotic leaks (LSG). Fortunately, this and other complications have decreased progressively with experience and improved surgical techniques and new material. We had one abscess in the wound after sleeve. Other complications did not occur at an increased rate. Weight loss was acceptable and resolution of comorbidities occurred as anticipated. With more experience, we perform more and more GBP procedures. At the very beginning we used circular stapler, now we are performing gastro entero anastomosis with a linear one.

6. Conclusions

Bariatric surgery has proven to be the best treatment for morbid obesity. AGB is the procedure with less complications, but it is not convenient for everyone. Good preoperative psychological evaluation has proven to be necessary. Super obese patients have a high risk of perioparative complications but AGB is not the best choice. We prefere LSG in such cases. The results suggest that the surgeons practicing bariatric surgery should make efforts to learn the skills for laparoscopic gastric bypass, because it is likely to become the standard of care for the surgical treatment of obesity.

Good results can be expected with interdisciplinary approach after the learning curve. After the operation, the results are significantly better when the patients are regularly monitored. Our study shows that results are the best when they participate in the support group of operated patients guided by a psychologist - especially in patients who underwent gastric banding.

7. References

Belachew M, Belva PH, Desaive C. Long-term results of laparoscopic adjustable gastric banding for the treatment of morbid obesity. Obes Surg. 2002;12:564–568. .

Belachew M, Legrand M, Vincent V, et al. L'approche coelioscopique dans le traitement chirurgical de l'obésité morbide. Technique et résultats. Ann Chir 1997; 51: 165-172.

Breznikar B, Dinevski D. Bariatric Surgery for Morbid Obesity: Pre-operative Assessment, Surgical Techniques and Post-operative Monitoring. JIMR 2009; 37(5) 8.

'Brien PE, Brown WA, Smith A, et al. Prospective study of a laparoscopically placed, adjustable gastric band in the treatment of morbid obesity. Br J Surg 1999; 86: 113-118.

Ceelen W, Walder J, Cardon A, et al. Surgical treatment of severe obesity with a low-pressure adjustable gastric band. Experimental data and clinical results in 625 patients. Ann Surg. 2003;237:10–16. .

Council on Scientific Affairs. Treatment of obesity in adoults. JAMA 1988; 260: 2547-51.

Flum DR, Dellinger EP. Impact of gastric bypass operation on survival: a population-based analysis. J Am Coll Surg. 2004;199:543–551. .

Gallagher SF, Banasiak M, Gonzalvo JP, et al. The impact of bariatric surgery on the Veterans Administration healthcare system: a cost analysis. Obesity Surgery. 2003;13:245–248.

Gravante G, Araco A, Araco F, Delogu D, De Lorenzo A, Cervelli V. Laparoscopic adjustable gastric bandings: a prospective randomized study of 400 operations performed with 2 different devices. Arch Surg. 2007 Oct;142(10):958-61.

Lara MD, Kothari SN, Sugerman HJ. Surgical management of obesity: a review of the evidence relating to the health benefits and risks. Treatments in Endocrinology. 2005;4:55–64.

Lippincott Williams, Wilkins. Laparoscopic Gastric Banding: A Minimally Invasive Surgical Treatment for Morbid Obesity, Ann Surg 237(1):1-9, 2003.

Mason EE, Tang S, Renquist KE, al. A decade of change in obesity surgery. Obesity Surg 1997;7: 189-197.

Miller K, Laparoscopic bariatric surgery in the treatment of morbid obesity. Endoscopic Rev. 2005;24:73-88.

Moy J, Pomp A, Dakin G, Parikh M, Gagner M. Laparoscopic sleeve gastrectomy for morbid obesity. Am J Surg. 2008 Nov;196(5):e56-9.

National Institute of Health, Health Implications of Obesity, 1985, 59.

National Institutes of Health Consensus Conference. Gastrointestinal surgery for severe obesity. Am J Clin Nutr 1992; 55: 487S-619S.

O'Brien PE, Dixon JB, Brown W, et al. The laparoscopic adjustable gastric band (Lapband®): a prospective study of medium-term effects on weight, health and quality of life. Obes Surg. 2002;12:652–660.

Oppert JM, Rolland-Cachera MF. Prévalence, évolution dans le temps et conséquences économiques de l'obésité. Med Sci 1998; 14: 939-943.

Oria EH, Moorehead KM. Baratric analysis and reporting outcome system (BAROS). Obes Surg 1998; 8: 487-497.

Perry Y, Courcoulas AP, Fernando HC, et al. Laparoscopic Roux-en-Y gastric bypass for recalcitrant gastroesophageal reflux disease in morbidly obese patients. Journal of the Society of Laparoendoscopic Surgeons. 2004;8:19–23.

Pories WJ. Who would have thought it? An operation proves to be the most effective therapy for adult-onset diabetes mellitus. Ann Surg 1995; 222: 339-352.

Schauer PR, Burguera B, Ikramuddin S, et al. Effect of laparoscopic Roux-en Y gastric bypass on type 2 diabetes mellitus. Ann Surg. 2003;238:467–484.

Schauer PR, Ikramuddin S, Gourash W, et al. Outcomes after laparoscopic Roux-en-Y gastric bypass for morbid obesity. Ann Surg 2000; 232: 515-529 Higa KD. Laparoscopic surgery for morbid obesity. In: Cameron JL, ed. Current Surgical Therapy. 8th ed. Philadelphia: Elsevier Mosby; 2004:1292- 1298.

Schirmer BD. Morbid obesity. In: Townsend CM Jr, Beauchamp RD, Evers BM, Mattox KL, eds. Sabiston Textbook of Surgery. 17th ed. Philadelphia: W.B. Saunders; 2004: 357-399

Sugerman HJ, Wolfe LG, Sica DA, et al. Diabetes and hypertension in severe obesity and effects of gastric bypass-induced weight loss. Ann Surg. 2003;237:751–756.

Wise MW, Martin LF, O'Leary JP. Morbid obesity. In: Cameron JL, ed. Current Surgical Therapy. 7th ed. St. Louis: Mosby; 2001:98-105.

Wittgrove AC, Clark GW, Tremblay LJ. Laparoscopic gastric bypass, Roux-en-Y: preliminary report of five cases. Obes Surg 1994; 4: 353–357.

Zinzindohoue F, Chevallier JM, Douard P, et al. Laparoscopic gastric banding: a minimally invasive surgical treatment for morbid obesity. Prospective study of 500 consecutive patients. Ann Surg. 2003;237:1–9.

8

BPD and BPD-DS Concerns and Results

Francesco Saverio Papadia, Hosam Elghadban, Andrea Weiss,
Corrado Parodi and Francesca Pagliardi
Genoa University,
Italy

1. Introduction

Biliopancreatic diversion (BPD) is considered one of the most effective surgical procedures in the treatment of obesity since its introduction in clinical practice by Professor Nicola Scopinaro in 1976. Nonetheless, it is, up until now, still largely the preserve of a selected group of bariatric surgeons, and faces frequently unjustified prejudices in its clinical acceptance.

In fact, despite the complexity of the operation (which is more apparent than real), its perceived operative risk (which is on the contrary probably even lower than operations such as sleeve gastrectomy) and the concerns regarding late metabolic sequelae (which can be extremely severe, but, with an adequate and in reality not particularly close follow-up are also extremely infrequent), biliopancreatic diversion with or without duodenal switch represents a formidable weapon in the most challenging cases, such as superobesity, uncontrolled metabolic syndrome, especially insulin-dependent diabetes type 2, and revisional surgery, in which it yields results that are far superior to those of any other bariatric operation. For these reasons, we believe that this operation should be in the armamentarium of every bariatric surgeon, to the point that no bariatric surgeon should be defined as such if he/she is not familiar with BPD and its patho-physiology.

In this chapter, we will briefly describe the development of the operation up to its latest modifications, highlight surgical technical points, detail the follow-up patients with BPD should be submitted to, explore early and late morbidity of the technique and describe the management of the complications. Finally, we will address the importance and ease of BPD as a revisional procedure.

1.1 Clinical development of BPD

The reduction of nutrient absorption was the first approach to surgical treatment of obesity. The early weight loss results with jejunoileal bypass (JIB) led to more than 100,000 of these operations performed in the USA through the years 1960's and 1970's. However, the analysis of late results and complications of JIB caused a drastic coolness of the initial enthusiasm. In addition to its complications, essentially due to indiscriminate malabsorption and the harmful effects of the long blind loop, the main problem with JIB is its narrow "therapeutic interval". In fact, the total length of the small bowel left in continuity is restrained within the range of 40 to 60 cm, a shorter or longer bypass resulting in life-threatening malabsorption or no weight reduction, respectively. On the other hand, the massive intestinal adaptation phenomena cause an increased absorptive surface leading out of the upper limits of the above range, with ensuing substantial recovery of energy absorption capacity (Scopinaro, 1974). This, in addition to the frequent need of restoration for major complications, ends in a high rate of failure with weight regain (Halverson et al, 1980; MacLean & Rhode, 1987). The high complication rate and the overall unsatisfactory weight loss results of jejunoileal bypass (JIB) during the years around 1980 led to general abandoning of the malabsorptive approach for obesity surgery, the gastric restriction procedures becoming those most frequently used.

Because of the absence of a blind loop and of the malabsorption essentially selective for fat and starch, biliopancreatic diversion (BPD) is largely free of many of the complications pertaining to JIB (Scopinaro et al, 1979a, 1979b). Moreover, BPD has a very wide "therapeutic interval" because by varying the length of the intestinal limbs, any degree of fat, starch and protein malabsorption can be created, thereby adapting the procedure to the population's or even the patient's characteristics, to obtain the best possible weight loss results with the minimum of complications (Scopinaro et al, 1996) . This extreme flexibility also allows us to neutralize the consequences of intestinal adaptation phenomena, which, on the other hand, are little effective in BPD.

BPD consists of a partial gastrectomy with a gastro-ileal anastomosis, which results in a temporary decrease of appetite and occurrence of postcibal syndrome, and thus a reduction of food intake during the early postoperative period. Gastrointestinal continuity is obtained by the construction of a long Roux-en-Y with an alimentary limb of variable length (usually between 200 and 250 cm) and a 50 cm common channel (Fig.1).

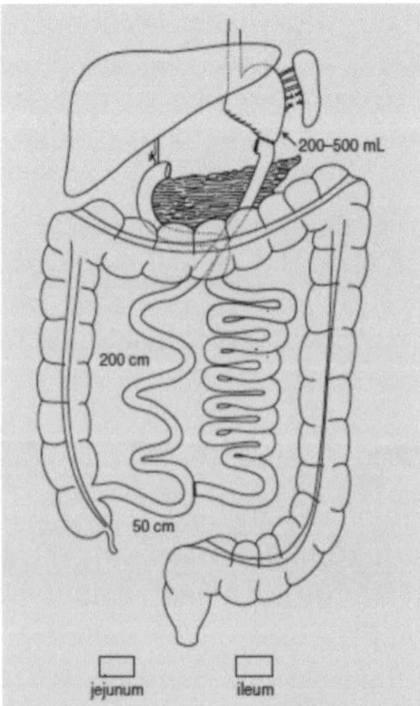

Fig. 1. Ad hoc stomach biliopancreatic diversion. Alimentary limb, from gastroenterostomy (GEA) to enteroenterostomy (EEA); biliopancreatic limb, from duodenum to EEA; and common limb, from EEA to ileocecal valve (ICV)

This anatomical arrangement creates malabsorption that is essentially selective for fat and starch, and ensures long-term weight maintenance. In our experience, the long-term results of this operation are represented by a mean reduction of approximately 75% of the initial excess weight (IEW), a weight loss which is maintained over 20 years.

2. BPD physiology

Through this part of the chapter we will try to explain the new physiology of the digestive apparatus after BPD and the specific effect of BPD on the metabolic syndrome.

2.1 Weight loss and maintenance

The initial weight loss is determined by the **temporary forced food limitation** that occurs immediately after operation. As a rule, the operated patient fully recovers appetite and eating capacity before the stabilization weight is attained. The final weight loss (the weight of stabilization) depends on **the amount of daily energy absorption** that the operation permits (a permanent mechanism), and influenced by the gastric volume, most likely because a smaller stomach, resulting in more rapid gastric emptying, accelerates intestinal transit, thereby reducing absorption (Scopinaro et al, 1999).

The original philosophy for limitation of digestion in BPD was to delay the meeting between food and biliopancreatic juice in order to confine the pancreatic digestion to a short segment of small bowel. The analysis of changes in weight loss and in protein intestinal absorption in the BPD models that followed each other in the evolution of the operation (Gianetta etal, 1980; Scopinaro et al, 1980; 1997) demonstrated that in the present model of BPD no pancreatic digestion occurs in the CL. Protein and starch digestion, which is only due to intestinal brush-border enzymes, occurs in the entire small bowel from the GEA to the ICV, while only fat absorption, which needs the presence of bile salts, is confined to the CL.

Some clinical-statistical observations on the modalities of this very long term weight maintenance indicate that body weight after BPD is essentially independent of individual and interindividual variations of food intake. This prompted us to investigate the relations between usual energy intake and energy intestinal absorption.

		Alimentary intake	Fecal loss	Apparent absorption	Apparent absorption (%)
energy (kcal/24h)	mean	3070	1329	1741	58
	range	1840-4060	210-2590	1012-2827	32-71
fat (g/24h)	mean	130	89	39	28
	range	88-185	22-251	13-94	12-59
nitrogen (g/24h)	mean	27	12	15	57
	range	15-48	2.5-36	6.7-20	25-82
calcium (mg/24h)	mean	1994	1443	551	26
	range	1037-3979	453-2565	251-1414	-24-69

Table 1. Energy, fat, nitrogen and calcium intestinal apparent absorption in 15 subjects (3 men) with stable body weight 2-3 years after BPD (mean ± s.d. body weight: at the time of the operation 119 ± 24 kg; at the time of the study 75 ± 14 kg).

An absorption study was carried out,(Scopinaro et al, 2000) the results of which are reported in Table -1, demonstrating that the BPD digestive/absorptive apparatus has a maximum transport capacity for fat and starch, and thus energy. Consequently, all the energy intake that exceeds the maximum transport threshold is not absorbed; therefore, assuming that daily energy intake is largely higher than the aforementioned threshold, daily energy absorption is constant for each subject. Therefore, in each BPD individual, the weight of stabilization cannot be modified by any increase or decrease of fat-starch intake, provided the intake is greater than the maximum transport threshold.

In conclusion, the original intestinal lengths and gastric volume being equal, the interindividual variability of the weight of stabilization in BPD subjects is accounted for by interindividual differences of; (1) Original energy intestinal digestive-absorptive capacity per unit of surface; (2) Intestinal adaptation phenomena; (3) Intestinal transit time (which, in addition to gastric volume, can be influenced by the intake of fluids); (4) Simple sugar intake; and (5) Energy expenditure per unit of body mass. In reality, since the intestinal carrier becomes rapidly desaturated after the passage of food, an increased number of meals per day can also increase energy absorption, and this is confirmed by clinical experience.

The aforementioned results were confirmed by **an overfeeding study**, where 10 long-term BPD subjects kept a strictly stable body weight when fed their usual diet for 15 days and the same diet plus 2,000 fat-starch kcal/day (without increasing the number of meals per day) for 15 more days (Table 2), without observing any increase in body weight, considering that, with a positive balance of 2000kcal/day for 15 days, the average increase in body weight should have been in excess of 2 kg (Forbes GB, 1987).

subjects	initial BW	BW on usual food intake	BW after overfeeding
1	77.7	78.0	78.0
2	90.0	90.5	89.2
3	97.0	96.5	95.7
4	73.0	72.7	73.4
5	89.1	88.8	90.3
6	68.5	68.0	68.5
7	102.8	103.5	103.0
8	87.0	87.0	86.5
9	66.5	66.0	66.0
10	70.5	70.0	71.0

Table 2. Overfeeding study in 10 subjects 3-9 years after BPD. Individual data of body weight (BW, kg) at the beginning of the study, after a 15 day period on usual food intake (mean: ~ 3800 kcal/day) and after a 15 day period of overfeeding (usual food intake plus 2000 fat/starch kcal/day).

3. Immediate morbidity and mortality

BPD is major abdominal surgery and, as for any other similar operation, its postoperative morbidity and mortality essentially depend on the frequency in its use. We do an average of about 100 open plus 100 laparoscopic operations per year, and our mortality rate is steadily

<0.5%. Similarly, general and major surgical complications tend to decrease with increasing surgical volumes and are reasonably low. Both the anastomoses are well vascularized and without tension, so leaks are exceptional.

3.1 Weight loss results

The 50-cm CL in BPD has proven to be the best compromise between fat absorption limitation and bile salt loss in the colon such as not to cause bile acid diarrhea. Lenghtening the common limb will increase fat and bile salt absorption; protein absorption needs an elongation of the total bowel length comprised between GEA and ICV. For the rest, the smaller the gastric volume and the shorter the small bowel between the GEA and the ICV, the lower the stabilization weight but the greater the risk of nutritional complications.

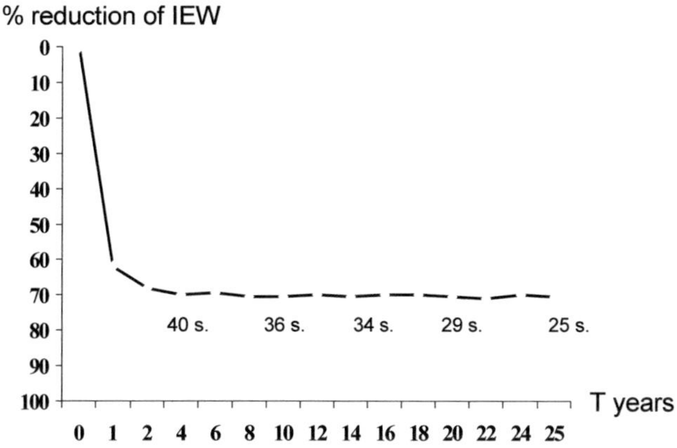

Fig. 2. Weight changes following "ad hoc stomach" BPD in operated subjects with minimum follow-up 5 years. Unpaired data: 2 years 2,371 patients; 20 years 427 patients.

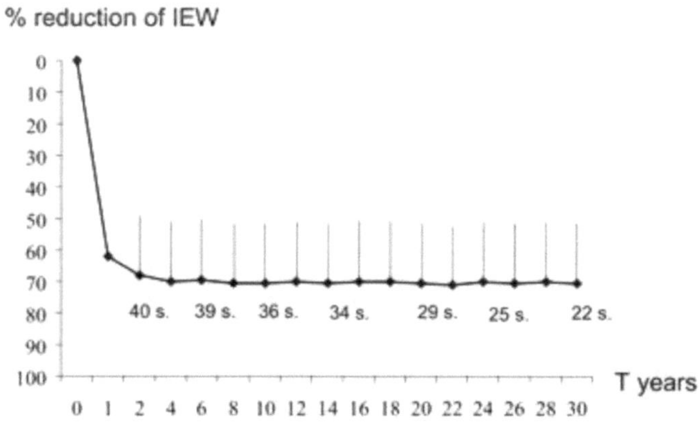

Fig. 3. Very long-term weight changes in a group of 40 subjects submitted to "half-half" BPD. Paired data.

The 20-year weight loss curve in **Fig. 2** (patients with a minimum follow-up of 5 years) goes from little more than 70% loss of the initial excess weight at 1 year to about 80 IEW%L at 20 years. This of course does not mean that the weight loss increases with time. Simply, the one with unpaired data in the graph shows that, by slowly increasing the gastric volume and the alimentary limb length, we reached the other extremely important compromise, the one between weight loss and protein nutritional complications. To make a long story brief, 25 years ago we had a wonderful 90% EWL, at the unacceptable price of protein malnutrition in ~30% of patients, which was recurrent in ~10%, and thus necessitated revision of the BPD consisting of elongation of the CL (obviously, at the expense of the BPL; see revision).

The real weight maintenance after BPD can be appreciated in **Fig. 3,** where weight loss paired data is reported for a group of 40 patients submitted to the original "half-half " model of BPD, 22 of whom who could be followed-up until the 30th year.

In conclusion, after BPD the weight maintenance is ensured by the existence of an intestinal energy transport threshold. The weight of stabilization depends partly on that threshold and partly on the changes of body composition consequent to the operation.

3.2 Other beneficial effect

The other benefits obtained after BPD are listed in **Table 3**. The percents of changes observed after the operation were calculated for each complication in patients with a

	minimum follow-up (mo)	disappeared (%)	improved (%)	unchanged (%)	impaired (%)
Pickwickian syndrome* (2%)	1	100	-	-	-
Somnolence† (6%)	1	100	-	-	-
Hypertension‡ (39%)	12	81	13	6	-
Fatty liver§ (46%)	24	87	9	4	-
Leg stasis• (31%)	12	45	39	16	-
Hypercholesterolemia¶ (55%)	1	100	-	-	-
Hypertriglyceridemia (33%)	12	95	5	-	-
Hyperglycemia (14%)	4	100	-	-	-
DM (6%)	4	100	-	-	-
DM requiring insulin (2%)	12	100	-	-	-
Hyperuricemia (16%)	4	94	-	3	3
Gout (2%)	4	100#	-	-	-

(%) percent of patients with condition.
*Somnolence with cyanosis, polycythemia, and hypercapnia
†In absence of one or more characteristics of pickwickian syndrome.
‡Systolic ≥ 155, diastolic ≥ 95 mmHg, or both.
§More than 10%.
•Moderate or severe.
¶More than 200 mg/mL (21% more than 240 mg/mL).
#Serum uric acid normalized, no more clinical symptoms.

Table 3. Other beneficial effects of AHS BPD.

minimum follow-up corresponding to the postoperative time after which there was generally no further substantial modification.

Recovery and improvement were considered only when favorable changes were essentially maintained at all subsequent reexaminations. The observed beneficial effects are obviously not attributable to the BPD itself, but to the weight loss and/or the reduced nutrient absorption, the only two exceptions being the effects on glucose and cholesterol metabolism (Scopinaro et al, 1997, Marinari et al, 1997).

3.3 Glucose homeostasis and antidiabetic effects of BPD

One of the most impressive benefits of BPD other than weight loss is certainly represented by the disappearance of type 2 diabetes mellitus (T2DM) in nearly 100% of the previously diabetic morbidly obese patients. This effect was observed both at short term in Buchwald meta-analyses (Buchwald et al, 2004, 2009) and as long as 10 years (Scopinaro et al, 2005) and even 20 years after BPD in very long-term series (Scopinaro et al, 2008).

It could be not surprising, considering that weight reduction, no matter how obtained, causes a decrease in insulin resistance (McAuley & Mann, 2006), thus explaining the beneficial effect on T2DM the greater and the more sustained depending on size and duration of weight reduction. Even the apparent resolution of T2DM occurring within days after operation could be easily explained keeping in mind that insulin resistance, which, due to the surgical stress, generally increases immediately after a surgical operation (Brandi et al, 1993, Thorell et al, 1999) is on the contrary postoperatively reduced in the diabetic patient (Adami et al, 2003, Wickremesekera et al, 2005). The early and late effect of BPD on T2DM could then be an aspecific consequence of weight loss and calorie deprivation, shared with all other bariatric operations. However, the normalization of insulin sensitivity after BPD is maintained after weight has stabilized around BMI 30 that is still in the obese range. Moreover, differently from other bariatric procedures, BPD has shown the ability to restore acute insulin response to intravenous glucose load (AIR) in morbidly obese patients, both at short (Briatore et al, 2008) and long term (Polyzogopoulou et al, 2003).

Furthermore, a group of preoperatively diabetic women after BPD never showed one single serum glucose value higher than normal during the whole pregnancy and delivered normal weight babies, thus demonstrating a beta-cell function adequate to the requirement (Adami et al, 2008). This restored insulin secretion capacity, which was never observed before, not only demonstrates that beta cell function is not irreversibly lost in T2DM patients but also indicates that BPD possesses a specific action, independent of weight loss and negative calorie balance, which, together with the normalized insulin sensitivity, fully accounts for the diabetes resolution after the operation.

Hypothetically, the BPD-specific action can be identified with the food-stimulated incretin GLP-1, produced by the distal ileum, where after BPD stomach directly empties, which was demonstrated able to improve beta-cell function (Doyle & Egan, 2007), stimulate beta-cell proliferation (Xu et al, 1999), and inhibit beta cell apoptosis (Farilla et al,2003). GLP-1 production was found increased after BPD both in rat (Borg et al, 2007) and in man (Valverde et al, 2005, Guidone et al, 2006). More than 90% of type 2 diabetic patients are not morbidly obese, being in the BMI range 25 to 35. Recently, with the aim to investigate if the BPD effect is maintained in the above BMI range, we submitted to BPD 30 T2DM patients belonging to that range, with the obvious rationale that, if the action of BPD is specific, and thus independent of weight loss, it should be maintained also in the patients who, being only mildly obese or simply overweight, lose little or no weight after operation (Scopinaro et al, 2011). The reason why BPD does not entail risk of excessive or undue weight loss is that there is a maximum energy absorption capacity after the operation, which corresponds to a weight of stabilization of about 85 kg for men and 70 kg for women (Scopinaro et al, 2000). The more starting weight, with the related energy intake, approaches these values, the less calorie imbalance, and thus weight loss, is to be expected after BPD. Patients with initial weight equal to or lower than those should absorb all energy they eat and consequently have no energy malabsorption or weight reduction at all.

Recently, our group published the first results of BPD in diabetic, non/morbidly obese patients BMI 25-34.9 kg/m^2. The main finding of this study was the striking difference between the effect of BPD on T2DM in the morbidly obese patients (BMI > 35) and the patients with BMI 25-34.9 kg/m^2. One year after the operation, this latter group had a control (HbA1c≥7%) rate of 83%, normal HbA1c (≥ 6.5%) was found in 63% of patients, whereas full remission (FSG ≥ 110 mg/dL) was shown by only 30% of patients, vs. nearly 100% in the morbidly obese group. Diabetic patients with BMI >35 showed then a much better response to BPD than those with BMI 25-34.9 kg/m^2, considered together.

Contrary to expectations, in this study mean serum triglyceride values remained essentially unchanged during the first postoperative year, whereas the percentage of abnormally high values showed a remarkable increase until the eighth postoperative month, followed by a nonsignificant reduction, ending up with values at 1 year double than preoperatively. An increase of serum triglyceride concentration following interruption of enterohepatic bile acid circulation by means of bile-acid-binding resins (cholestyramine or colestipol) was demonstrated almost 30 years ago (Beil et al, 1980, Ast & Frishman, 1990). Since an important interruption of the enterohepatic bile acid circulation also occurs after BPD, our hypothesis is that, due to increased liver bile acid neosynthesis aimed at compensating for intestinal loss, cholesterol pool is depleted, and very low-density lipoprotein synthesis is stimulated, with consequent VLDL-triglyceride parallel increase. Indeed, an elongation of the common limb up to 100 cm, which entails a greater bile acid absorption in the distal ileum, led to normalization of postoperative serum triglyceride levels up until now in a small series of diabetic patients with BMI< 30. Incidentally, this elongation determines a significant amelioration in bowel habits.

3.4 Cholesterol homeostasis

Two specific actions of BPD account for the permanent serum cholesterol normalization in 100% of operated patients: the first is the calibrated interruption of the enterohepatic bile salt circulation (bile acids are electively absorbed by the distal ileum) that causes enhanced synthesis of bile acids at the expense of the cholesterol pool; the second specific action is the strongly reduced absorption of endogenous cholesterol consequent to the limitation of fat absorption.

The serum cholesterol level shows a stable mean reduction of approximately 30% in patients with normal preoperative values and 45% in patients who were hypercholesterolemic before the operation (Gianetta et al, 1985). High-density lipoprotein (HDL) cholesterol remains unchanged, the reduction being entirely at the expense of low-density lipoprotein (LDL) and very lowdensity lipoprotein (VLDL) cholesterol (Montagna et al, 1987). These results were maintained at long term, the HDL cholesterol showing a significant increase, in 51 BPD subjects at 6 years (total serum cholesterol: preop. 210 ± 46 mg/dL, postop. 124 ± 25 mg/dL, Student's t test, $p < 0.0001$; HDL cholesterol: preop. 44±12 mg/dL, postop. 50±15 mg/dL, Student's t test, $p < 0.03$) and at very long termin the 10HHBPD subjects whose values were available 15–20 years after operation (Table 4).With the National Institutes of Health criterion of 200 mg/dL as the upper recommended limit for serum cholesterol, of the 2,888 (total series) obese patients submitted to BPD with a minimum follow-up of 1 month, 1,542 had hypercholesterolemia (612 had values higher than 240 mg/dL and 110 had values higher than 300 mg/dL). All of these patients had serum cholesterol values lower than 200 mg/dL 1 month after operation, and the values remained below that level at all subsequent examinations.

		serum cholesterol 15-20 years after HH BPD	
subjects	preoperative total serum cholesterol	total	HDL
1	205	116	47
2	140	125	38
3	150	140	52
4	210	158	65
5	280	158	73
6	230	127	61
7	180	118	35
8	285	120	36
9	189	130	59
10	260	171	33
mean	213	136 *	50

Table 4. Serum cholesterol (mg/dl) in ten subjects before and 15-20 years after HH BPD.

4. Patient selection and perioperative preparation

Patients who undergo either BPD or DS must be prepared for the consequences of a malabsorptive operation. In very simple words, it must be made clear to the patient that he/she will trade one illness (severe obesity with or without its complications) with another one, less morbid and easier to control, malabsorption. Once this clear, it is probably easier to understand the necessity for lifelong chronic follow-up.

There is no clear consensus on indications and contraindications to BPD in the bariatric surgical community. Absolute contraindications are chronic diarrhea, alcoholism, inflammatory bowel disease, uncontrolled psychiatric illnesses, chronic renal failure, severe liver cirrhosis, and endogenous protein loss (protein losing enteropathy, nephrotic syndrome, etc.).Other relative contraindications for the procedure are significant geographic distance from the surgeon, lack of financial means to afford supplements, inability or unwillingness to undergo lifelong chronic follow-up.

On the other hand, BPD is a very useful tool for those patients with superobesity, severe metabolic syndrome especially uncontrolled T2DM, and as a surgical option for revision of failed other bariatric operations. Finally, although still investigational, promising preliminary reports have been given by our group for BPD in the surgical approach to type 2 diabetes mellitus in patients with a BMI between 35 and 25 as mentioned above.

Patient selection begins in the outpatient office. Particular attention has to be put on the patients' eating habits and behavior, because a protein-rich postoperative diet is required. The postoperative daily minimum oral protein requirements are approximately 80 g/day, which are easily met in most European and North-American diets, but that could be challenging e.g. in vegetarians or in patients less prone to eating meat or protein in general. Therefore, some basic nutritional skills are required in the surgeons' hands, in order to discriminate patients with an obviously bad outcome. It is in fact to be expected that the patient will not change his/her habits, and therefore the operation will have to be tailored to the patient, and not the patient to the operation.

Furthermore, false expectations and realistic goals have to be discussed openly with the patient: mean postoperative % excess weight loss is 70%, and any greater degree of weight loss is likely to be associated with complications. Finally, bowel habits change have to be discussed very clearly. Bowel movements will be increased in the vast majority of patients, slight modifications of eating habits may be necessary to achieve the best results and minimize side effects: milk, simple sugars, large amounts of fruits and vegetables should be avoided in order to prevent weight regain and reduce flatulence and frequency of stools. It is nonetheless to be remarked that sweet-eaters and nibblers have bad outcomes with any operation.

Being a choice for superobese and bariatric revisional cases, BPD candidates usually present with co-morbidities that are much more severe than the usual bariatric candidate. A multi-disciplinary approach comprising sleep-apnea studies, pulmonary and respiratory function tests, arterial blood gases, cardiologic consultation should be easily available. In case of abnormal arterial blood gases or sleep apnea studies, outpatient C-PAP prescription is mandatory to improve respiratory function. Any coexisting co-morbidity should, if possible, be treated, always with the aim to reduce perioperative morbidity.

Preoperative weight loss is always desirable, nonetheless it is very difficult to achieve in practice. A two-step approach is feasible for BPD with duodenal switch, but it is impossible for standard BPD, where intragastric balloon placement and subsequent surgery can be offered.

On top of the routine preoperative laboratory investigations, we usually stress upon vitamin A, D and E and PTH determinations, in order to have a baseline value upon which to compare the subsequent follow-up values. Preoperative investigations should reasonably rule out pregnancy and chronic renal or liver disease, either by biochemical tests, or by ultrasound. Whereas frankly abnormal liver function tests may highlight an undiagnosed NASH, which benefits from the operation, patients with abnormal platelet counts, low albumin, high creatinine or any frankly abnormal finding on abdominal ultrasound should be put on hold or excluded from the operation.

Upper GI radiology and endoscopy are not routinely used, except for revisional cases, because the routine distal gastric resection eliminates the problem of the unexplored distal gastric stump, which is on the contrary of concern in gastric bypass.

After admission, routine antithrombotic prophylaxis is started, usually with 4000 to 6000 units of low-molecular weight heparin. No bowel preparation is necessary: the patient is kept on a liquid diet the day before the operation. A single dose of second-generation cephalosporin is administered as an ultra-short-term antibiotic prophylaxis half an hour before skin incision.

5. Surgical technique

5.1 Position of the patient and operating table

The operating table should be specific for bariatric surgery, and must allow tilting and extreme inclination in total safety. We must pay especially close attention to the pressure areas, since, due to the patient's weight there is a greater risk of ischemic, venous, and nervous injuries. For the laparoscopic approach, the patient is placed with legs wide apart; the operator stands between the patient's legs, the cameraman [assistant] generally to his right and 2nd assistant to his left. The laparoscopy monitor should be placed to the right of the patient, next to the head of the table.

An urinary catheter is routinely placed, and kept for the first 24 hours. A central venous line is not mandatory, but in practical terms useful especially for high-risk patients. Invasive pressure monitoring is not used routinely, but fiberoptic conscious sedation intubation is used in difficult patients, according to the anesthesiologists' preference.

5.2 Trocar position

The pneumoperitoneum is usually performed through Trocar 1 supraumbilical midline 10/12 mm port done through open procedure with Hasson technique [safe]. In morbidly obese patients, the umbilical scar should never be used as an anatomic point of reference for the introduction of the trocars. CO_2 pressure should be maintained at 15 mm/Hg during the procedure. Once the 30 degree optical system has been inserted, an additional 4-5 trocars are placed under direct vision according to the following diagram (Fig.5.).

Trocar 2 (10/12 mm) along the left midclavicular line, about 6 cm below the costal margin.
Trocar 3 (10/12 mm) along the right midclavicular line, about 6 cm below the costal margin
Trocar 4 (10/12 mm) on the midline, 3 cm below the xiphoid.
Trocar 5 (5mm) on the left costal margin, along the left middle axillary line.

Occasionally, if the intestinal measurement or the entero-enterostomy appears difficult, an additional 5 mm trocar is introduced in the left iliac fossa. The procedure is entirely done with a 10-mm and 30° optical camera.

5.3 Operative steps (laparoscopic approach)

5.3.1 First phase: cholecystectomy and gastric resection

Cholecystectomy [prophylactic or therapeutic] is carried out first and the gallbladder is left in the right hypochondrium over the liver to be removed from the abdominal cavity at the end of the surgery. With the surgeon between the patient's legs and the operating table slight head up, the optical system stays in portal 1; the first assistant uses the grasping

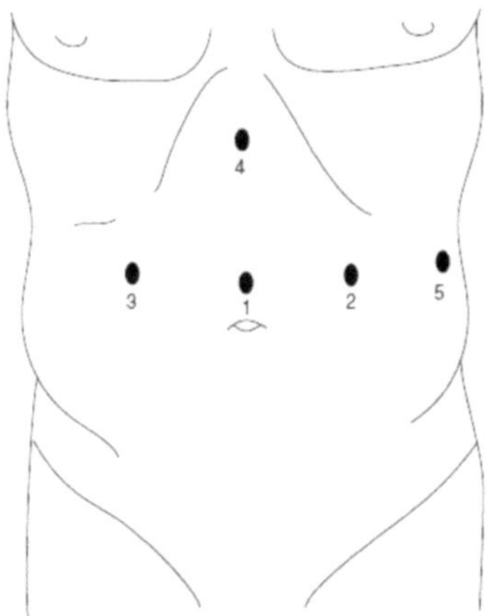

Fig. 5. Trocar position in laparoscopic standard biliopancreatic diversion. 1: supraumbilical (10–12 mm), on the midline, 3–4 cm above the superior margin of the umbilicus; 2: left hypondriac (10–12 mm), along the left midclavicular line, about 6 cm below the costal margin; 3 right hypondriac (10–12 mm), along the right midclavicular line, about 6 cm below the costal margin; 4: xiphoid (10–12 mm), on the midline, 3 cm below the xiphoid; 5: left subcostal (5 mm), on the left costal margin, along the left middle axillary line.

forceps in portal 5 to expose the stomach. The surgeon uses portal 2 for the harmonic scalpel and portal 3 for the grasping forceps, thus exposing and dissecting the stomach. The second assistant pushes the liver away by means of portal 4.

The gastrectomy is made in the caudo-cranial direction following the great curvature, starting in the middle and ending up dissection after division of the first two short gastric vessels. Aim of the dissection is to fully mobilize the gastric fundus, so that the stapler can be safely fired about 15 cm below the angle of His. This dissection is always made with the harmonic scalpel, and close to the gastric wall, aiming at reducing bleeding, and it extends down to 2 cm distal from the pylorus. Subsequently, the lesser omentum is incised, and the right gastric vessels are ligated close to the pylorus. Next, the duodenum is transected with a linear endostapler: we usually use a 45 or 60 mm stapler with a blue cartridge introduced through the port 3.

After the duodenal transection, the stomach is pulled caudally and to the left in order to facilitate the dissection of the lesser gastric curvature, which is made up to the level of the left gastric artery, always close to the gastric wall, so as to prevent bleeding. Once the level of the left gastric artery is reached, the gastric resection is carried out by repeated firing of endoGIA 45 or 60, blue and green cartridges, starting from the greater curve, at approximately 15 cm from the angle of His, towards the lesser curve, at the end of the dissection, about 7 cm caudally from the cardias. A landmark of 15 cm on the greater curve corresponds to a gastric volume of about 300mL; a distance of 20 cm corresponds to a volume of about 500mL. The divided stomach is left in the patient's left hypochondrium to be removed at the end of surgery together with the gallbladder.

5.3.2 Second phase: intestinal measurement and enteroenterostomy

The operating table is rotated approximately 15º degree to the left with a slight Trendelenburg position. The surgeon positions himself at the level of the patient's left flank, having the first assistant on his left and the second assistant on his right, at the level of the patient's head. The optical system is placed in portal 2 by the first assistant.

The surgeon uses portals 5 and 6 by grasping forceps for measuring the intestinal loops. Both forceps have a mark at 10 cm from the distal extremity. The small bowel is measured backwardws from the cecum, fully stretched, using the two forceps in alternating movements. A mark is left at 50 cm. The measurement of the loop continues up to 250 or 300 cm from the ileocecal valve, at which level it is divided using the linear endoGIA, which is introduced through portal 5. At this point the alimentary limb should be identified by a stitch, and the mesentery is sectioned in depth with the ultrasonic scissors. Care should be taken to arrange the alimentary limb to the patient's right side and the biliopancreatic limb to the left side to avoid twist.

Next, the stitch left 50 cm from the ileocecal valve is identified, and the biliopancreatic limb is brought next to it. The correct orientation and positioning of the limbs has to be checked before stapler firing to ensure that there is no twist in the mesentery. If The enteroanastomosis is performed in a laterolateral, isoperistatic technique. This is done first by opening a small orifice into both loops with the harmonic scalpel and passing a linear endostapler through them. The enterotomies are then closed in a running seromuscular suture.

5.3.3 Third phase: gastroenterostomy, liver biopsy and drain placement

The surgeons return back to the primary position, with the surgeon between the patient's legs, and the assistants to his left and right. The transverse mesocolon is elevated up until identification of Treitz's ligament, and a small opening is performed with the harmonic scalpel just above it. The surgeon then pulls the left angle of the gastric stump though it into the submesocolic space. The distal intestinal stump (alimentary limb) is identified and perforated with the ultrasonic scissors at a distance from the suture line equal to the operative length of the endoGIA 45 or 60. Of extreme importance at this pont is the final check of the correct orientation of the intestinal limbs. The alimentary limb should lie on the right of the patient,, adherent to the transverse mesocolon and the root of the mesentery. It should be traced from its most cranial stump up until the entero-enterostomy, and no additional bowel loops should be interposed: this is an unequivocal sign of twist.

Next, a laterolateral isoperistaltic gastro-enterostomy is performed on the posterior wall of the stomach, as close as possible to the distal angle and at midway between the suture line and the greater curve, with manual closure of the conjoined defect. A methylene blue test of the anastomosis is performed in the end.

Liver biosy is taken for baseline analysis of the liver condition. This data is useful in order to identify patients with severe liver pathology, in whom rapid weight loss may be hazardous.

One closed suction drain on top of the duodenal stump is placed. Stomach stump and gallbladder are extracted through the supra-umbilical port. Fascia is closed on the supra-umbilical port only, with interrupted slowly-absorbable 0-stitches.

5.4 Operative technique (open approach)

Through an upper midline incision and after abdominal exploration, the first step is the intestinal measurement. The small bowel is measured backwards from the cecum to the ligament of Treitz and marking stitches are placed at 50 and 300 cm. It is very important that the small bowel is measured fully stretched, to make intestinal measurements reproducible in all hands. The ratio between the same small bowel fully loose and fully stretched is approximately 1-2. The small bowel is then transected at the 250 or 300-cm from the ileo-cecal valve and the ileal mesentery is sectioned in depth. The EEA can be done with any technique, bringing the BPL to the left side, and the AL to the right of the abdomen.

The distal gastrectomy is done, the duodenal stump is closed, the gallbladder is removed, and a wedge liver biopsy is obtained. We are used to cutting the stomach on a TA 90 linear stapler placed as oblique as possible, in order to compensate for the shortness of the ileal mesentery. As with the laparoscopic technique, the first two short gastric vessels on the greate curve are ligated and sectioned, whereas the dissection reaches up to the left gastric artery on the lesser curve. If the transaction is performed along those landmarks, a gastric volume of around 400 mL will be obtained. In any case, actual measurement of the gastric volume may be useful during the surgeon's learning curve.

The mesocolon is incised and the AL is brought into the supramesocolic space, checking for possible twist. Any technique can be used for the GEA. We prefer to do it end-to side, by cutting away the left corner of the gastric stump. The GEA is then anchored by two stitches to the mesocolic rent, to avoid intestinal kinkings and internal hernias. We always close the distal mesenteric defect and never the proximal.

The last maneuver is the final intestinal check, starting from the ICV, with the surgeon following the alimentary limb and the first assistant following the biliopancreatic limb. The fascia is closed with continuous suture. Drains are put as in the laparoscopic technique. A subcutaneous suction drain is controversial, and in any case used only for patients with very thick subcutaneous fat.

6. Postoperative care

Routine intensive care admission is not mandatory. Only very selected cases, with severe respiratory co-morbidities are sent to ICU in our practice, as discussed preoperatively with the anesthesiologist. Analgesia is performed via continuous infusion of opiates, NSAIDs and anti-emetics. Usually, 100 ml/h of fluids are administered in the first 24 hours.

The morning after the operation, bloods are checked, in particular, CPK and myoglobin, in order to detect rhabdomyolysis. With CPK values above 1000 U/dl, an aggressive protocol is started, with infusion of 200ml/h of saline, 100 mg bid fuorsemide, and 100 ml 8.4% HCO_3^-, with close monitoring of urine output, and daily check of CPK values. Hyperhydration is stopped when CPK values are steadily dropping and/or below 500 U/dl. The urinary catheter is usually kept until rhabdomyolysis is ruled out or resolved.

Preoperative antithrombotic prophylaxis is continued postoperatively up until 30 days from the operation. An upper GI radiology may be useful but is not mandatory. The naso-gastric tube is removed on the first postoperative day. Oral liquid diet and drain removal is performed on the third postoperative day. If tolerated, the diet is the progressed to soft diet first and, on the fifth or sixth postoperative day, to a free diet.

6.1 Patient instructions

Patients undergoing BPD must be aware that for the rest of their lives they will absorb minimal fat, (Gianetta et al, 1981; Scopinaro et al, 1987) little starch, sufficient protein, (Scopinaro et al, 1987;Gianetta et al, 1981) and nearly all mono- and disaccharides, short-chain triglycerides, and alcohol (i.e., the energy content of sugar, fruit, sweets, soft drinks, milk, and alcoholic beverages). They must also understand that when their body weight will have reached the level of stabilization the intake of these aliments may be varied as needed for individual weight adjustments.

All patients undergoing BPD have reduced appetite, early satiety and occasionally in association with epigastric pain and/or vomiting. These symptoms characterize the postcibal syndrome and are caused by rapid gastric emptying with subsequent distention of the postanastomotic loop and early food stimulation of the ileum. All these symptoms, which are more intense and last longer the smaller the gastric volume is, rapidly regress with time, most likely due to intestinal adaptation.

One year after operation, the appetite and the eating capacity are fully restored and the patient's mean self-reported food intake is one and a half times as much as preoperatively, independently of gastric volume.

Interestingly, the vasomotory phenomena characterizing the dumping syndrome are always absent after BPD, this indicating the lack of the specific receptors and/or the vasoactive gut hormones in the ileum that are thought to be implicated in the pathogenesis of dumping syndrome.

6.2 Home medication and diet program

Anti-thrombotic prophylaxis is continued up until 30 days after the operation. Patients are prescribed 30 to 60 mg/day of PPI for the first year. Oral multivitamin supplementation is started at discharge, whereas calcium and iron supplementation are begun one month after the operation, when appetite is starting to resume.

Patients are advised to assume a protein-rich diet, in small, frequent meals. In practice, little amounts of bread and pasta may be allowed, whereas milk, vegetables and fruit should be avoided for the first weeks. Frequent vomiting should be immediately reported, because it may be sign of gastric outlet obstruction due to early ulcer, and necessitate not only aggressive PPI treatment, but sometimes also endoscopic dilation, and, to prevent vitamin B1 deficiency and Wernicke's encephalopathy, aggressive vitamin B complex supplementation. In case of near-starvation, we administer intra-muscular vitamin B1 (as cocarboxylase) 38 mg, pyridoxin chloridrate (Vit. B6) 300 mg, and hydroxocobalamine (Vit. B12) 5000 mcg per day for five to ten days.

The first follow-up visit is scheduled 30-45 days after uncomplicated surgery. Although extremely rare, we encountered three cases of early postoperative porto-mesenteric vein thrombosis, which presented as severe, unexplained abdominal pain one week after an otherwise normal discharge. Unexplained severe, unremitting postoperative abdominal pain should therefore be investigated and not attributed to unspecific complaints.

6.3 Bowel habits

After full resumption of food intake, BPD subjects generally have two to four daily bowel movements of soft stools. Most have foul-smelling stools and flatulence. These phenomena, which can be reduced by modifying eating habits or by neomycin or metronidazole or pancreatic enzyme administration, tend to decrease with time along with a reduction of bowel movement frequency and increased stool consistency.

Diarrhea usually appears only in the context of postcibal syndrome, and then it rapidly disappears, being practically absent by the fourth month (Scopinaro et al, 1996). Sporadic acute gastroenterocolitis, generally lasting not more than a few days, may be observed, especially during the summer.

6.4 Follow/up care

Standard follow/up visits are scheduled at one, four and twelve months, and early afterwards. At each outpatient visit, the patient has to check blood exams according to Table. 5 Furthermore, any abnormal clinical condition is annotated and dealt with. In the long term, PTH and vitamins A, D, E are of particular importance, to prevent metabolic bone disease (with adequate oral calcium and parenteral vitamin D supplementation) and emeralopia (vitamin A deficiency)or peripheral neurpathy (vitamin E deficiency). Prompt detection of low values ensures early supplementation and absence of severe symproms.

Postoperative biochemical examination
Complete blood count
Total protein and differential
Na, K, Ca, Cl, P, Ma
Ferritin, Transferritin
Glycated haemoglobin
Serum cholesterol level, LDL, HDL, Triglycerides
Bilirubin (total and direct)
Fibrinogin
Transaminases
LDH, Gamma glutamile transferase
APTT
Amylase
Uricic acid
Creatinine
HBV and HCV marker only after 4th month
PTH, vitamine A, D, E one year after the operation and yearly after
Other exams; complete urine analysis

Table 5. Postoperative laboratory examinations and their frequency.

6.5 Standard supplementation would be

Oral calcium carbonate, 2g per day, increasing or decreasing the dose according to PTH values (and not, in the firs instance, serum calcium levels: Oral "over the counter" multivitamins.

Oral iron sulfate, 500 mg/day, and 1000 mg/day in menstruating women. Oral Vitamin A and E, 30.000 U and 70 mg per day, respectively. Vitamin D is administered on occasional basis when a deficiency is detected

7. Late complications

7.1 Specific complications

7.1.1 Anemia

The exclusion of the primary site for iron absorption in the alimentary tract causes this unavoidable complication. More rarely, the anemia is due to folate deficiency and, exceptionally, to vitamin B12 deficiency (Schilling test gives normal results short term after BPD (Scopinaro et al, 1987, Civalleri et al, 1982). Anemia appears only in BPD patients with chronic physiologic (menstruation) or pathologic (hemorrhoids, stomal ulcer) bleeding. Reflecting the cause of the anemia, most cases are **microcytic**, fewer are **normocytic**, and a few are **macrocytic**. The general incidence of anemia after BPD in our population would probably be around 40%, but chronic supplementation with iron, folate, or both can reduce its occurrence to less than 15%.

7.1.2 Stomal ulcer

BPD is a potentially ulcerogenic procedure. Since the beginning of experimental work in dogs,(Scopinaro et al, 1979) distal gastrectomy was preferred to gastric bypass (Mason & Ito, 1967) because it was thought to be more effective in preventing stomal ulcer (Storer et al, 1950) and because of the concern for the fate of the bypassed stomach (Scopinaro et al, 1992). The incidence of stomal ulcer was initially rather high (12.5% with the HH BPD) because of the large residual parietal cell mass. Considering only the ulcers diagnosed in the first two postoperative years in order to allow comparisons among groups, the incidence was successively reduced to 9.1% in the first 132 consecutive patients submitted to AHS BPD, simply due to the reduced stomach size (Civalleri et al, 1986).

Some changes of surgical technique, namely preserving as much as possible of the gastrolienal ligament with its sympathetic nerve fibers (Scopinaro et al, 1982) and shifting from end-to-end to end-to-side GEA, the latter being better vascularized and less prone to stenosis,(Gianetta et al, 1987) led to further progressive reduction (5.8% in the subsequent 650 cases). In the following group of 640 AHS patients operated on from January 1991 to March 1999 with a minimum follow-up of 2 years, thanks to H2-blockers' oral prophylaxis (Adami et al, 1991) during the first postoperative year in patients at risk (see below), started at the beginning of 1991, the incidence of stomal ulcer in the first 2 years was further reduced to 3.3%.

If the totality of stomal ulcers in the first two groups are considered, they were significantly more frequent in men (14.4%) than in women (5.2%). Differently than what was reported in previous articles, (Scopinaro et al, 1992, 1996, 1998) the incidence of stomal ulcer appeared ***unaffected*** by alcohol consumption, increased in men (though not significantly) by cigarette smoking, and significantly increased, more in women than in men, by the association of alcohol and smoke. Stomal ulcers responded well to medical treatment (100% healing with PPI) and they showed no tendency to recur, provided the patient refrained from smoking. Endoscopic evidence of stomal ulcer was obtained in 52% of cases within the first postoperative year, in 26% of cases within the second year, and in 22% of cases, with progressively decreasing frequency, between the third and the tenth year.

However, it must be considered that (1) most patients diagnosed in the second and the third year were symptomatic already in the first one; (2) most patients diagnosed at a greater distance from the operation had been treated (one or more times) previously because of specific symptoms; (3) many patients once or repeatedly treated because of specific symptoms had refused endoscopy at all instances; (4) in some cases operated patients with no endoscopic diagnosis had received PPI therapy from their family doctors; and (5) with few exceptions, all patients with specific symptoms appearing after the second postoperative year were smokers, or smokers and drinkers. The consideration of all the above facts leads to the conclusions that (1) for BPD patients, not smokers or smokers/drinkers, the risk of developing a peptic ulcer is essentially confined to the first postoperative year and (b) the real incidence of stomal ulcer after BPD is certainly higher than that reported above.

For all these reasons, prophylactic PPIs should be given to all patients for the first year, and probably discontinued in the non/smokers only.

7.1.3 Bone demineralization

The duodenum and proximal jejunum are selective sites for calcium absorption. However, our study on calcium intestinal absorption showed a more than sufficient mean apparent absorption in the 15 subjects on a free diet. Moreover, intestinal absorption as an absolute value was positively correlated with the intake (Kendall rank test: $p < 0.03$), which means that, unlike fat and energy and similarly to protein, an increase of calcium intake results in increased absorption. Therefore, all of our patients are encouraged to maintain an oral calcium intake of 2 g/day (with tablets supplementation, if needed), while the daily requirement of vitamin D, as well as of all other vitamins and trace elements, is contained in a multi-integrator that all patients are recommended to take for all life.

When natural history of bone disease was investigated by us in obese patients and operated subjects not taking any supplementations 1–10 years after BPD, histomorphologic signs of mild to severe bone demineralization (cross-sectional study on 252 transiliac bone biopsies after double-labeling with tetracycline, 58 of which preoperatively) were present in 28% of the obese patients and 62% of the operated subjects. Slightly low levels of serum calcium and high levels of alkaline phosphatase were found in about 20% of the subjects in that study, with no significant differences between obese patients and operated subjects or between operated subjects with and without bone alterations.

Serum magnesium, phosphorus, and 25-hydroxyvitamin D levels were essentially normal both prior to and after operation. The prevalence and severity of metabolic bone disease

(MBD) increased after BPD until the fourth year [prevalence: preop. 16/58, at 4 year 15/21, chi-square test $p < 0.001$; severity (subjects with moderate or severe MBD): preop. 7/58, at 4 year 8/21; chisquare test $p < 0.01$], at which point they tended to regress.

Long-term (6–10 year) mineralization status was not significantly worse than that observed before operation. Patients with the most severe preoperative alterations, i.e., the older and the heavier patients, showed a sharp improvement in bone mineralization status compared to their preoperative status (prevalence of moderate or severe MBD in patients over 45-year-old: preop. 25%, at 1-2 year 29%, at 3-5 year 33%, and at 6–10 year 11%; in patients with an IEW greater than 120% these values were, respectively, 24%, 28%, 53%, and 14%) (Scopinaro et al, 1987, Compston et al, 1984, Adami et al, 1987). The histomorphology data were in total agreement with the clinical findings. Bone pain attributable to demineralization (with prompt regression after calcium, vitamin D only when needed, and diphosphonate therapy) was observed in 6% of patients, generally between the second and fifth postoperative years (maximum prevalence: 2.4% during the fourth year) and more rarely on long term(10–20 years).

The pathogenesis of bone demineralization in obese patients is unclear. The bone problems caused by BPD do not seem to differ substantially from those reported in 25%–35% of postgastrectomy subjects with duodenal exclusion for peptic ulcer (Williams, 1964, Eddy, 1984, Fisher, 1984) and in one-third of patients with gastric bypass for obesity (Crowley et al, 1986). The mechanism is very likely a decreased calcium absorption causing an augmented parathyroid hormone (PTH) release which is generally sufficient to normalize serum calcium level at the expense of bone calcium content. During the first postoperative years, the adverse effect of reduced calcium absorption seems to prevail over the beneficial one of the weight loss, whereas the opposite happens at long term, this being more evident in the subjects with the most severe preoperative alterations.

Recently, it has been suggested that low albumin level is also implicated in the pathogenesis of MBD after BPD (Marceau et al, 2002). In our experience, oral calcium supplementation seems to be able both to prevent and to cure bone alterations caused by BPD, monitored by computerized bone mineralometry. Still, great differences in calcium requirement and metabolism exist among populations and individuals in the same population. Vitamin D synthesis in the skin at different latitudes probably also plays a major role. It is important to remember that parenteral vitamin D supplementation should not be used in the treatment of MBD unless low serum levels have been documented. In fact, an excess of vitamin D can cause bone damage similar to that caused by its deficiency.

7.1.4 Neurological complications

Peripheral neuropathy and Wernicke's encephalopathy, early complications caused by excessive food limitation(Primavera et al, 1987) have now totally disappeared (none in the last consecutive 1,969 operated subjects of the total series with a minimum follow-up of 1 year) because of prompt administration of large doses of thiamin to patients at risk, i.e., those reporting a very small food intake during the early postoperative weeks.

A more insidious cause of peripheral neuropathy is vitamin E deficiency, which can lead to various degrees of impairment, up to ataxia in the most severe cases. Patients reporting paresthesia, especially if long-term after the operation and not well supplemented, should be checked for vitamin E levels and promptly corrected in necessary.

7.1.5 Protein malnutrition

Protein malnutrition (PM), with its classic symptoms, is the most severe possible complication of BPD, and it may require hospitalization with parenteral nutrition. It can be early episodic (1st postoperative year) due to patient non-compliance with alimentary rules to be followed during the first postoperative months, or late recurrent due to insufficient protein intake or intestinal absorption, generally requiring elongation of the CL. Protein absorption after BPD corresponds to ~70% of a meal containing 60 grams of protein.

Unfortunately, our study on protein absorption also showed a five-fold increase in endogenous nitrogen loss, which doubles daily protein requirement and accounts for possible occurrence of PM. This complication in our hands was frequent many years ago, when, with the aim of obtaining greater weight loss, we explored the formidable power of the small stomach volume. The evolution of BPD, essentially consisting of increasing the stomach volume and the length of the AL, eventually led to near disappearance of PM, both in the early and recurrent form. However, as the operation is active for life, sporadic PM can occur at any time after BPD, if there is prolonged diarrhea or reduced food intake for any reason.

Therapy for early or late PM must be aimed at eliminating PEM and restoring normal nutritional status, with parenteral feeding that includes both the nitrogen and the energy necessary to restore the amino acid pool, reestablish the anabolic condition, and resynthesize deficient visceral protein.

In addition to the increased endogenous nitrogen loss, with its impact on daily protein requirement, important phenomenon acting in the same direction is the overgrowth of colonic bacterial flora. Overgrown bacterial flora, the synthesis of which partly or totally occurs at the expense of alimentary protein escaped to absorption in the small bowel, reduces protein absorption by the colonic mucosa, thus increasing protein malabsorption and protein requirement.

Correlation between stomach volume (gastric restriction) and protein malnutrition, At a remote phase of BPD development, in an attempt to accelerate and increase the weight loss, we drastically reduced mean gastric volume to about 150 mL, obtaining, in addition to excellent weight reduction (near 90% of the IEW at 2 years), a catastrophic approximate 30% incidence of PM with 10% recurrence rate .With the aim of decreasing the PM incidence without losing the benefit of the small stomach, the gastric volume was adapted to the patient's initial EW (AHS BPD, June 1984). In fact, the original philosophy of the AHS was to confine the risk of PM to patients who required greater weight loss. It resulted in a 17.1% incidence of PM with 8.3% recurrence, and the mean weight reduction remained at a very satisfactory 77% of the IEW (initial 192 AHS BPD patients with a minimum follow-up of 2 years), the higher weight of stabilization being evidently due to the larger mean stomach volume (about 350 mL) with the consequent slower intestinal transit and greater energy absorption.

Further mean increases in gastric volume to about 400 mL, and of alimentary limb length (up to 250 or 300 cm) led to a further decrease of incidence in protein malnutrition to the present 3% (1% recurrent cases). Interestingly, there is a strong correlation between stomach volume, stabilization weight and protein malnutrition incidence. The smaller the gastric volume, the lower the stabilization weight, and the higher the likelihood of protein malnutrition. These data are an explicit warning against trying to combine gastric restriction with malabsorption.

7.2 Minor or rare late complications

Among the 2756 AHS BPD patients with a minimum follow up of 2 years, the following minor or rare complications were observed or reported: 284 (9%) cases of impairment or appearance of hemorrhoids, 110 (4%) cases of anal rhagades, 55 (2%) cases of perianal abscess, 88 (3.2%) cases of acne, 61 (2.2%) cases of inguino-perineal furuncolosis, 207 (7.5%) cases of night blindness, 4 cases of lipothymias from hypoglycemia, 2 cases of transient dumping syndrome, 1 case of bypass arthritis, and 1 case of gallstone ileus.

These complications showed a decreasing incidence in our population of operated patients. Anyway, they occur more rarely as time passes and tend to disappear in the long term. Halitosis after BPD could be due either to food stagnation in a virtually achloridric stomach, which can be avoided by correct execution of the GEA, or to pulmonary expiration of ill-smelling substances resulting from malabsorption, the oral administration of pancreatic enzymes being of use in these cases. This unpleasant side effect has also become less common in our series, currently affecting less than 5% of the operated patients.

BPD causes oxalate hyperabsorption, but not hyperoxaluria, though oxalate urinary excretion in the operated patients is significantly higher than in controls (Hofmann et al, 1981). The procedure can then be considered a remote cause of kidney stone formation, keeping in mind that not even hyperoxaluria can cause this complication in the absence of cofactors, the first of which is decreased urinary volume from dehydration. The incidence of kidney stones in our series (5/1,804 or 0.3%) does not differ from that of the general population. Thirty-two needle kidney biopsies obtained at long-term relaparotomy in BPD patients failed to demonstrate any microscopic or ultrastructural alterations (unpublished data: study in cooperation with Dr. Thomas Stanley, VA Hospital, Los Angeles, CA, 1984).

7.3 Late mortality

Specific late mortality is essentially attributable to the consequences of untreated protein malnutrition in lately presented or inadequately treated cases.

8. Revision of BPD

8.1 Options available

All specific late reoperations after biliopancreatic diversion (BPD) consisted of;
Elongations of the common limb (CL) which can be done either:
Along the biliopancreatic limb or
Along the alimentary limb
Restorations of intestinal continuity with either

Sparing the duodenum from the alimentary continuity
Putting the duodenum in the alimentary continuity

8.2 Indications to revision of BPD are

1. Recurrent protein malnutrition with or without poor protein intake
2. Excessive Weight loss with normal food intake
3. Excessive Foul Smelling of the stool and Flatulence
4. Diarrhea
5. Intractable severe bone demineralization
6. Occurrence of a disease whose consequences would be worsened by malabsorption
7. Intolerance of the operation

The revision is generally implemented to correct an excess of effect of the original operation, and, because it entails a permanent modification of intestinal absorption, it is critical to ensure that intestinal adaptation mechanisms have been substantially completed, which require at least 1 year. If the problems persist and reoperation is then indicated, the risk of having a premature reoperation with a consequent overcorrection and undue weight regain is minimal.

8.3 Post-revision physiology

Protein, simple sugar and starch absorption depend on the total bowel length between the gastro-enterostomy and the ileo-cecal valve. Fat and bile acid absorption depend on the length of the common limb. Bile acid absorption also depends on the length of ileum which is exposed to bile acid transit.

a. Elongation of the common limb along the biliopancreatic limb leads to an increase of the total intestinal length from the gastroenterostomy to the ileocecal valve, which in turn increases protein, energy and water absorption.
b. Elongation of the common limb along the alimentary limb leads to an increase of bile salt absorption without a direct increase in protein, energy and water absorption, because the total bowel length between the gastroenterostomy and the ileo-cecal valve remains unchanged. Energy absorption increase is also minimal, because only fat absorption is increased.
c. Restoration of intestinal continuity with a bypass of the duodenum allows the resumption of normal protein-energy absorption, still partially preserving both the specific effects of BPD on glucose and cholesterol metabolism.
d. Restoration of the intestinal continuity with re-canalization of the duodenum in the alimentary pathway will sacrifice the effect on glucose metabolism; the effect on cholesterol metabolism is preserved if the alimentary limb is kept interposed between the stomach and the duodenum, because it still entails a reduction of the ileum exposed to bile acid transit (Figure 34–5).

8.4 Problem solving

A recurrent Protein malnutrition (PM) (with or without additional problems) is the condition to be cured in the vast majority of cases. In this case, PM is due to insufficient protein intestinal absorption, either *absolute* (insufficient absorption capacity per unit of intestinal length, too rapid intestinal transit due to excessively little stomach) or *relative* (insufficient protein content of ingested food, excessive loss of endogenous nitrogen).

In both cases the aim of the surgical revision is to increase protein absorption, and this (keeping in mind the physiology of the operation), would not be obtained by elongating the CL along the alimentary one. Since, as said above, protein absorption after BPD substantially depends on the total intestinal length from the GEA to the ICV, the elongation of the CL for correction of a recurrent PM must be performed at the expense of the biliopancreatic limb, the length which in our experience has proven effective in all cases being 150 cm, with the result of a total of 400 cm of small bowel in the food stream (Fig 5).

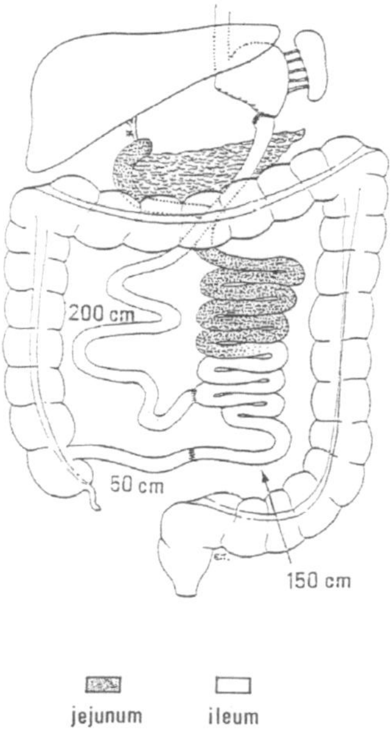

Fig. 5. Elongation of the CL along the BPL.

Excessive weight loss in presence of a normal food intake, problems of *foul-smelling stools and flatulence and diarrhea* due to excessive fluid intake are conditions which can be corrected by elongation of the common limb along the biliopancreatic limb.

Rarely, *diarrhea* is due to excessive reduction of ileal bile salt absorption. This condition can be easily diagnosed by cholestyramine administration, and it represents the only indication to the elongation of the CL along the alimentary one, 100 cm being sufficient in our experience (Fig. 6).

Restoration of the intestinal continuity is specifically indicated in presence of a recurrent PM and/or an excessive weight loss due to permanence of the food limitation effect with or without poor protein intake. The goal in these cases is to restore a normal intestinal absorption capacity in a subject who will maintain his/her weight reduction because of the permanently reduced food intake. This can be obtained with different operations, ranging from a simple high side-to-side enteroenterostomy to the complete reconstruction of the gastrointestinal tract, with a 50-cm ileal loop being interposed between the stomach and the duodenum (Fig. 7).

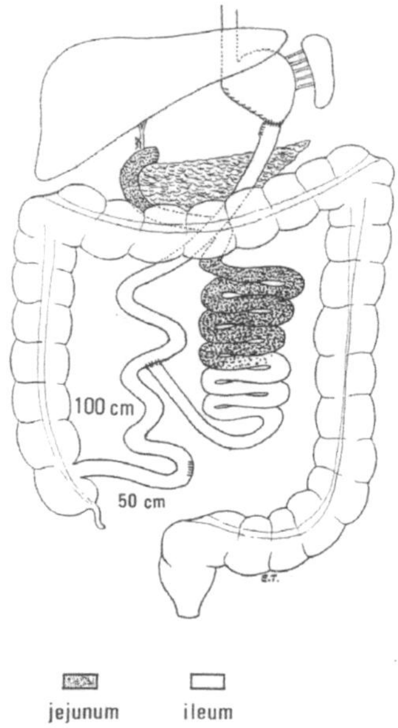

Fig. 6. Elongation of the CL along the AL.

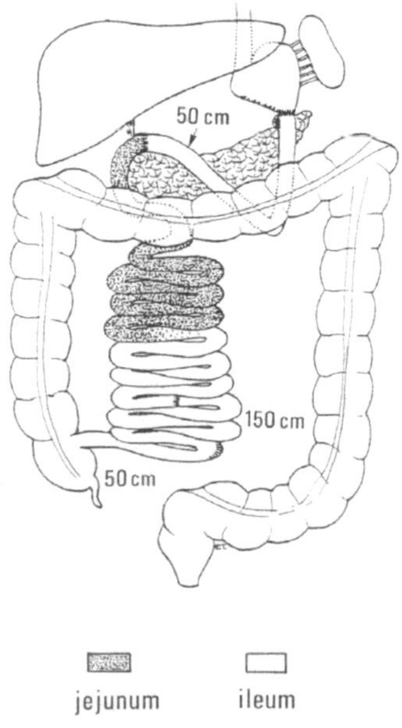

Fig. 7. Full restoration of intestinal continuity.

We prefer to section the alimentary limb (AL) immediately proximal to the enteroenterostomy (EEA) and join the ileal stump to the jejunum, immediately distal to the ligament of Treitz. This type of restoration allows the resumption of a normal protein-energy absorption, still partially preserving both the specific effects of BPD on glucose and cholesterol metabolism (Fig. 8).

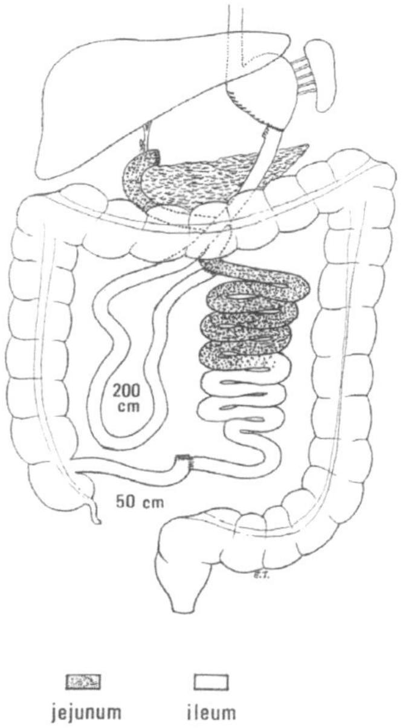

Fig. 8. Restoration bringing the AL to the ligament of Treitz.

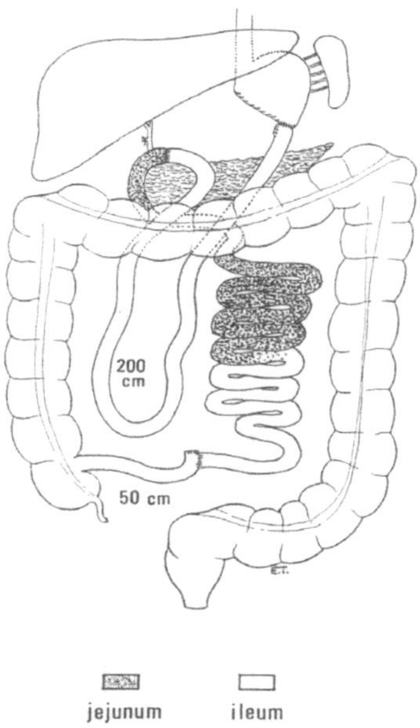

Fig. 9. Restoration bringing the AL to the duodenum.

Restoration may be necessary if **a disease occurs whose consequences would be worsened by malabsorption**, e.g., liver cirrhosis, nephrotic syndrome, chronic inflammatory bowel disease, malignancy, or psychosis. It may also be requested by the BPD subject instead of the elongation after a long period of recurrent PM, or for different reasons, e.g., intolerance of the stool/gas problems, or psychological intolerance of the environmental problems originated by the changed body shape, or what we simply call **"intolerance of the operation."**

Only in case of **intractable severe bone demineralization**, or of moderate bone demineralization associated with a condition that indicates the restoration, we accept the sacrifice of the effect on glucose metabolism by putting the duodenum in the alimentary continuity, which can be accomplished as shown in Figure 34-3, or, if the effect on cholesterol metabolism is to be preserved, by keeping the entire AL interposed between the stomach and the duodenum (Fig. 9).

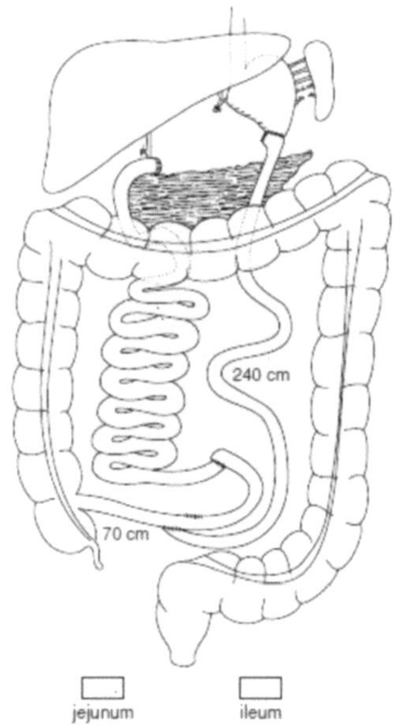

Fig. 10. Shorting of both alimentary and the common.

Exceptionally, a shortening of the intestinal limbs may be considered. The most common cause for **weight regain** after BPD is excessive intake of simple sugar. Only if this type of **patient's noncompliance** can be reasonably excluded, an excess of the adaptive phenomena leading to late energy absorption increase may be suspected. A preliminary measurement of alimentary protein intestinal absorption is, in our opinion, mandatory. More than 90% absorption on the one hand confirms the excessive adaptation, on the other hand it means that there is a wide margin for shortening without causing excessive protein malabsorption.

In two cases, both with 370-cm AL, we resected the proximal part of the AL exceeding the 240cm which, as a mean of the intestinal measurements taken at late reoperations for any cause, result after adaptation, with redo of GEA. Since these two patients failed to lose weight, we thought it could be due to the highly consuming small bowel removed, which compensated for the decreased absorption. In a third case, with 520-cm AL and 80-cm CL, we sectioned the AL 240 cm distal to the GEA, detached the biliopancreatic limb (BPL) from the distal ileum, and then anastomosed the BPL to the distal stump of the AL section and the proximal stump to the distal ileum, thus creating a CL of 70 cm (mean CL length after adaptation), as shown in Figure 9. The patient slowly lost all the excessive weight previously regained. The same operation was subsequently successfully used in another case that had been submitted to BPD elsewhere and had had minimal weight reduction. Both the CL and the AL were excessively long, and this most probably was due to wrong intestinal measurement, even if a rapidly occurring excessive intestinal adaptation could not be ruled out.

8.5 Timing

The total number of revisions in the last consecutive 1000 AHS-AHAL BPD patients with a minimum follow-up of 1 year was 10 or 1.0%, 4 (0.4%) being elongation of the CL and 6 (0.6%) restorations of intestinal continuity. The latter cases presented with ensuing medical problems, unrelated to the operation, which necessitated resumption of normal protein absorption

8.6 Secondary effects

All problems of recurrent PM, excessive weight loss, diarrhea, stool/gas, and bone demineralization permanently disappeared after revisions. While no recurrences of hypercholesterolemia were ever observed, there were two cases of mild hyperglycemia in previously diabetic patients after elongation.

8.7 Weight regain

Since protein and starch digestion/absorption occur in the entire small bowel between the GEA and the ICV, and fat absorption in the intestinal segment between the EEA and the ICV, the elongation of the CL along the BPL which is necessary to increase protein absorption also causes an increase of starch and fat absorption. This obviously results in a higher energy absorption threshold, which explains the restabilization at a higher body weight of the subjects undergoing elongation of the CL for recurrent PM and/or excessive weight loss.

The subjects who were elongated along the AL because of diarrhea from excessive bile salt malabsorption had and maintained a food intake equal to the preoperative one, and they did not gain any weight in a 6- and 11-year follow-up, respectively.

The weight changes after BPD revisions indicate that, when the indication was correctly given by us according to the physiology of the operation, the revised subjects had a moderate weight regain with restabilization, the success being maintained, while in the other cases they regained weight progressively toward failure.

A final consideration regards the mean weight loss at the time of revision, which was in most cases lower than the average in our series. Any degree of weight reduction can be obtained with BPD, but, as we learned at our expenses, the greater the mean weight loss, the greater the number of problems. Unless a surgeon has an experience sufficient to enable him to tailor the operation on each single subject, any mean reduction of the IEW greater than 70% should be considered potentially dangerous. Weight maintenance, not weight loss, is the real magic of BPD.

9. Revision to BPD

The superior results of BPD both in weight maintenance and control of component of metabolic syndrome make this operation a good choice for revision of failed other types of bariatric procedures. Furthermore, revision to BPD often enables the surgeon to avoid scarred tissue high up in the stomach, thus simplifying reoperation and reducing perioperative morbidity.

Revisional Bariatric surgery is technically challenging and becoming more common due to the rapid increase in patients undergoing surgery for morbid obesity. Unfortunately, there is no sufficient evidence to help the surgeon deciding which revisional procedure to choose based. There are several factors that need to be considered when unsatisfactory outcomes after bariatric surgery are obtained.

The extent of weight loss may not be the only factor to be considered while evaluating the results of a bariatric restrictive procedure, because the major goal of bariatric procedures is the cure or control of comorbidities along with the weight loss. With this idea in mind, a borderline weight loss with a successful control of comorbidities (eg, easier hypertension or diabetes control, disappearance of articular pain or swelling, cure of sleep apnea, etc.) in a high-risk patient without surgery-related complications should probably be considered a good outcome, and the patient could avoid additional surgery. These issues should be clarified with the patient when discussing risks and benefits of the reoperation.

Both patient and surgeon need to be aware that a new operation will be a difficult task, and realistic goals have to be presented to the patient. There is a higher risk of complications, and a possibility that a new bariatric procedure may not be completed in one intervention as planned owing to inflammation, scarring, and bleeding. Patients must know that more than one intervention may be required. Unlike gastric restrictive revisional surgery, revision to BPD usually does not impair final weight loss results.

9.1 Indications for revision

1. Insufficient weight loss.
2. Weight regain.
3. Complications of previous the procedure.

9.2 Patient evaluation

Surgeons should consider that failure of specific restrictive bariatric procedures is owing to many factors. One of these factors is patient's compliance with the dietary program, and when required, with behavioral modifications after the primary procedure. Patients may not need a second surgery but a close follow-up and behavior counseling before deciding on a more drastic intervention.

9.3 Approach to the patient

Detailed evaluation of the preoperative data of the these patients, operative notes and postoperative BMI and complications through a Pre-operative check-list;

1. History and Physical examination;
   BMI
   Symptoms of dysmotility
   Symptoms of acid hypersecretion
   Screening for eating disorders
   Psychological evaluation if positive
2. Review old operative notes and videos if possible
3. Barium swallow to document anatomy
4. EGD if patient has symptoms of GERD

Imaging and endoscopic studies are necessary to study the problem and give an accurate map of the existing anatomy. As restrictive bariatric procedures are practiced following different techniques with modifications of some of the originally described steps, it is advisable to read the operative note or to discuss the case with the surgeon who carried out the index surgery.

9.4 General considerations

Revisional bariatric surgery is technically demanding. There are technical aspects common to any reoperation after gastric surgeries that need to be taken into account to minimize complications.

Adhesions are likely to be present and they may be anywhere. Therefore, access to the cavity should be attained by open technique, or alternatively using an optical trocar, trying to prevent visceral injuries.

Once in the cavity, following ports should be placed in an order that allows dividing the adhesions from the best point of view. In addition, liver retraction should be done delicately, and only after its adhesions have been addressed, because any sudden movement or excessive force could produce a tear, and bleeding will obscure the surgical field, reducing visibility and causing delays.

Division of gastric vessels should only be carried out after the gastric vascular supply has been assessed. Restrictive procedures usually preserve lesser curvature vessels, and therefore these should be preserved at all costs. If the left gastric artery or its branches need to be cut at some stage, the condition of the stomach must to be carefully observed to rule out ischemia leading to gastric resection.

Intraoperative endoscopy is a valuable tool when during the procedure it is difficult to accurately characterize the anatomic changes seen during the laparoscopy. It should be scheduled beforehand to avoid delays in a possibly long intervention.

9.5 Open versus laparoscopic approach

Laparoscopic surgery has had a major impact on obesity surgery the last decade. All bariatric procedures have been proven to be technically feasible via laparoscopy (Buchwald et al, 2004). There is also evidence that the laparoscopic approach is advantageous, since it is associated with less perioperative morbidity and faster recovery (The Society of American Gastrointestinal and Endoscopic Surgeons (SAGES) Guidelines Committee , 2008; Weller

Rosati, 2008) . Laparoscopic approach to malabsorption procedures, such as the BPD or the duodenal switch operation (DS), is more complex and technically difficult (Scopinaro et al, 2002; Baltasar et al, 2002; Weiner et al, 2004). Several reports have demonstrated the efficacy of laparoscopic revisional bariatric surgery (Gumbs et al, 2007). However, laparoscopic re-do surgery, after failed primary bariatric procedures, should be handled cautiously. Van Dessel et al, 2008 reported recently that the threshold for conversion to open approach should be low.

In patients after failed or complicated bariatric operations, it is the surgical management that eventually matters and not the approach.

9.6 Which type of revision? And why BPD?

Surgeons differ in their management of failed bariatric procedures, depending on their individual experience and resultant choice of surgical operation or operations. Revision of failed gastric restrictive operation is a common problem today, and is likely to increase in the near future (Sarr, 2007). In our opinion, the conversion of a restrictive operation to a malabsorptive one appears for some patients as the only alternative to cope with poor weight loss results. Such conversions, after unsuccessful weight loss, have been previously described (Fox, 1991; Keshishian et al, 2004; Di Betta et al, 2006). Since gastric bypass relies primarily on restriction, a different surgical approach, based essentially on malabsorption was employed as the final option in this cohort of patients with multiple previous bariatric interventions. In a recent report, (Topart et al, 2007) demonstrated that BPD with duodenal switch resulted in greater weight loss compared to Roux-en-Y gastric bypass after failed gastric banding. However, BPD-DS resulted in a higher early complication rate. When compared to RYGB, BPD and BPD-DS procedures are suggested to create superior weight loss and more accurately, superior weight loss maintenance (DeMaria, 2004).

In a recent analysis, it was demonstrated that obesity surgery results depend on the performed technique. BPD was proven to be the only operation that kept excellent weight results in time but unfortunately, with increased morbidity (Gracia et al, 2009). So far, no adequate prospective trial has been done to adequately answer the question of "which revisional bariatric procedure to do" in the setting of inadequate weight loss or excessive weight regain (Gumbs et al, 2007).

Furthermore, failed RYGB represent a subset of particularly challenging cases, in which only BPD can provide adequate results. Conversion from RYGB to biliopancreatic diversion with duodenal switch (BPD-DS) might provide the most durable weight loss of all revision procedures currently available. Revision to BPD-DS can be done laparoscopically in 1 or 2 stages and involves 4 anastomoses: gastrogastrostomy, duodenoileostomy, ileoileostomy, and jejunojejunostomy (to reconnect the old Roux limb).

10. Duodenal switch

Duodenal Switch (DS), is the malabsorptive procedure that is usually performed in North America for treatment of morbid obesity. In 1987, DeMeester, in some experimental studies conducted on biliary gastritis, showed that keeping even a short duodenal limb could significantly reduce the incidence of anastomotic ulcers. By transferring these observations to bariatric context, the goal of the Duodenal Switch (DS) variation of Biliopancreatic Diversion (BPD) proposed by Douglas Hess and Picard Marceau was to reduce the complications correlated with Scopinaro's original procedure while maintaining its long-term effectiveness on weight loss and co-morbidities resolution.

10.1 Modifications

The modifications adopted in DS are: modifying the distal gastrectomy of the BPD with a vertical gastrectomy along the greater curvature (sleeve gastrectomy). Further modification foresaw the lengthening of the common channel to 100cm, thus doubling the length of the absorbent common ileal segment, for greater control of the number of daily bowel movements. Some procedures that are consensual to BPD, like cholecystectomy, appendectomy and liver biopsies were routinely performed by different authors even in the DS variation. These modifications have led, according to the same authors, to the reduction in the incidence of dumping syndrome, anastomotic ulcer, and proteins malabsorption.

Analysing the results of open BPD vs. DS, Marceau reports fewer daily evacuations, less diarrhea, vomiting and bone pain following DS associated with higher serum levels of ferritin, calcium and Vitamin A.

Whether this report is simply the result of a progressive learning curve (standard BPD had been adopted in the early experience, and BPD with DS had been further developed in later years), or if the longer length of the common channel, by increasing bile acid absorption, and thus lowering the degree of steatorrhea, leads to fewer bowel movements per day, and, consequently, to less endogenous nitrogen loss, has never been studied in a prospective fashion. In fact, most recent publications report very similar results and side effects for both operations. Just as for standard BPD, BPD- DS primarily induces malabsorption of fats due to the diversion of bile and pancreatic enzymes to the common limb. Therefore, the length of the alimentary limb and the common limb is of the fundamental importance; if the common channel is too long, the malabsorption of fats might not be sufficient to guarantee an adequate weight loss over the long term; an excessively long alimentary limb leads to insufficient weight loss for insufficient malabsorption of starch.

Duodenal switch might nonetheless be a better option in revision of failed sleeve gastrectomies, as the latter operation had in fact been introduced in clinical practice as the first stage of BPD-DS in super-superobese patients.

10.2 Peri- and postoperative complications

10.2.1 Fistula

Suture line dehiscence can occur at the gastric suture after sleeve gastrectomy, at both anastomoses and at the duodenal stump. The incidence of suture-line leak after sleeve gastrectomy ranges between 1.3% and 4.6% (Hess, 1998, Lee et al, 2007). The critical areas for leak are the top of the suture line and the transition point between sequential cartridges. To prevent leak many authors suggest reinforcing the long suture line with buttress material, a running suture or fibrin glue. The suture line fistula can be managed by percutaneous drainage plus total parenteral nutrition and antibiotics associated, in selected cases, with endoscopic stenting.

Anastomotic leak seems to have the same incidence rate in LapBPD-DS as in the open series (2.5%) (Marceau et al, 1998, Ren et al, 2000, Lee et al, 2007). The clinical presentations involves tachycardia (heart rate >120 beats /minute), fever, abdominal pain, hypotension and mental deadness. To make the correct diagnosis an upper GI X-ray can be useful, but a negative contrast X-ray study does not exclude a fistula.

Therefore, a spiral angioCT scan is the most accurate diagnostic tool in doubtful cases. In case of low output fitulas and when there are no signs of haemodynamic instability, management could be conservative. Failure of nonoperative management or signs of peritonitis, a laparoscopic or laparoscopic reoperation is indicated. Options includes suture of the anastomotic dehiscence, wide drainage and/or with the creation of a jejunostomy in the biliopancreatic limb for decompression and for enteral nutrition and supportive care. Compared to the most recent series of standard BPD, fistula incidence after BPD-DS seems higher.

11. Conclusions

BPD yields the best results obtained in the treatment of obesity and metabolic syndrome. The reasons why, although in use for more than 35 years, this operation still has relatively minimal diffusion in the world are many, and they have little to do with its effectiveness and safety. However, this is to be considered a favorable event: BPD would cause dramatic damages if improperly used, and this would certainly happen if the operation had a rapid diffusion among the average bariatric surgeon. For the same reason, being able to master BPD and its complications, and understanding its pathophysiology, is extremely important for a committed bariatric surgeon, because, *at the very least*, it represents a very powerful and effective weapon in difficult revisional cases and in the metabolically highly compromised patient. To be limited to a slowly increasing number of good hands is the main guarantee of safety for biliopancreatic diversion.

12. References

Adami GF, Compston JE, Gianetta E, et al.(1987) Changes in bone histomorphometry following biliopancreatic diversion. In: *Proceedings of the III International Symposium on Obesity Surgery,* Genoa, Italy, September 1987.

Adami GF, Gandolfo P, Esposito M, et al. (1991). Orally-administered serum ranitidine concentration after biliopancreatic diversion. Obes Surg, 1, 293–294.

Adami GF, Cordera R, Camerini G, et al. (2003) Recovery of Insulin Sensitivity in Obese Patients at Short Term after Biliopancreatic Diversion.J Surg Res.113, 217–221.

Adami GF, Murelli F, Briatore L, et al. (2008). Pregnancy in Formerly Type 2 Diabetes Obese Women Following Biliopancreatic Diversion for Obesity. Obes Surg.18, 1109–1111.

Ast M, Frishman WH. (1990) Bile acid sequestrants. J Clin Pharmacol.30, 99–106.

Baltasar A, Bou R, Miró J, et al. (2002)Laparoscopic biliopancreatic diversion with duodenal switch: technique and initial experience. Obes Surg.12, 245–248.

Beil U, Crouse JR, Einarsson K, et al. (1982) Effects of interruption of the enterohepatic circulation of bile acids on the transport of very low density-lipoprotein triglycerides. Metabolism.31, 438–444.

Borg CM, le Roux CW, Ghatei MA, et al. (2007) Biliopancreatic Diversion in Rats is Associated with Intestinal Hypertrophy and with Increased GLP-1, GLP-2 and PYY levels. Obes Surg.17, 1193–1198.

Brandi LS, Santoro D, Natali A, et al. (1993) Insulin Resistance of Stress: Sites and Mechanisms. Clin Sci (Lond).85, 525–535.

Briatore L, Salani B, Andraghetti G, et al. (2008) Restoration of Acute Insulin Response in T2DM Subjects 1 Month after Biliopancreatic Diversion. Obesity.16, 77–81.

Buchwald H, Avidor Y, Braunwald E, et al. (2004)Bariatric surgery: a systematic review and meta-analysis. JAMA. 292, 1724- 1737.

Buchwald H, Estok R, Fahrbach K, et al. (2009) Weight and Type 2 Diabetes after Bariatric Surgery: Systematic Review and Meta analysis. Am J Med.122, 248–256.

Civalleri D, Scopinaro G, Gianetta E, et al. (1982)Assorbimento della vitamina B12 dopo bypass biliopancreatico per l'obesit`a. Min Diet Gastroenterol. 28, 181–188.

Civalleri D, Gianetta E, FriedmanD, et al. (1986): Changes of gastric acid secretion after partial biliopancreatic bypass. Clin Nutr, 5 (Suppl), 215- 220.

Compston JE,Vedi S, Gianetta E, et al. (1984) Bone histomorphometry and vitamin D status after biliopancreatic bypass for obesity. Gastroenterology, 87, 350–356.

Crowley LV, Seay J, Mullin GT Jr, et al. (1986). Long term hematopoietic and skeletal effects of gastric bypass. Clin Nutr, 5(Suppl),185–187.

DeMaria EJ. (2004) Is gastric bypass superior for the surgical treatment of obesity compared with malabsorptive procedures? J Gastrointest Surg, 8, 401–403.

Di Betta E, Mittempergher F, Di Fabio F, et al. (2006) Duodenal switch without gastric resection after failed gastric restrictive surgery for morbid obesity. Obes Surg, 16, 258–261.

Doyle ME, Egan JM. (2007). Mechanisms of Action of Glucagone-like Peptide 1 in the Pancreas. Pharmacol Ther,113, 546–593.

Eddy RL: (1984) Metabolic bone disease after gastrectomy. AmJMed, 8, 293–302.

Farilla L, Bulotta A, Hirshberg B, et al. (2003) Glucagon-like Peptide 1 Inhibits Cell Apoptosis and Improve Glucose Responsiveness of Freshly Isolated Human Islets. Endocrinology,144, 5149- 5158.

Fisher AB: (1984). Twenty-five years after Billroth II gastrectomy for duodenal ulcer.World J Surg 8:293–302,.

Forbes GB. (1987). Human Body composition; Growth, aging and nutrition and activity. Springer Verlag New York, 1987.

Fox SR. (1991) The use of biliopancreatic diversion as a treatment for failed gastric partitioning in the morbidly obese. Obes Surg, 1, 89–93.

Gianetta E, Civalleri D, Bonalumi U, et al. (1980). Studio dell'assorbimento proteico dopo bypass bilio-pancreatico per l'obesit`a. MinDiet e Gastr, 26, 251–256.

Gianetta E, Civalleri D, Bonalumi U, et al. (1981). Studio dell'assorbimento lipidico dopo bypass biliopancreatico per l'obesit`a. Min Diet e Gastr, 27, 65–70.

Gianetta E, Friedman D, Adami GF, et al. (1985). Effects of biliopancreatic bypass on hypercholesterolemia and hypertriglyceridemia. In: Proceedings of the Second Annual Meeting of the American Society forBariatric Surgery, Iowa City, IA, June 1985.

Gianetta E, Friedman D, Adami GF, et al. (1987). Present status of biliopancreatic diversion (BPD). In: Proceedings of the Third International Symposium on Obesity Surgery. Genoa, Italy, September, 1987.

GriffenWO, Printen KJ (eds.). (1987) Surgical Management of Morbid Obesity. Marcel Dekker, New York.

Guidone C, Manco M, Valera-Mora E, et al. (2006) Mechanisms of Recovery from Type 2 Diabetes after Malabsorptive Bariatric Surgery. Diabetes,55, 2025–2031.

Gumbs AA, Pomp A, Gagner M. (2007) Revisional bariatric surgery for inadequate weight loss. Obes Surg, 17, 1137–1145.

Halverson JD, Scheff RJ, Gentry K, et al. (1980). Jeunoileal bypass. Late metabolic sequelae and weight gain. Am J Surg, 140, 347–350.

Hess DW. (1998) Biliopancreatic Diversion with a Duodenal Switch, Obes Surg, 8, 267-282.

Hofmann AF, Schnuck G, Scopinaro N, et al. (1981) Hyperoxaluria associated with intestinal bypass surgery for morbid obesity: Occurrence, pathogenesis and approaches to treatment. Int J Obes, 5 , 513–518.

Keshishian A, Zahriya K, Hartoonian T, et al. (2004) Duodenal switch is a safe operation for patients who have failed other bariatric operations. Obes Surg, 14, 1187–1192.

Lee CM, Cirangle PT, Jossart GH; (2007), Vertical gastrectomy for morbid obesity in 216 patients report of two years. Surg Endosc, 21 ,1810-1816.

Marceau P, Hould FS, Simart S, et al.(1998). Biliopancreatic Diversion with Duodenal Switch, World J Surg, 22 , 947-954.

Marceau P, Biron S, Lebel S, et al. (2002). Does bone change after biliopancreatic diversion? J Gastrointest Surg, 6 , 690–698.

Marinari G, Adami GF, Camerini G, et al.(1997). The effect of biliopancreatic diversion on serum cholesterol. Obes Surg, 7 , 297.

Mason EE, Ito C: (1967) Gastric bypass in obesity. Surg Clin North Am, 47 ,1345–1352.

McAuley K, Mann J. (2006) Thematic Review Series: Patient Oriented Research. Nutritional Determinants of Insulin Resistance. J Lipid Res, 47, 1668–1676.

Montagna G, Gianetta E, Elicio N, et al.(1987).Plasma lipid and apoprotein pattern in patients with morbid obesity before and after biliopancreatic bypass. Atheroscl Cardiovasc Dis, 3 ,1069–1074.

Polyzogopoulou EV, Kalfarentzos F, Vagenakis AG, et al.(2003). Restoration of Euglycemia and Normal Acute Insulin Response to Glucose in Obese Subjects with Type 2 Diabetes Following Bariatric Surgery. Diabetes, 52 ,1098–1103.

Primavera A, Schenone A, Simonetti S, et al.: (1987) Neurological disorders following biliopancreatic diversion. In: Proceedings of the Third International Symposium on Obesity Surgery, Genoa, Italy, September, 1987.

Ren CJ, Patterson E, Gagner M. (2000) early results of biliopancreatic diversion with duodenal switch; a case series of 40 consecutive patients. Obes surg, 10 , 514-523.

SAGES Guidelines Committee. SAGES guideline for clinical application of laparoscopic bariatric surgery. Surg Endosc. 2008; 22:2281–300.

SarrMG. (2007) Reoperative bariatric surgery. Surg Endosc, 21 ,1909–1913.

Scopinaro N: (1974) Intervento in Tavola rotonda su: Trattamento medicochirurgico della obesit`a grave. Accad Med, 88–89 ,215–234.

Scopinaro N, Gianetta E, Civalleri D, et al. (1979) . Bilio-pancreatic by-pass for obesity, I: An experimental study in dogs. Br J Surg , 66 , 613–617.

Scopinaro N, Gianetta E, Civalleri D, et al. (1979) . Bilio-pancreatic by-pass for obesity, II: Initial experience in man. Br J Surg , 66 , 619-620.

Scopinaro N, Gianetta E, Civalleri D, et al. (1980) . Two years of clinical experience with biliopancreatic bypass for obesity. Amer J Clin Nutr, 33 , 506-514.

ScopinaroN, Gianetta E, FriedmanD, et al. (1992) . Biliopancreatic diversion for obesity. Probl Gen Surg , 9 , 362-379.

Scopinaro N, Gianetta E, Adami GF, et al. (1996) . Biliopancreatic diversion for obesity at eighteen years. Surgery, 119 , 261-268.

Scopinaro N, Adami GF, Marinari G, et al. (1997) . The effect of biliopancreatic diversion on glucose metabolism. Obes Surg, 7 , 296-297.

Scopinaro N, Marinari GM, Gianetta E, et al. (1997) . The respective importance of the alimentary limb (AL) and the common limb (CL) in protein absorption (PA) after BPD. Obes Surg, 7 , 108.

Scopinaro N, Adami GF, Marinari GM, et al. (1998) . Biliopancreatic diversion. World J Surg, 22 , 936-946.

Scopinaro N, Marinari GM, Adami GF, et al. (1999) . The influence of gastric volume on energy and protein absorption after BPD. Obes Surg , 2 , 125-126.

Scopinaro N, Marinari GM, Camerini G, et al. (2000) . Energy and nitrogen absorption after biliopancreatic diversion. Obes Surg , 10 , 436-441.

Scopinaro N, Marinari GM, Camerini G. (2002) . Laparoscopic standard biliopancreatic diversion: technique and preliminary results. Obes Surg , 12 , 241-244.

Scopinaro N, Marinari GM, Camerini GB, et al. (2005) . Specific Effects of Biliopancreatic Diversion on the Major Components of Metabolic Syndrome: A Long-term Follow-up Study. Diabetes Care , 28 , 2406-2411.

Scopinaro N, Papadia F, Camerini G, et al. (2008) . A Comparison of a Personal Series of Biliopancreatic Diversion and Literature Data on Gastric Bypass Help to Explain the Mechanisms of Resolution of Type 2 Diabetes by the Two Operations. Obes Surg ,18 ,1035-1038.

Scopinaro N, Adami GF, Papadia FS, et al. (2011) . Effects of biliopancreatic diversion on type 2 diabetes in patients with BMI 25-35. Ann Surg , 253 , 699-703.

Storer EH,Woodward ER, Dragstedt LR: (1950) . The effect of vagotomy and antrum resection on the Mann-Williamson ulcer. Surgery , 27 , 526- 530.

Thorell A, Nygren J, Ljungqvist O. (1999) Insulin Resistance: A Marker of Surgical Stress. Curr Opin Clin Nutr Metab Care , 2 , 69-78.

Topart P, Becouarn G, Ritz P. (2007) . Biliopancreatic diversion with duodenal switch or gastric bypass for failed gastric banding: retrospective study from two institutions with preliminary results. Surg Obes Relat Dis , 3 , 521-525.

Valverde I, Puente J,Martín-Duce A, et al. (2005) Changes in Glucagon-like Peptide-1 (GLP-1) Secretion after Biliopancreatic Diversion or Vertical Banded Gastroplasty in Obese Subjects. Obes Surg ,15 , 387-397.

Van Dessel E, Hubens G, Ruppert M, et al. (2008). Roux-en-Y gastric bypass as a re-do procedure for failed restricive gastric surgery. Surg Endosc , 22 , 1014-1018.

Weiner RA, Blanco-Engert R, Weiner S, et al. (2004) . Laparoscopic biliopancreatic diversion with duodenal switch: three different duodeno-ileal anastomotic techniques and initial experience. Obes Surg , 14 ,334-340.

Weller WE, Rosati C. (2008) . Comparing outcomes of laparoscopic versus open bariatric surgery. Ann Surg , 248 , 10-5.

Wickremesekera K, Miller G, Naotunne TD, et al. (2005) Loss of Insulin Resistance after Roux-en-Y Gastric Bypass Surgery: A Time Course Study. Obes Surg ,15 , 474-481.

Williams JA: (1964) Effects of upper gastro-intestinal surgery on blood formation and bone metabolism. Br J Surg , 51 , 125-134.

Xu G, Stoffers DA, Habener JF, et al. (1999) . Exendin-4 Stimulates Both Beta-cell Replication and Neogenesis, Resulting in Increased Beta-cell Mass. Diabetes ,48 , 2270-2276.

Body Weight and Energy Intake and Expenditure in Bariatric Surgery

Maria Rita Marques de Oliveira, Patrícia Fátima Sousa Novais, Karina Rodrigues Quesada, Carolina Leandro de Souza, Irineu Rasera Junior and Celso Vieira de Souza Leite
UNESP - Universidade Estadual Paulista – Botucatu-SP, Clinica Bariátrica – Hospital dos Fornecedores de Cana, Piracicaba-SP, Brazil

1. Introduction

Body weight is ultimately determined by energy homeostasis, a complex process of regulation. Homeostasis is one of the greatest challenges for understanding the etiology, treatment and prevention of obesity (Hill, 2006). The high rate of weight regain in individuals who undergo weight loss treatments is proof of this (Melo et al., 2008). Even among morbidly obese individuals submitted to more radical treatments, such as surgery, weight regain sometimes occurs [Fogaça, 2009]. In this sense, energy intake and expenditure assessments represent extremely important factors, both for studies and as an aid in the process of caring for the obese.

Given the premise that all obesity treatment methods are based on reducing food intake and increasing energy metabolism, the present chapter intends to discuss the variables in the energy balance equation using the results from works of the research group *Bariatric Surgery and Metabolism* of Paulista State University - UNESP, Campus Botucatu, São Paulo, Brazil, and of the Bariatric C.inic of Piracicaba, São Paulo, Brazil, as reference. Components of energy metabolism and indirect calorimetry will be discussed.

Indirect calorimetry is a reference method that has been used for almost 100 years for measuring energy intake in humans during resting or physical activity. Studies using indirect calorimetry allow assessing the effects of energy intake, physical activity and other factors involved in the energy metabolism on the total body mass of obese individuals or its compartments. Here, indirect calorimetry was used to assess the agreement between itself and prediction formulas, to discuss the effects of food restriction and to assess energy intake underreporting by obese women submitted to food intake surveys. Indirect calorimetry data also allow one to discuss the effects of weight loss and body mass index on energy expenditure and biochemical indicators of glucose and fat metabolism. These studies allowed the elucidation of some energy metabolism particularities of individuals who undergo bariatric surgery, as well as the proposition of some hypotheses for new studies.

2. Energy expenditure and food restriction

Daily total energy expenditure (TEE) is the term used for defining the amount of energy necessary for an organism to perform its vital functions and activities of daily living. TEE consists of the resting energy expenditure (REE), which is the energy used by the body during rest, that is, in bed, under comfortable environmental conditions (60-75% do TEE), by food-induced thermogenesis, which is the heat effect of foods (5-15% do GET) and by energy spent on physical activities, considered the most variable component of the TEE and which can contribute to a significant amount of the energy spent by very active individuals (Meirelles & Gomes, 2004, Prentice, 2007).

Indirect calorimetry is a noninvasive technique used to measure the volume and concentration of the gases inhaled by the lungs and allows the calculation of the amount of oxygen (O_2) consumed and the production of carbonic gas (CO_2). These values may stem from the baseline energy expenditure (BEE), the REE and the respiratory quotient (RQ), given by the equation: exhaled CO_2 /inhaled O_2 (Simyrnios & Curley, as in Rippe et al., 1996). There is a difference between BEE and REE. The BEE corresponds to the energy expenditure that occurs during a 12- to 14-hour fast and with the individual resting in the supine position, awake and immobile, under comfortable environmental conditions. This standardized metabolic state corresponds to the situation in which foods and physical activity have the least influence on metabolism (Institute of Medicine, 2005). Meanwhile, REE is obtained while the individual is awake in the supine position and includes the energy used during awakeness plus the energy used for food metabolism, or thermogenesis (Institute of Medicine, 2005). Both BEE and REE are influenced by gender, age, nutritional status and endocrine problems.

Thermogenesis, or thermal effect of foods, corresponds to the increase in energy expenditure after food intake for digestion to occur and for the substrates to be transformed and stored. It represents roughly 5 to 10% of the TEE (Institute of Medicine, 2005; Prentice, 2007). Thermogenesis intensity and duration are determined primarily by the amount and composition of the foods consumed (Flatt, as cited in Bray, 1978). The use of proteins demands more energy than the use of carbohydrates, which demands more energy than the use of fats (Institute of Medicine, 2005, 1998, Larson et al., 1995). High-fat diets promote a low RQ. For carbohydrates, the RQ equals 1.00; for proteins, 0.82; and for fats, 0.70. For mixed diets, the RQ of 0.85 is usually used (Rosado & Monteiro, 2001).

Physical activity is the most variable component of energy expenditure, varying both from individual to individual and from one day to the next. In inactive individuals, it represents roughly 15% of the TEE, while in active individuals it may exceed 30% of the TEE (World Health Organization, 1998). Physical activity can lead to steep increases in TEE because of the energy cost to perform the exercise and to recover from the exercise, or in the long-term, by changing the REE by increasing the amount of lean mass (Hill et al., 1995). The level of physical activity is commonly described as the ratio between TEE and REE (TEE:REE). This ratio is known as the level of physical activity level (PAL) and is used to asses physical activity habits as a component of daily energy expenditure (Institute of Medicine, 2005).

The doubly-labeled water with deuterium and oxygen-18 technique, although less accessible, has been used increasingly for TEE assessment. The method, based on the principle of isotope dilution, consists in the ingestion of water containing ^2H_2O and $H_2{}^{18}O$.

The labeled elements are then measured in organic fluids, namely blood and urine. The equations for predicting the energy requirements proposed by the Institute of Medicine (2005) in the Dietary Reference Intakes (DRI) stemmed from studies using doubly-labeled water in normal weight, pre-obese and obese populations. Studies with doubly-labeled water have made the generalized low-metabolism hypothesis associated with obesity less evident.

Many researchers have observed that obese individuals, contrary to the expected, present a high REE, that is, their metabolic rate is not low (Das et al., 2004; Prentice, 2007). Obese individuals present a higher amount of lean mass, the main REE determinant (Prentice et al., 1986; Prentice, 2007; Ravussin et al., 1986). The occurrence of less energy expenditure in other components of the energy metabolism has also been studied in obese individuals. Danforth (1985) noticed reduced thermogenesis from foods. Other authors have showed that REE is influenced by regular physical activity, diet, blood pressure, as well as hormones and cytokines (Trayhurn et al., 1995; Hardie et al., 1996). Genetic predisposition must also be considered a determinant of energy expenditure.

Many genes of the molecular components of physiological systems that regulate energy balance are involved in obesity (Duarte et al., 2007; Yurtcu et al., 2009). Examples of this are the polymorphisms found in genes of the uncoupling proteins 2 and 3 (UCP2 and UCP3) and in leptin receptors (LEPR) (Jacobson et al., 2006). Polymorphism Gln223Arg of the gene LEPR, for example, has already been associated with obesity in a sample of the Brazilian population, and it presented a strong association with body mass index - BMI (Duarte et al., 2007). Studies with rats show that leptin can reduce adiposity both by promoting changes in eating habits and by increasing energy expenditure (Halaas et al., 1995). Ghrelin, a gastric peptide involved in the regulation of satiety and oxidation of energy substrates, is of interest for genetic studies on the weight loss mechanisms promoted by bariatric surgery (Marzullo et al., 2004). The regulation of ghrelin effects on hypothalamic neurons has been suggested as the most important mechanism by which leptin controls energy intake and body weight (Sahu, 2004).

In some people, low energy expenditure could be explained by adaptive thermogenesis, which would occur naturally or as a consequence of dietary restrictions. There is evidence that low energy intake is a predictor of weight gain and that, in individuals who undergo weight loss therapies, decreased REE is associated with weight regain over time (Doucet et al. 2000). In this sense, food restriction promotes adaptive physiological mechanisms that serve as a defense of the body to maintain body weight, resulting in less energy expenditure (Negrão & Licino, 2000). Hence, food restriction produces weight loss under adaptive conditions. The Institute of Medicine (2005), in the energy DRI assumes a reduction of 7.2 Kcal for each lost gram, which corresponds to 16.6 Kcal of TEE reduction at each kilogram lost. Furthermore, it considers a reduction of 8.4% of the TEE after 10 weeks of food restriction because of the adaptation to food restriction. In our studies, we have observed that in fact there is not a linear relationship between energy intake and body weight homeostasis. As shown by Figure 1, there is no correlation between total dietary energy and weight loss among obese women but there is a weak correlation between the reduced proportion of the total energy (TE) intake. This shows how relevant it is to personalize the diet plan considering the adaptation of the energy metabolism to restrictive diets. Caution is also warranted when prescribing excessively restrictive diets. Another relevant finding of our study group that corroborates this statement was that there is a negative correlation between the reported number of attempts of losing weight and the resting energy expenditure measured by indirect calorimetry, assessed in 100 women in the waiting line for bariatric surgery.

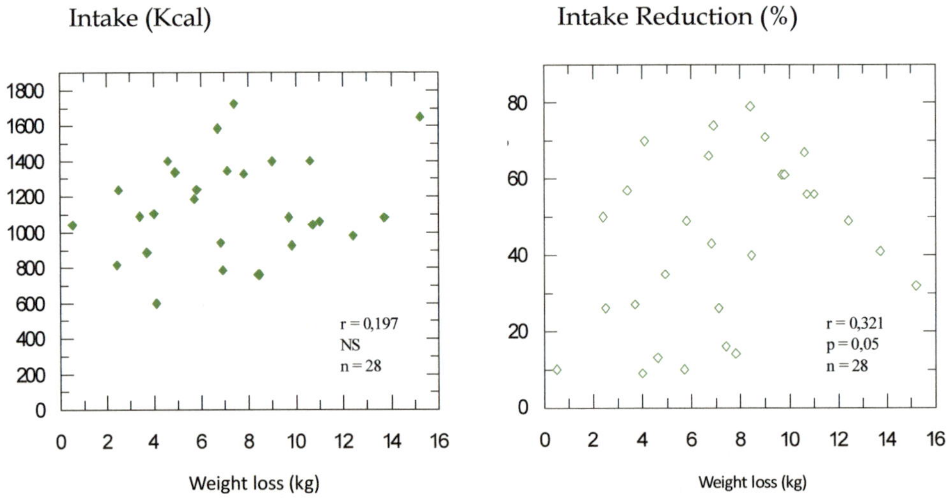

Fig. 1. Correlation between the absolute value (left) and the proportion of reduction of the habitually consumed energy in obese women after 2 months of a low-calorie diet (n = 28). SPEARMAN and RANK tests, with probability considered significant when $p < 0.05$.

In studies done in the region of Piracicaba, São Paulo, Brazil (Dallemole, 2006; Souza, 2006; Fogaça, 2009) with women recruited from the general population and those who had undergone bariatric surgery, as shown in Chart 1, energy expenditure increases with body weight. However, in relative terms, there is less energy expenditure by unit of weight as weight increases. Operated women present absolute and relative REE lower than the other women.

Since the first equation proposed by Harris and Benedict in 1919, many equations to predict REE were developed based on indirect calorimetry, and also to estimate TEE by combining the expenditure with physical activities with REE. The formulas used for predicting energy requirements have been widely used in clinical practice.

A cross-sectional study was done by our group with 51 women aged from 28 to 61 years submitted to banded or not bariatric surgery (Roux-en-Y gastric bypass, RYGB) 5.1±1.7 years before the study, all of them with stable weight. The measured REE was confronted with the values of the respective predictive equations obtained from regression studies in a number of different populations (Harris & Benedict, 1919; Schofield, 1985; Food and Agriculture Organization, World Health Organization & Organização das Nações Unidas, 1985; Owen et al., 1986; Mifflin et al., 1990, Luis et al., 2006). When the measurements were compared (Figure 2), the values obtained by indirect calorimetry were below those obtained by the equations, and when the results were organized in increasing order of the value obtained by calorimetry (Figure 3), there was great similarity in the behavior of the lines constructed with the sequence of the results of the equations, but they diverged from those constructed with the results of calorimetry. Thirty-one (77.5%) women presented a median REE measured by indirect calorimetry below the REE estimated by the Harris & Benedict (1919) equation, indicating some women in the group had low metabolism. Weijs & Vansant

(2010) assessed 27 prediction equations in relation to the indirect calorimetry data from Belgium women and concluded that more specific equations are necessary for women whose BMI > 30 Kg/m^2.

Population	BMI Kg/m^2	n	REE Mean±SD	REE/BW Mean±SD	Reference
Surgery-naive	< 25	22	1216±214	22±3	Dallemole, 2006
	25-30	11	1322±212	23±3	Dallemole, 2006
	30-35	13	1425±167	19±3	Dallemole, 2006
	> 35	35	1600±430	16±4	Souza, 2006
Before and 3 months after surgery	46±6	21	2006±376	17±4	Cesar et al., 2008
	39±6	21	1763±310	18±3	César et al., 2008
2 or more years after surgery	< 30	18	1046±264	15±4	Fogaça, 2009
	> 30	27	1270±252	15±3	Fogaça, 2009

Chart 1. Energy expenditure determined by indirect calorimetry in women recruited in Piracicaba, São Paulo, Brazil.

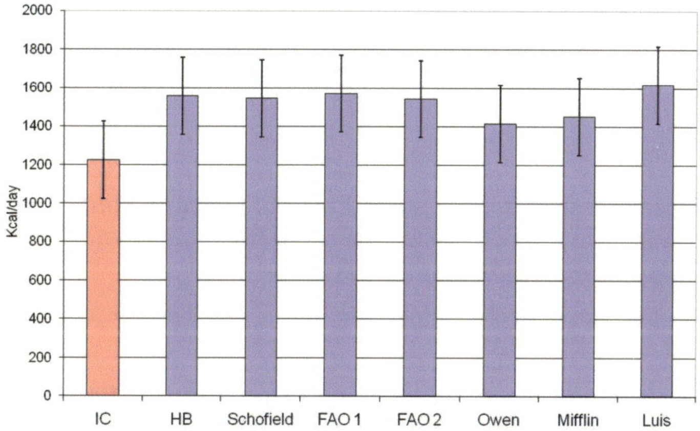

Fig. 2. **Comparison of the resting energy expenditure measured by indirect calorimetry (IC) and estimated by different equation in women after two years of bariatric surgery** (HB= Harris & Benedict; p<0.01 means compared with ANOVA; *p<0.01 others compared with the Tukey test; **p<0.05 in the comparison with FAO 1 and Luis by the Tukey test).

The metabolic state can be classified as normal, high or low, by comparing the measured REE with the estimated REE according to the mean of a reference population, using a variation coefficient of 15% (Food and Agriculture Organization, World Health Organization & Organização das Nações Unidas, 1985). In this sense, very low REE values deserve better investigations regarding adaptation to metabolic restriction after bariatric surgery.

These equations are based on body mass, height, age, gender and specific body composition markers, such as body surface area, lean mass, fat mass, total body potassium, among others (Rocha et al., 2005). The equations have been used in underweight, overweight, obese and morbidly obese individuals and also in those with specific diseases. However, interpersonal variation shows that much caution is necessary for estimating REE by the existing prediction equations, since it has been shown that they do not always estimate REE correctly (Frankenfield & Yousey, 2005) resulting in errors when estimating the energy requirements of individuals and populations (Duarte et al., 2007). More studies are necessary to state if the proportion of women with low metabolism who underwent bariatric surgery was in fact greater than that of the surgery-naive population, obese or otherwise, since there are not enough data from the population who lives in the same environmental conditions as that of the present study.

Although much has been done since Harris & Benedict (1919), the current formulas for estimating REE and TEE (that takes into account the energy spent in physical activities) are very limited and tend to overestimate the results.

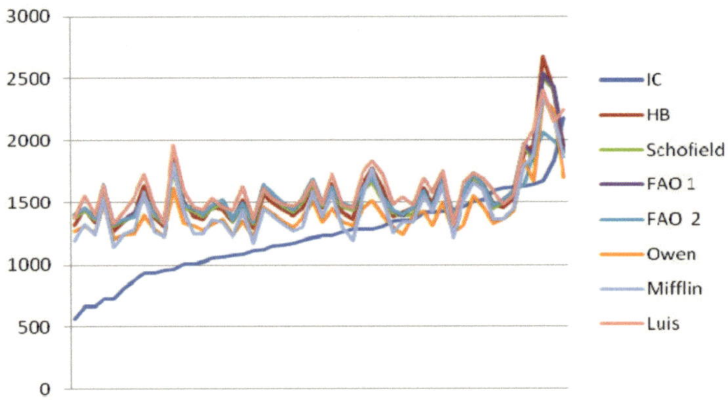

Fig. 3. Illustration of the resting energy expenditure, in increasing order, measured by indirect calorimetry (IC), in relation to that estimated by different equations among women two years or more after bariatric surgery (n=51).

3. Energy intake

One of the most challenging aspects of the science and practice of nutrition and dietetics is the measurement of energy and nutrient intakes, given the limitations of the methods to correctly measure food intake (Subar et al., 2006). Dietary surveys are used as indirect methods for assessing nutritional status. However, these instruments are subject to mistakes inherent to the individual and data analysis and use (Beaton, 1994; Slater et al., 2004). Individual quantitative and qualitative food intake may be estimated by different diet survey methods. There are retrospective methods where individuals recall the foods they have eaten, such as the Food Frequency Questionnaire (FFQ) and the 24-hour Recall (24hR). And the methods in which the individual records, when he eats, all the foods he ate, thereby creating a food diary (Gibson, 2005).

Intraindividual error sources, because of the variability of the food intake pattern, or interindividual error sources, stemming from the distribution of the population's requirements, together with a small number of days of observation, have a great impact on the reliability of food intake data analysis (Nusser et al., 1996). Hence, intake assessment studies will always be reporting the apparent intake of the individual and not the real intake, but they can be statistically adjusted to approximate the actual intake (Institute of Medicine, 2005).

Possible error sources can distort information about food intake, such as the perception of what is eaten, the interviewee's memory, the effects stemming from age, gender and interview environment, daily diet variation and seasonality, submission to data collection can affect the intake pattern and veracity of the information, the ability of the interviewer to obtain information and the disposition to collaborate with the investigation (Witschi, as in Willett, 1990). Practically, all dietary assessment studies are based on self-reporting of food intake, which can be biased, resulting in under- or overreporting of real energy intake (Black et al., 1991; Black, 2000), being able to seriously distort the interpretation of the study results (Rennie et al., 2006).

Underreporting has been associated with a number of different individual characteristics, including gender, body mass index, age, ethnicity, race, smoking, education level, social class, depression and physical activity (Johansson, et al., 2001; Scagliusi, et al., 2003; Scagliusi et al., 2008; Maurer et al., 2006, Maurer et al., 2008; Mendez et al., 2011). The desire to be socially accepted and body dissatisfaction have also been associated with underreporting of food intake (Tooze et al., 2004; Maurer et al., 2006; Scagliusi, 2007). Excess weight may be one of the greatest determinants of subnotification (Johansson et al., 2001; Johnson, 2002; Huang, et al., 2005; Bazanelli et al., 2010).

In individuals who are in energy balance, energy intake should correspond to the TEE. Thus, the doubly labeled water can be used to validate the energy obtained through dietary surveys. However, this method is unviable in large studies because of its cost and because it is technically challenging for use in routine validation of energy intake (Schoeller, 1999; Livingstone & Black, 2003).

As an alternative, other methods for identifying underreporting can be used, such as the comparison between reported energy intake (EI_{rep}) with TEE, when both are expressed in multiples of the REE, using a confidence interval for statistically comparing EI_{rep}:REE with the level of PAL. During weight stabilization, EI_{rep}:REE theoretically is equal to TEE:REE. The ratio TEE:REE is also known as PAL, then the equation may be rewritten as EI_{rep}:REE = PAL (Goldberg, et al., 1991).

As described by Black 2000, the cut-off point of the ratio EI_{rep}:REE should be calculated for the group being studied, since below this level it is statistically unlikely that the mean energy intake reported represents the real consumption, according to the equation below:

$$\text{Cut-off point} = \text{PAL} \times \exp\left[\text{SD}_{\text{min}} \times \frac{(S/100)}{\sqrt{n}}\right]$$

Where SD is the standard deviation. When 95% of the confidence interval is used (SD_{min} =-2) or 99.7% (SD_{min} = - 3); **n** is the number of individuals in the study, but when this formula is used to individually detect underreporting, n=1. **S** is the factor that takes into consideration the variation of all components of the equation and is given by:

$$S = \sqrt{\left[\left(\frac{CV^2_{EIrep}}{d}\right) + \left(CV^2_{REE}\right) + \left(CV^2_{PAL}\right)\right]}$$

Where VC_{EIrep} is the intra-individual energy intake variation coefficient; **d** is the number of days that the survey was administered; VC_{REE} is the intra-individual variation coefficient of repeated REE measurements and CV_{PAL} is the intra-individual variation coefficient of the level of physical activity.

Recently, other authors (Huang, 2005; Mendez, et al., 2011), assessed the underreporting phenomenon comparing EI_{rep} with estimated TEE using the DRI equations (Institute of Medicine, 2005), adjusting the intra-individual variation of the equation components. The cut-off point is calculated for the study group in percentage (%EI:TEE).

Energy and macronutrients	Before surgery n=37			After surgery n=35			p
	median	25%	75%	median	25%	75%	
Energy (Kcal)	2780	1037	6338	1346	673	2981	0.000
Carbohydrates (g)	320	115	1031	166	68	428	0.000
Fats (g)	110	28	395	51	20	104	0.000
Proteins (g)	104	38	302	51	15	89	0.000
Energy distribution							
Carbohydrates (%)	50	28	72	51	38	61	0.387
Fats (%)	38	14	56	34	25	49	0.034
Proteins (%)	16	9	23	15	8	25	0.226

p = Mann Whitney test used for comparing energy and macronutrient intakes before and after surgery

Table 1. The energy and macronutrient intakes of women before surgery and two or more years after surgery, Pircacicaba-SP, Brazil.

	Mean	Standard deviation	Median	First Quartile (25%)	Third Quartile (75%)
EI_{rep}	1428	523	1334	1147	1678
ER	2786*	524	2812	2389	3036
Harris&Benedict (1919)	1445*	152	1445	1376	1604
REE	1188	276	1209	1023	1376
PAL_{est}	1,45	0,22	1,42	1,28	1,56
EI_{rep} :REE	1,27	0,57	1,08	0,86	1,66

EI_{rep} = reported energy intake, ER = estimated energy requirement, REE = measured resting energy expenditure, PAL_{est} = estimated level of physical activity.
*$p<0.000$ in the paired t-test between EI_{rep} and ER and between Harris & Benedict (1919) and $REE_{measured}$.

Table 2. Energy intake and expenditure variables in women more than two years after bariatric surgery (n=40).

Among the bariatric patients we studied, mean reported energy intake before surgery corresponds to half the intake reported after surgery (Table 1). In the comparison, the proportion of macronutrients in the energy of the diet varied little. The operated women consumed a fat proportion in the daily intake a little smaller than those in the waiting line for surgery. Those in the waiting line for surgery reported consuming a fat proportion above the recommended proportion (Institute of Medicine, 2005), while the operated women reported consuming a proportion close to the upper limit. About the data presented by Table 1, one may ask how much they correspond to reality based on the analysis presented by Table 2 given the discrepancy between the measured expenditure and reported intake. The data presented in Table 1 were obtained from 24-hour recalls on nonconsecutive days, one of the days being on a weekend. The data in Table 2 stem from indirect calorimetry, and the total energy requirement was calculated by the DRI formula (Institute of Medicine, 2005). Among these women, the EI_{rep}:REE and PAL values that, in theory should agree, present only a small correlation (Figure 4)

Our data (Table 2 and Figure 3) show that energy intake divided by resting energy expenditure (EI_{rep}:REE) was not compatible with the level of physical activity (PAL_{est}) of the studied population. On the other hand, this can be explained by overestimating the reported physical activity which composes the PAL_{est} calculation. It may also be related to a substantially greater energy intake than that reported. Although one may not expect absolute agreement on this datum, since there are measurement errors in all elements of the equation (EI_{rep}:REE = PAL). The fact is that the studied women were in a stable weight condition and reported consuming half the estimated energy requirement (RE). This leads us to the generalization that the scale is still the best instrument for assessing the adequacy of energy intake. That is, if the individual is involuntarily gaining weight, it is because he is consuming more energy than he needs. However, it is not convenient to give up trying to solve this difficult issue, which is to know the values of the two sides of this balance, which for now remain obscure. This information can help to explain, for example, weight recovery after bariatric surgery, which, in most cases, is accompanied by intake underreporting.

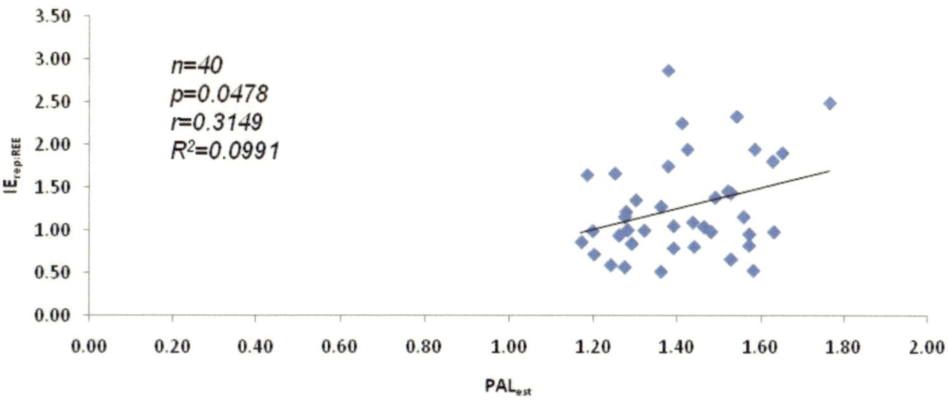

Fig. 4. **Correlation between the estimated level of physical activity** (PAL_{est}) and the ratio Energy Intake/Resting Energy Expenditure (EI_{rep}/REE) in women more than two years after bariatric surgery (n=40).

4. Body mass

There is a consensus that lean mass (LM) is the greatest determinant of energy expenditure, since it is metabolically more active than fat mass (Ravussin et al., 1986). Meanwhile, the differences in the volume of fat mass (FM), age and gender would have little effect on energy expenditure (Ravussin et al., 1986). Much has been discussed if an REE reduction could precede obesity; however, some researchers have rejected this hypothesis (Prentice, 2007). On the contrary, obese individuals present a high REE, that is, they do not have a low metabolism (Das et al., 2004; Hams et al., 2009; Prentice, 2007). This may occur because these individuals present a greater amount of lean mass, main determinant of the REE (Prentice, 2007; Prentice et al., 1986; Ravussin et al., 1986). Libel et al. (1995) assessed the energy expenditure during 24 hours and the REE in obese individuals and individuals who had never been obese in their habitual weights; after gaining 10% of the body weight by consuming a hypercaloric diet; or after losing 10 to 20% of the body weight by consuming a hypocaloric diet. They found that energy expenditure changed in both groups, of obese and nonobese individuals, after the change in the body weight. A 10% increase or reduction in habitual body weight causes an increase or reduction, respectively, of 15% in the 24-hour energy expenditure corrected for body weight. They also verified that TEE presented a positive correlation with LM and FM. The positive correlation between the total body mass of obese individuals and TEE has been explained by the increase in energy necessary for moving this mass (Institute of Medicine, 2005).

Reduction of LM associated with weight loss is also discussed, and that the reduction of LM would result in a reduction of TEE, thus the importance of exercising during weight loss. Tamboli et al. (2010) found a LM loss in the order of 27.8% one year after Roux-em-Y gastric bypass and associated this loss with the reduction of the TEE of these patients. In another study done in obese individuals after weight loss, concomitantly with REE reduction, there was a significant reduction of LM (Hill et al., 1987).

Active individuals present a significantly higher REE than inactive individuals of the same weight (Matzinger et al., 2002). There is the hypothesis that this occurs because of the amount of LM, which is greater in active individuals (Tappy et al., 2003). The REE differences in body weight in many individuals like men, women or athletes normally disappear when REE is considered in relation to LM (Institute of Medicine, 2005).

Based on these studies it is possible to verify that body composition, especially LM, significantly affects REE and TEE, both in obese and nonobese individuals. Current knowledge allows us to state that there is little difference between energy expenditure by unit of body mass of an underweight individual and an obese individual, but there is individual variation in the energy expenditure by unit of body mass of individuals in general, which in practice limits the use of formulas that predict energy requirement. In relation to surgery, studies that use more sensitive methods are needed to confirm the hypothesis that the REE adjusted for LM after surgery does not decrease, by adaptation or modification mechanisms of body composition in LM no matter how long after surgery.

Type of fat tissue also appears to have a strong influence on energy expenditure. White fat tissue, in addition to working as a primary site for energy storage, produces a series of substances that act on many places of the body, modulating the general metabolism. Excess white fat tissue results in obesity. Meanwhile, brown fat tissue is highly specialized and is capable of regulating energy expenditure by adaptive thermogenesis. This process depends on UCP-1 expression (Cinti et al., 1997). White fat tissue is responsible for most of the leptin produced (Cinti et al., 1997), although the action of this peptide occurs in the hypothalamus, which is where most of its receptors are found (Schwartz et al., 1996).

The total LM in the body is the factor that is most closely associated with leptin concentrations in the blood and so BMI, which is an indirect measurement of body fat, is also strongly and positively associated with the concentration of circulating leptin (Considine et al., 1996; Jeon et al., 2003; Kennedy et al., 1997). In a study done by our research group, the positive correlation between BMI and serum concentration of leptin was confirmed (Figure 5). This study assessed 45 women, of which 27 had less than 10% of weight regain 2 or more years after surgery and 18 presented an appropriate weight loss.

Another theme of interest relative to body composition is the role of FM by itself on the improvement of the comorbidities associated with obesity. Lowering of blood glucose (improvement of diabetes) in morbidly obese individuals after surgery occurs even before an important weight loss has been achieved and has been attributed to the modulation of the gastrointestinal hormonal response which acts in the recovery of the first phase of insulin secretion and improves its peripheral resistance (Polyzogopolou et al., 2003; Cummings et al., 2004). The important association of BMI with insulin and leptin concentrations in nondiabetic operated women (Figure 5) confirms the relevance of body weight reduction and maintenance for obtaining benefits after surgery. There was also a correlation of BMI with glucose concentration in women in the late postoperative period. Among the biochemical markers of lipid metabolism, an association between the concentrations of serum triglycerides with BMI was found, but not with total cholesterol and its fractions. The reduction of serum leptin that accompanies the reduction in body weight after bariatric surgery was inversely associated with the secretion of VLDL in studies of particle kinetics (Magkos, 2010), showing that the triglyceride metabolism has an important relationship with BMI.

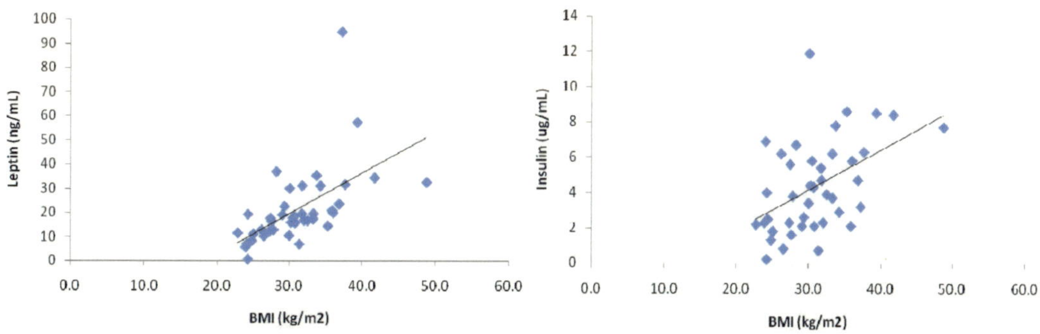

Fig. 5. Correlation of the serum leptin concentrations and insulin with body mass index (BMI) in women in the late postoperative period after Roux-en-Y gastric bypass (*n=41, r=0.729; R^2=0.531; p = 0.000*), (Fogaça, 2009).

Finally, an aspect of great relevance associated with obesity and insulin resistance is the distribution of body fat. Not all obese individual are insulin-resistant, and it has been shown that predominantly abdominal obesity is more strongly associated with insulin resistance. Inflammation of the omental adipose tissue is an important determining factor of insulin resistance (Hardy, 2011).

5. Conclusions

Energy balance is determined by energy intake and expenditure variables. Among the energy expenditure variables, REE and the expenditure with physical activities are responsible for roughly 90% of the TEE. Based on calorimetry studies, we have noticed that there is an important interpersonal variation in REE of women submitted to bariatric surgery. To know the magnitude of the effect of surgery on REE, we are conducting a prospective study to assess the interpersonal variation before surgery and after different lengths of postoperative time. Another aspect that needs to be better elucidated is the magnitude of the effect of physical exercise on REE in different lengths of postoperative periods.

In the energy requirement assessment, the use of prediction REE formulas does not seem adequate for the bariatric population and should be done with caution.

Physical activity is an important component of total energy expenditure and TEE assessment depends on precise information regarding the type and duration of each activity. As the energy intake registry, the registry of physical activity must be detailed and as close as possible of the real energy intake. This is a challenging task since among the obese, overestimation of the reported intake usually happens.

If, on the one hand, physical activities are usually overestimated, on the other hand, and more strikingly, food intake reports are usually underestimated. Among obese women, intake reports can be below the $REE_{measured}$, which is completely implausible. This observation challenges us in the development of more appropriate methods to assess food intake.

BMI is an important indicator of the result of bariatric surgery and more studies are necessary on the effects of the distribution and type of body fat and the surgery results on the comorbidities associated with obesity.

6. References

Bazanelli, AP., Kamimura, MA., Vasselai, P., Draibe, SA. & Cuppari, L. (2010). Underreporting of energy intake in peritoneal dialysis patients. *Journal of Renal Nutrition*, Vol. 20, No. 4, pp. 263-269, ISSN 1051-2276.

Beaton, GH. (1994). Approaches to analysis of dietary data: relationship between planned analyses and choice of methodology. *The American Journal of Clinical Nutrition*, Vol. 59, Supl. 1, pp. 253-261, ISSN 0002-9165.

Black, AE. (2000). Critical evaluation of energy intake using the Goldberg cut-off for energy intake: basal metabolic rate. A practical guide to its calculation, use and limitations. *International Journal of Obesity*, Vol. 24, No. 9, pp. 1119-1130, ISSN 0307-0565.

Black, AE. & Cole, TJ. (2001). Biased over-or under-reporting is characteristic of individuals wheter over time or by different assessment methods. *Journal of the American Dietetic Association*, Vol. 101, No. 1, pp. 70-80, ISSN 0307-0565.

Black, AE., Goldberg, GR., Jebb, SA., Livingstone, MB., Cole TJ. & Prentice AM. (1991). Critical evaluation of energy intake data using fundamental principles of energy physiology: 2. Evaluating the results of published surveys. *European Journal of Clinical Nutrition*, Vol. 45, No.12, pp. 583-599, ISSN 0954-3007.

Carriquiry, RH., Jensen, HH., Fuller, WA. & Guenther, P. (1994). Methods for estimating usual intake distributions. *The American Journal of Clinical Nutrition*, Vol. 59, Suppl.1, pp. 305, ISSN 0002-9165.

Cesar, MC., Montebelo, MIL., Rasera, I., Oliveira, AV., Gonelli, RG. & Cardoso, GA. (2008). Effects of Roux-en-Y Gastric Bypass on Resting Energy Expenditure in Women. Obesity Surgery, Vol.18, No 11, pp. 1376-1380, ISSN 0960-8923

Cinti, S., Frederich, RC., Zingaretti, MC., De Matteis, R., Flier, JS. & Lowell, BB. (1997). Imunohistochemical localization of leptin and uncoupling protein in white and brown adipose tissue. Endocrinology, Vol. 138, pp. 797-804, ISSN 0013-7227

Considine, RV., Sinha, MK., Heiman, ML.; Kriauciunas, A., Stephens, TW. NYCE, MR., Ohannesian, JP., Marco, CC., Mckee, LJ., Bauer, TL. & Caro, JF. (1996). Serum immunoreactive leptin concentrations in normalweight and obese humans. *The New England Journal of Medicine*, Vol. 334, No. 5, pp. 292-295, ISSN 1533-4406.

Cowley, MA., Smith RG., Diano, S., Tschöp, M., Pronchuk, N., Grove, KL et al. (2003). The distribution and mechanism of action of ghrelin in the CNS demonstrates a novel hypothalamic circuit regulating energy homeostasis. *Neuron*, Vol. 37, No. 4, pp. 649–661, ISSN 0896-6273.

Cummings, DE., Overduin, J. & Foster-Schubert, KE. (2004). Gastric bypass for obesity: mechanisms of weight loss and diabetes resolution. *The Journal of Clinical Endocrinology & Metabolism*, Vol. 89, No. 6, pp. 2608-15. ISSN 0021-972X.

Dallemole, C. (2006). *Avaliação da composição corporal e da taxa metabólica de repouso de mulheres jovens residentes no interior do estado de São Paulo/Brasil*. 120 f. Dissertação (Mestrado em Educação Física - Performance Humana) - Universidade Metodista de Piracicaba/UNIMEP, Piracicaba/ SP.

Danforth, JE. (1985). Diet and obesity. *The American Journal of Clinical Nutrition*, Vol. 41, pp. 1132-1145, ISSN 1938- 3207.

Das, SK., Saltzman, E., McCrory, MA., Hsu, LK., Shikora, SA., Dolnikowski, G., Kehayias, JJ. & Roberts SB. (2004). Energy expenditure in very high in extremely obese women. *The Journal of Nutrition*, Vol. 134, No. 6, pp. 1412-1416, ISSN 1541-6100.

Doucet, E., Pierre, S., Alméras, N., Mauriège, P., Richard, D. & Tremblay, A. (2000). Changes in Energy Expenditure and Substrate Oxidation Resulting from Weight Loss in Obese Men and Women: Is There an Important Contribution of Leptin? *The Journal of Clinical Endocrinology & Metabolism*, Vol. 85, No. 4. pp.1550–1556, ISSN 1945-7197.

Duarte, SFP., Francischetti, EA., Genelhu, VA., Duarte, SF., Francischetti, EA., Genelhu, VA., Cabello, PH. & Pimentel MM. (2007). LEPR p.Q223R, *β3-AR* p.W64R and *LEP* c.-2548G>A gene variants in obese brazilian subjects. *Genetics and Molecular Research*, Vol. 6, No. 4, pp. 1035-1043, ISSN 1676-5680.

Flatt, JP. The biochemistry of energy expenditure. In: Bray, GA. (1978). *RecentAdvances in Obesity Research*. Newman, London.

Flatt, JP. & Tremblay, A. Energy expenditure and substrate oxidation. In: Bray, GA., Bouchard, C. & James, WPT. (1998). *Handbook of obesity*. Marcel Dekker, New York.

Fogaça, KCP. (2009). *Investigação de Fatores envolvidos na Recuperação de Peso após Derivação Gástrica*. 121 f. Tese (Doutorado em Alimentos e Nutrição) - Universidade Estadual Paulista "Julio de Mesquita Filho"/UNESP, Araraquara/SP.

Food and Agriculture Organization, World Health Organization & Organização das Nações Unidas (1985). *Energy and protein requeriments*. World Health Organization, WHO, Technical Report Series, 724, ISBN 92 4 120724 8. Geneva.

Frankenfield, D., Yousey, LR. & Compher, C. (2005). Comparison of predictive equations for resting metabolic rate in healthy nonobese and obese adults: a systematic review. *Journal of the American Dietetic Association*, Vol. 105, No. 5, pp. 775-789, ISSN 0002-8223.

Gibson, RS. (2ed.). (2005). *Principles of nutritional assessment,* Oxford University, ISBN-10 0195171691, New York.

Goldberg, GR., Black, AE., Jebb, SA., Cole, TJ., Murgatroyd, PR., Coward, WA. & Prentice, AM. (1991). Critical evaluation of energy intake data using fundamental principles of energy physiology: 1. Derivation of cut-off limits to identify under-recording. *European Journal of Clinical Nutrition,* Vol. 45, No. 12, pp. 569-581, ISSN 0954-3007.

Halaas, JL., Gajiwala, KS., Maffei, M., Cohen, SL., Chait, BT., Rabinowitz, D. et al. (1995). Weight-reducing effects of the plasma protein encoded by the obese gene. *Science,* Vol. 269, No. 5223, pp. 543-546, ISSN 1095-9203.

Hardie, LJ., Rayner, DV., Holmes, S. & Trayhunr, P. (1996). Circulating leptin levels are modulated by fasting, cold exposure and insulin administration in lean but not Zucker (fa/fa) rats as measured by ELISA. *Biochemical and Biophysical Research Communications,* Vol. 223, No. 3, pp. 660-665, ISSN 0006-291X.

Hardy, OT., Perugini, RA., Nicoloro, SM., Gallagher-Dorval, K., Puri, V., Straubhaar, J. & Czech, MP. (2011). Body mass index-independent inflammation in omental adipose tissue associated with insulin resistence in morbid obesity. *Surgery for Obesity and Related,* Vol. 7, No. 1, pp. 60-67, ISSN 1708-0428.

Harris, JA. & Benedict, FA. (1919). A biometric study of basal metabolism in man, Carnegie Institution of Washington, Boston.

Hill, JO. (2006). Understanding and addressing the epidemic of obesity: an energy balance perpective. *Endocrine Reviews,* Vol. 27, No 7, pp. 750-761, ISSN 1945-7189.

Hill, JO., Sparling, PB., Shields, TW. & Heller, PA. (1987). Effects of exercise and food restriction on body composition and metabolic rate in obese women. *The American Journal of Clinical Nutrition,* Vol. 46, No. 4, pp. 622-630, ISSN 1938- 3207.

Hill, JO., Melby, C., Johnson, SL. & Peters, JC. (1995). Physical activity and energy requirements. *The American Journal of Clinical Nutrition,* Vol. 62, Suppl., pp. 1059S-1066S, ISSN 1938- 3207.

Huang, TTK., Roberts, SR., Howarth, NC. & McCrory, MA. (2005). Effect of screening out implausible energy intake reports on relationships between diet and BMI. *Obesity Research,* Vol. 13, No. 7, pp. 1205-1217, ISSN 1071-7323.

Institute of Medicine - IOM. (2005). Food and Nutrition Board. Dietary Reference Intakes (DRIs): *Dietary Reference Intakes for Energy, Carbohydrates, Fiber, Fat, Protein and Amino Acids (Macronutrients).* National Academy Press, Washington, D.C.

Jacobson, P., Rankinen, T., Tremblay, A., Pérusse, L., Chagnon, YC. & Bouchard C. (2006). Resting metabolic rate and respiratory quotient: results from a genome-wide scan in the Quebec Family Study. *The American Journal of Clinical Nutrition* Vol. 84, No. 6, pp. 1527-1533, ISSN 0002-9165.

Jeon, JY., Steadward, RD., Wheeler, GD., Bell, g., Mccargar, L. & Harber, V. (2003). Intact Sympathetic Nervous System Is Required for Leptin Effects on Resting Metabolic Rate in People with Spinal Cord Injury. *The Journal of Clinical Endocrinology & Metabolism,* Vol. 88, No. 1, pp. 402-407, ISSN 1945-7197.

Johansson, G., Wikman, A., Ahrén, AM., Hallmans, G. & Johansson, I. (2001). Underreporting of energy intake in repeated 24 - hour recalls related to gender, age, weight status, day of interview, educational level, reported food intake, smoking habits and area of living. *Public Health Nutrition,* Vol. 4, No. 4, pp. 919-927, ISSN 1368-9800.

Johansson, L., Solvoll, K., Björneoe, GE., & Drevon, C. (1998). Under- and overreporting of energy intake related to weight status and lifestyle in a nationwide sample. *The American Journal of Clinical Nutrition*, Vol. 68, No. 2, pp. 266-274, ISSN 0002-9165.

Johnson, RK. (2002). Dietary intake - how do we measure what people are really eating? *Obesity Research*, Vol. 10, Suppl. 1, pp. 63-68, ISSN 1071-7323.

Kamegai, J., Tamura, H., Shimizu, T., Ishii S, Sugihara H & Wakabayashi I. (2001). Chronic central infusion of ghrelin increases hypothalamic neuropeptide Y and Agouti-related protein mRNA levels and body weight in rats. *Diabetes*, Vol. 50, No. 11, pp. 2438-2443, ISSN 0012-1797.

Kennedy, A., Gettys, T., Watson, P., Wallace, P., Ganaway, E., Pan, Q. & Garvey, WT. (1997). The metabolic significance of leptin in humans: gender-based differences in relationship to adiposity, insulinsensitivity, and energy expenditure. *The Journal of Clinical Endocrinology & Metabolism*, Vol. 82, No. 4, pp. 1293-1300, ISSN 1945-7197.

Körtzinger, I., Bierwag, A., Mast, M. & Muller M.J. (1997). Dietary underreporting: validity of dietary measurements of energy intake using a 7-days dietary record and a diet history in non-obese subjects. *Annals of Nutrition and Metabolism*, Vol. 41, No. 1, pp. 37-44, ISSN 0250-6807.

Larson, DE., Tataranni, PA., Ferraro, RT., & Ravussin, E. (1995). *Ad libitum* food intake on a "cafeteria diet" in native American women: relations with body composition and 24-h energy expenditure. *The American Journal of Clinical Nutrition*, Vol. 62, No. 5, pp. 911-917, ISSN 1938- 3207.

Leibel, RL., Rosenbaum, M. & Hirsch, J. (1995). Changes in energy expenditure resulting from altered body weight. *The New England Journal of Medicine*, Vol. 332, No. 10, pp. 621-8, ISSN 1533-4406.

Livingstone, MB. & Black, AE. (2003). Markers of the validity of reported energy intake. *The Journal of Nutrition*, Vol. 133, Suppl 3, pp. 895-920, ISSN 1541-6100.

Luis, DA., Aller, R., Izaola, O. & Romero, E. (2006). Prediction equation of resting energy expenditure in adult Spanish of obese adult population. *Annals of Nutrition and Metabolism*, Vol. 50, No. 3, pp. 193-196, ISSN-1421-9697.

Magkos, F., Fabbrini, E., McCrea, J., Patterson, BW., Eagon, JC &, Klein, S. (2010). Decrease in hepatic very-density lipoprotein-triglyceride secretion affer weight loss is inversely associated with changes in circulating leptin. *Diabetes, Obesity and Metabolism*, Vol. 12, No. 7, pp. 584-590, ISSN 1463-1326.

Marzullo, P., Verti, B., Savia, G., Walker, GE., Guzzaloni, G., Tagliaferri, M., et al. (2004). The relationship between active ghrelin levels and human obesity involves alterations in resting energy expenditure. *The Journal of Clinical Endocrinology & Metabolism*, Vol. 89, No. 2, pp. 936–939, ISSN 1945-7197.

Masuda, Y., Tanaka, T., Inomata, N., Ohnuma, N., Tanaka, S., Itoh, Z. et al. (2000). Ghrelin stimulates gastric adic secretion and motility in rats. *Biochemical and Biophysical Research Communications*, Vol. 276, No. 3, pp. 905-908, ISSN 0006-291X.

Mattevi, VS., Zembrzuski, VM. & Hutz, MH (2002). Association analysis of genes involved in the leptin signaling pathway with obesity in Brazil. *International Journal of Obesity*, Vol. 26, No. 9, pp. 1179–1185, ISSN 0307-0565.

Matzinger, O., Schneiter, P. & Tappy, L. (2002). Effects of fatty acids on exercise plus insulin-induced glucose utilization in trained and sedentary subjects. *American Journal of Physiology Endocrinology and Metabolism*, Vol. 282, pp. E125–E131, ISSN 1522-1555.

Maurer, J., Taren, D.L., Teixeira, PJ., Thomson, C., Lohman, TG., Going, SB. & Houtkooper, LB. (2006). The psychosocial and behavioral characteristics related to energy misreporting. *Nutrition Reviews*, Vol. 64, No. 2, pp. 53-66, ISSN 1753-4887.

Maurer, J., Thomson, C., Ranger-Moore, J., Teixeira, PJ., Lohman, TG., Taren, DL., Cussler, E., Going, SB. & Houtkooper, LB. (2008). Psychosocial and behavioral profile and preditors of self-reported energy underreporting in obese middle-aged women. *Journal of the American Dietetic Association*, Vol. 108, No. 1, pp.114-119, ISSN 0002-8223.

Meirelles, CM. & Gomes, PSC. (2004). Efeitos agudos da atividade contraresistência sobre o gasto energético: revisitando o impacto das principais variáveis. *Revista Brasileira de Medicina do Esporte*, Vol. 10, No. 2, pp. 122-130, ISSN 1806-9940.

Mela, DJ. & Rogers, PJ. (1998). *Food, eating and obesity*.Chapman & Hall, London.

Melo, CM., Tirapegui, J. & Ribeiro, SML. (2008). Gasto energético corporal: conceitos, formas de avaliação e sua relação com a obesidade, *Arquivos Brasileiros de Endocrinologia & Metabologia*, Vol. 52, No 3, pp. 452-464, ISSN 0004- 2730.

Mendez, MA., Popkin, BM., Buckland, G., Schroder, H., Amiano, P., Barricarte, A., Huerta, JM., Quirós, JR., Sánches, MJ. & Gonzáles, CA. (2011). Alternative methods of accounting for underreporting and overreporting when measuring dietary intake-obesity relations. *American Journal of Epidemiology*, Vol. 173, No. 4, pp. 448-458, ISSN 1476-6256.

Mifflin, MD., Jeor, ST., Hill, LA., Scott, BJ., Daugherty, SA. & Koh, YO. (1990). A new predictive equation for resting energy expenditure in healthy individuals. *The American Journal of Clinical Nutrition,* Vol. 51, No. 2, pp. 241-247, ISSN 1938- 3207.

Negrão, AB. & Licinio, J. (2000.) Leptina: o diálogo entre adipócitos e neurônios. *Arquivos Brasileiros de Endocrinologia & Metabologia*, Vol. 44, No. 3, pp. 205-214, ISSN 0004-2730.

Nusser, SM., Carriquiry, AL., Dood, KW. & Fuller, WA. (1996). A semiparametric transformation approach to estimating usual daily intake distribuitions. *Journal of American Statistical Association*, Vol. 436, No. 91, pp. 1440-1449, ISSN 0162-1459.

Olafsdottir, AS., Thorsdottir, I., Gunnarsdottir, I., Thorgeirsdottir, H. & Steingrimsdottir, L. (2006). Comparison of women`s diet assessed by FFQs and 24-hour recalls whith and without underreporters: association with biomarkers. *Annals of Nutrition and Metabolism*, Vol. 50, No. 5, pp. 450-460, ISSN 1421-9697.

Owen, OE., Kavle, E., Owen, RS., Polansky, M., Caprio, S., Mozzoli, MA., et al. (1986). A reappraisal of caloric requeriments in healthy women. *The American Journal of Clinical Nutrition*, Vol. 44, No. 1, pp. 1-19, ISSN-1938- 3207.

Polyzogopolou, EV., Kalfarentzos, F., Vagenakis, AG. & Alexandrides, TK. (2003). Restoration of euglycemia and normal acute insulin response to glucose in obese subjects with type 2 diabetes following bariatric surgery. *Diabetes*. Vol. 52, No. 5, pp.1098-1103, ISSN 0012-1797.

Prentice, AM., Black, AE, Coward., WA, Davies, HL., Goldberg, GR., Murgatroyd, PR., Ashford, J., Sawyer, M. & Whitehead RG. (1986). High levels of energy expenditure in obese women. *British Medical Journal*, Vol. 292, pp. 983-987, ISSN 0959 8138.

Prentice, AM. Are defects in energy expenditure involved in the causation of obesity? (2007).*Obesity Reviews*, Vol. 8, suppl. 1, pp. 89-91, ISSN 1467-789X.

Probst, Y. & Tapsell, L. (2007). Over-and underreporting of energy intake by patients with metabolic syndrome using an automated dietary assessment website. *Nutrition & Dietetics*, Vol. 64, pp. 280-284, ISSN 1747-0080.

Ravussin, E., Lillioja, S. & Anderson, T. (1986). Determinants of 24-hour energy expenditure in man: methods and results using a respiratory chamber. *The Journal of Clinical Investigation*, Vol. 78, No. 6, pp. 1568-1578, ISSN 0021-9738.

Rennie, KL., Siervo, M. & Jebb, SA. (2006). Can self-reported dieting and dietary restraint identify underreporters of energy intake in dietary surveys. *Journal of the American Dietetic Association*, Vol. 106, No. 10, p. 1667-1672, ISSN 0002-8223.

Rocha, EEM., Alves, VGF., Silva, MHN., Chiesa, CA. & Fonseca, RBV. (2005). Can measured resting energy expenditure be estimated by formulae in daily clinical nutrition practice? *Current Opinion in Clinical Nutrition & Metabolic Care*, Vol. 8, No. 3, pp. 319-328, ISSN 1363-1950.

Rosado, EL. & Monteiro, JBR. (2001). Obesidade e a substituição de macronutrientes da dieta. *Revista de Nutrição*, Vol. 14, No. 2, pp. 145-152, ISSN 1415-5273.

Rutanen, J., Pihlajamäki, J., Karhapää, P., Vauhkonen, I., Kuusisto, J., Moilanen Mykkänen, L. & Laakso, M. (2004). The Val103Ile Polymorphism of Melanocortin-4 Receptor Regulates Energy Expenditure and Weight Gain. *Obesity Reasearch*, Vol. 12, No. 7, pp. 1060 –1066, ISSN 1071-7323.

Sahu, A. Leptin signaling in the hypothalamus: emphasis on energy homeostasis and leptin resistance. (2004). *Frontiers in Neuroendocrinology*, Vol. 24, No. 4, pp. 225–53, ISSN 0091-3022.

Samaras, K.; Kelly, PJ. & Campbell, LV. Dietary underreporting is prevalent in middleaged British women and is not related to adiposity (percentage body fat). (1999). *International Journal of Obesity*, Vol. 23, No. 8, pp. 881-888, ISSN 0307-0565.

Scagliusi, FB. *Validade das estimativas de ingestão energética de três métodos de avaliação do consumo alimentar, em relação a água duplamente marcada.* (2007). 185 f. Tese (Doutorado em Educação Física e Esporte) - Universidade de São Paulo/USP, São Paulo.

Scagliusi, FB., Ferrioli, E., Pfrimer, K., Laureano, C., Cunha CS., Gualano, B., Lourenço, BH. & Lancha, AH. (2008). Underreporting of energy intake in Brazilian women varies according to dietary assessment: a cross-sectional study using doubly labeled water. *Journal of the American Dietetic Association*, Vol. 108, No. 12, pp. 2031-2040, ISSN 0002-8223.

Scagliusi, FB., Polacow, VO., Artioli, GG., Benatti, FB. & Lancha, AH. (2003). Selective underreporting of energy intake in women: magnitude, determinants, and effect of training. *Journal of the American Dietetic Association*, Vol. 103, No. 10, pp. 1306-1313, ISSN 0002-8223.

Schoeller, DA. How accurate is self-reported dietary energy intake? (1990). *Nutrition Reviews*, Vol. 48, No 10, pp. 373-379, ISSN 1753-4887.

Schoeller, DA. Recent advances from application of doubly labeled water to mensurement of human energy expenditure. (1999). *The Journal of Nutrition*, Vol. 129, No. pp. 1765-1768, ISSN 1541-6100.

Schoeller, DA., & Fjeld, CR. (1991). Human energy metabolism: what have we learned from the doubly labeled water method? *Annual Review of Nutrition*, Vol. 11, pp. 355-373, ISSN 0199-9885.

Schofield, WN. (1985). Predicting basal metabolic rate, new standards and review of previous work. *Clinical Nutrition*, Vol.39C (suppl), No1, pp. 5-41, ISSN 0261-5614.

Schwartz, MW., Seeley, RJ., Campfield, LA., Burn, P. & Baskin, DG. Identification of targets of leptin action in rat hypothalamus (1996). J Clin Invest, Vol. 98, pp.1101-6, ISSN 0021-9738.

Slater, B., Marchioni, DL. & Fisberg, RM. (2004). Estimando a prevalência da ingestão inadequada de nutrientes. *Revista de Saúde Pública,* Vol. 38, No. 4, pp. 599-605, ISSN 1518-8787.

Smyrnios, NA. & Curley, FJ. Indirect calorimetry. *In* Rippe, JM., Irwin, RS., Fink, MP. & Cerra, FB. (1996). *Intensive care medicine,* 3a ed., Little, Brown. Boston.

Souza, CL. (2009). *Fatores relacionados ao gasto e consumo energético de mulheres obesas com e sem síndrome metabólica.* 121 f. Dissertação (Mestrado em Alimentos e Nutrição) - Universidade Estadual Paulista. "Júlio de Mesquita Filho"/ UNESP, Araraquara/ SP.

Subar, AF., Dood, KW., Guenther, PM., Kipnis, V., Midthune, D., Mcdowell, M. *et al.* (2006). The food propensity questionnaire: concept, development, and validation for use as a covariate in a model to estimate usual food intake. *Journal of the American Dietetic Association,* Vol. 106, No. 10, pp. 1556-1563, ISSN 0002-8223.

Svendsen, M. & Tonstad, S. (2006). Accuracy of food intake reporting in obese subjects with metabolic risk factors. *British Journal of Nutrition,* Vol. 95, No.3, pp. 640-649, ISSN 1475-2662.

Tamboli, RA., Hossain, HA., Marks, PA., Eckhauser, AW., Rathmacher, JA., Philips, SE., Buchowski, MS., Chen, KY. & Abumrad, NN. (2010). Body composition energy metabolism following Roux-en-Y gastric bypass surgery. *Obesity,* Vol. 18, No. 9, pp. 1718-1724, ISSN 1467-789X.

Tappy, L., Binnert, C. & Schneiter, P. (2003). Energy expenditure, physical activity and body-weight control. Proceedings Nutrition Society, Vol. 62, No 3, pp. 663-6, ISSN 1475-2719.

Tooze, JA., Subar, AF., Thompson, FE., Troiano, R., Schatzkin, A. & Kipnis V. (2004). Psychosocial predictors of energy underreporting in a large doubly labeled water study. *The American Journal of Clinical Nutrition,* Vol. 79, No. 5, pp. 795-804, ISSN 1938- 3207.

Tortorella, C., Macchi, C., Spinazzi, R., Malendowicz, LK., Trejter, M. & Nussdorfer, GG. (2003). Ghrelin, an endogenous ligand for the growth hormone-secretagogue receptor, is expressed in the human adrenal cortex. *International Journal of Molecular Medicine,* Vol. 12, No 2, pp. 213–217, ISSN 1791-244X.

Trayhurn, P., Thomas, ME., Duncan, JS. & Rayner, DV. (1995). Effects of fasting and refeeding on ob gene expression in white adipose tissue of lean and obese (ob/ob) mice. *FEBS Letters,* Vol. 368, No. 3, pp. 488-490, ISSN 0014-5793.

Yurtcu, E., Yilmaz, A., Ozkurt, Z., Yurtcu, E., Yilmaz, A., Ozkurt, Z., Kolukisa, E., Yilmaz, M., Keles, H., Ergun, MA., Yetkin, I. & Menevse A. (2009). Melanocortin-4 Receptor Gene Polymorphisms in Obese Patients. *Biochemical Genetics,* Vol. 47, No. 3, pp. 295-300, ISSN 0006-2928.

Weijs, PJ. & Vansant, GA. Validity of preditive equations for resting energy expenditura in Belgian normal weight to morbid obese women. (2010) *Clinical Nutrition;* Vol. 29, No. 3, pp. 347-351, ISSN 0261-5614.

Witschi JC. Short-term dietary recall and recording methods. In: Willett, W. (1990). *Nutritional epidemiology.* Oxford University Press, New York.

World Health Organization - WHO. (1998). *Life in the 21st century: a vision for all.* WHO, Geneve.

10

Origins for Micronutrient Deficiencies

Anyea S. Lovette[1], Timothy R. Shope[2] and Timothy R. Koch[3]
[1]Departments of Pharmacy, [2]Surgery and [3]Medicine,
Center for Advanced Laparoscopic & Bariatric Surgery Washington Hospital Center
and Georgetown University School of Medicine Washington,
USA

1. Introduction

Dietary and activity programs result in poor weight loss or poor maintenance of weight loss, and bariatric surgery therefore remains the major treatment option for patients with medically-complicated obesity. There are now over 220,000 bariatric surgical procedures performed each year in the United States and Canada. The 'divided' or 'isolated' Roux-en-Y gastric bypass remains the most commonly performed bariatric surgical procedure in the United States and Canada for surgical treatment of patients with medically-complicated obesity.

Micronutrients in human physiology include essentials minerals such as iron, water soluble vitamins (such as the B vitamins and vitamin C), fat soluble vitamins (A, D, E, and K), and trace elements (zinc, copper, selenium, manganese, and likely chromium). Understanding the origins for micronutrient deficiencies in patient who have undergone bariatric surgery should permit better screening and maintenance techniques to prevent and discover underlying deficiencies. As a first step, the importance of preoperative evaluation for identification of micronutrient deficiencies is under evaluation. The importance of this preventative approach is supported by recent reports of major or fatal nutritional complications occurring more than 20 years after bariatric surgery.

In this chapter, dietary methods including food journals are shown to be important for examining pre-operative diets in order to predict potential micronutrient deficiencies. The relatively insufficient intake of specific micronutrients in those patients instructed post-operatively on a high protein diet is discussed.

The surgical origins for micronutrient deficiencies that are induced by bypass of physiologically relevant segments of the gastrointestinal tract are summarized. This chapter includes a discussion of the pre-operative medically-induced origins for micronutrient deficiencies including the importance of chronic gastric infection with *Helicobacter pylori* and small intestinal bacterial overgrowth related to diabetic gut autonomic neuropathy. Post-operative medical conditions that lead to micronutrient deficiencies including small intestinal bacterial overgrowth induced by achlorhydria of the gastric pouch are described.

Clinical presentations of micronutrient deficiencies after bariatric surgery are summarized. Common micronutrient deficiencies considered after bariatric surgery include iron deficiency, vitamin D deficiency and thiamine deficiency. Vitamin D deficiency with metabolic bone disease remains common after gastric bypass and recent results suggest that the present postoperative supplements of calcium and Vitamin D are inadequate. The potential role of copper deficiency as an origin for visual disorders and neurological disorders after gastric bypass is discussed. A major goal of ongoing clinical studies is a better understanding of whether blood levels of micronutrients are sufficient to exclude underlying deficiency states or whether clinical symptoms must be identified and categorized in patients who have undergone bariatric surgery.

2. Micronutrients

Macronutrients including fat, protein, and carbohydrates are important dietary components for conversion into chemical energy and for tissue and cellular structure. By contrast, micronutrients are essential dietary factors required for biochemical and cellular processes (please see Table 1). Specific micronutrients are required in microgram or milligram quantities in a diverse group of biochemical pathways and metabolic processes. Micronutrients include trace elements (chromium, copper, manganese, selenium and zinc), essential minerals (including calcium, iodine, iron, and magnesium), water-soluble vitamins (including B vitamins and vitamin C) and fat-soluble vitamins (vitamins A, D, E, and K).

Water Soluble Vitamin	**Cofactor In**
Thiamine (Vitamin B1)	Thiamine Pyrophosphate
Riboflavin (Vitamin B2)	Flavin Adenine Dinucleotide
Niacin (Vitamin B3)	Nicotinamide Adenine Dinucleotide
Folic Acid	Tetrahydrofolate
Pyridoxine (Vitamin B6)	Pyridoxal Phosphate
Cobalamin (Vitamin B12)	5'-Deoxyadenosyl-Cobalamine
Ascorbic Acid (Vitamin C)	
Trace Elements	**Cofactor In**
Chromium	Uncertain
Copper	Cytosolic Superoxide Dismutase & Cytochrome Oxidase
Manganese	Mitochondrial Superoxide Dismutase
Selenium	Glutathione Peroxidase
Zinc	Cytosolic Superoxide Dismutase & Hundreds of Proteins
Essential Minerals	**Cofactor In**
Calcium	
Iodine	Thyroid Hormone
Iron	Catalase & Hemoglobin
Magnesium	
Fat-Soluble Vitamins	
Vitamin A	
Vitamin D	
Vitamin E	
Vitamin K	

Table 1. Micronutrients and their roles as cofactors

Many bariatric programs recommend taking a comprehensive multivitamin with minerals twice daily after a malabsorptive procedure, and a daily calcium supplement (≥1.2 g/day elemental calcium). It is not certain whether these suggestions are sufficient to prevent micronutrient deficiencies after Roux-en-Y gastric bypass. This level of supplementation is unlikely to be adequate after a biliopancreatic diversion.

3. Dietary origins for micronutrient deficiencies

3.1 Statement of the problem

Body mass index (BMI; in kg/m2) is used to classify underweight (BMI <18.5), normal weight (BMI 18.5-24.9), overweight (25-29.9), obese (BMI 30-39.9), and extreme obesity (BMI > 40). Over the last 20 years, there has been a dramatic increase in obesity in the United States. Data from two National Health and Nutrition Examination Surveys (NHANES) show that among adults aged 20-74 years, the prevalence of obesity increased from 23%, in the 1988-1994 survey, to 33.8% in the 2007-2008 survey (1). Since the prevalence of obesity is increasing rapidly, it is important to find effective weight control or weight loss strategies for these individuals. This is of international concern as it appears that other developed countries are also facing increases in the prevalence of obesity.

Lifestyle interventions that involve diet, exercise, and behavior change strategies can result in an average weight loss of 7-10% of initial body weight after 6 months of treatment (2, 3). The most effective treatment for obesity, on the other hand, is bariatric surgery. The average mean excess weight loss (%EWL) is 50% for the adjustable gastric band and 68% for Roux-en-Y gastric bypass. This dramatic weight loss not only improves quality of life, but also reduces the risk of developing health conditions and may even improve existing health problems. Although weight loss improves health, surgical treatments for severe obesity may make pre-existing nutritional deficiencies worse or produce new ones, depending on dietary intake, adherence to supplementation and the degree of malabsorption associated with the bariatric procedure performed (4). As the popularity of bariatric surgery continues to increase, it is important for clinicians working with these individuals to identify and treat preexisting nutritional deficiencies.

3.2 Proposed origins

It has been proposed that the major causes of obesity include a combination of lack of physical activity, a high-fat, high-caloric Western diet, increased portion sizes, and low socioeconomic status (5-8). Regarding diet, data from four NHANES conducted between 1971 and 2002 for trends in self-reported food intake showed that energy intake, amount of food, and carbohydrate energy have significantly increased in all race and gender groups. Findings from a study published by Neilson (7) illustrate how energy intake has increased by increasing portion sizes. They found that between 1977 and 1996, portions inside and outside the home increased for salty snacks (by 93 Kcals), soft drinks (by 49 Kcals), hamburgers (by 97 Kcals), French fries (by 68 Kcals), and Mexican food (by 133 Kcals). Clearly, this increase growth in portion sizes mirrors our growing waistlines.

In addition to diet and increasing portion sizes, socioeconomic status and the environment must also be considered as contributors to the growing problem of obesity. Fruits, vegetables, low-fat dairy, nuts and legumes, and lean proteins are considered unprocessed, nutrient–dense foods, which contribute most of the vitamins and minerals necessary for health. While foods that are processed such as prepackaged convenience foods, sweets, and snack goods provide a high amount of calories but are nutrient-poor and lack proteins, vitamins, minerals, and fiber. These energy-dense, nutrient-poor foods are often more affordable than foods of lower energy-density or higher nutrient-density such as fruits, vegetables, and whole grains (9, 10). Poverty can lead to food insecurity and one outcome of food insecurity is obesity (11). It has been found that households characterized as food insecure also have the highest body mass index and prevalence of obesity (12). When a household runs out of food and is uncertain about the ability to obtain enough food, the quality of the diet becomes compromised and leads to an increase in the intake of energy from foods that are higher in fat and carbohydrate, but lower in nutrients (11). This may be one of the reasons why we see so many nutritional deficiencies in obese persons.

3.3 Micronutrient deficiencies and dietary intake

Studies are demonstrating that micronutrient deficiencies are common in obese people even before bariatric surgery (13, 14). As discussed above, one cause of these nutritional deficiencies in overweight and obese individuals may be due to a high intake of processed foods that are calorically dense, but nutritionally-poor. Additionally, obese individuals may have altered bioavailability of many nutrients, a condition that has been called "high calorie malnutrition" (15). The combination of low preoperative vitamin status and the malabsorption that follows bariatric surgery may leave these patients at risk for many severe vitamin deficiencies. Typical nutritional deficiencies associated with obesity include antioxidants, vitamin A, vitamin D, B-complex vitamins, calcium, iron, and zinc (16). In a retrospective study of 379 patients planning for gastric bypass, significant deficiencies were identified for thiamine (29%), iron (44%), and 25-hydroxyvitamin D (68%). A second study also examined cross-sectional data from NHANES III and found that obese subjects (n = 3831), particularly premenopausal women, were more likely to have low levels of various micronutrients than were normal-weight adults in the same sex/age category (17). Among women, low biochemical micronutrient levels were associated with increasing BMI categories for vitamin E, alpha-carotene, beta-carotene, beta-cryptoxanthin, lutein/zeaxanthin, lycopene, total carotenoids, vitamin C, selenium (premenopausal), vitamin D, and folate. And among men, low biochemical micronutrient levels were associated with increasing BMI categories for alpha-carotene, beta-carotene, beta-cryptoxanthin, lutein/zeaxanthin, total carotenoids, vitamin C, selenium, and folate. Since nutritional deficiencies are so common in the obese population, it will remain important to conduct trials involving preoperative testing with treatment of micronutrient deficiencies prior to surgery, in order to look for improved postoperative outcomes.

Behavioral weight loss programs often involve a reduced calorie diet, increased energy expenditure, and use of behavior strategies such as goal setting and self-monitoring (18). Self-monitoring has been described as the cornerstone of behavioral treatment for weight loss (19, 20). Usual techniques for self-monitoring involve keeping food, weight, and activity diaries. One recent randomized-controlled trial compared the effectiveness of self-monitoring with a paper diary versus two types of personal digital assistants (PDA) (21, 22). After 6 months, they found that, compared to the paper diary group, both PDA groups were more adherent to self-monitoring and that self-monitoring of diet in this group had a significant indirect effect on percent weight loss. The use of food diaries not only improves ones chances for weight loss, but it also gives clinicians a tool to assess food intake and dietary patterns. In addition, it may help to identify possible nutritional deficiencies both before and after weight loss surgery.

When considering what nutritional deficiencies may be present before surgery it is important to look at what we are eating as a nation. NHANES is a continuous, cross-sectional survey designed to monitor the health and nutritional status of the civilian, noninstitutionalized U.S. population (23). Based on the most recent 2007-2008 NHANES data, adults over age 20 are not meeting the minimum recommended intakes for fruit, vegetables, and low-fat dairy and thus had diets that that did not meet the dietary reference intakes (DRIs) in fiber, vitamin A, vitamin D, vitamin E, vitamin K (men only), calcium, magnesium (women only) and potassium (24). It is interesting to note that over one-third (36.8% for men and 35.5% for women) of the total daily caloric intake for adults comes from solid fats, added sugars, and alcohol (SoFAS). This is well above the highest recommended limit and may be one answer to the growing obesity problem in America. MyPyramid recommends calories from SoFAS to range from 132-512 per day based on height, weight, gender, and activity level. According to the 2007-2008 NHANES data, the mean intake of calories from SoFAS in adult men was 923 calories/day and for women it was 624 calories/day.

Another recent study analyzed 2-day, 24-hour recall data from the 2003–2004 NHANES and found that fewer than 1 in 10 Americans met the MyPyramid recommendations for fruit and vegetable intake (25). Only 0.9% of adolescents, 2.2% of adult men, and 3.5% of adult women met the recommendations for both fruit and vegetables. A higher percentage of participants met fruit recommendations alone, 6.2% (adolescents), 8.6% (adult men), and 12.3% (adult women). Adolescents consumed less whole fruit and more juice than adults and the largest contributor to fruit intake was orange juice. Only 5.8% of adolescents, 14.7% of adult men and 18.6% of adult women met recommendations for vegetable intake. Interestingly, when fried potatoes were excluded only 2.2% of adolescents, 9% of adult men and 13.4% of adult women met recommendations for vegetable intake. The percentage meeting recommendations for vegetable subtypes for all groups was lowest for dark green vegetables, orange vegetables, and legumes but higher for starchy and other vegetables. This data makes it clear that we are not meeting the recommended intakes for low-calorie, nutrient-dense foods. And when we are choosing vegetables, they are likely to be fried starchy vegetables with added fats and thus contribute excessive calories in the diet. It is also important to consider the amount of calories we are consuming from the beverages we are drinking when looking at the obesity problem. One recent report based on NHANES data between 2005-2008, states that 50% of the population consumes sugary drinks on any given day, while 25% consumes some sugary drinks but less than 200 kcal (more than one 12-oz can of cola), and 5% consumes at least 567 kcal from sugar drinks per day (more than four 12-oz cans of cola) (26). Consumption of sugary drinks is lowest among the oldest females (42 kcal per day) and highest among males aged 12–19 (273 kcal per day). Among adults aged 20 and over, it was found that non-Hispanic white persons consume fewer sugary-drink calories as a percentage of total daily calories (5.3%) than do non-Hispanic black (8.6%) or Mexican-American persons (8.2%). Low-income individuals tend to consume more sugary beverages than higher-income individuals. Among adults living below 130% of the poverty line, they report that mean calories from sugary drinks makes up 8.8% of total calories; among those living between 130% and 350% of the poverty line, mean calories from sugary drinks is 6.2% of total calories; and among those at or above 350% of the poverty line, mean calories from sugary beverages is 4.4% of total calories. This data is alarming since consuming sweetened beverages has been linked to poor diet quality, weight gain, obesity, and, in adults, type 2 diabetes (27, 28). Since a good portion of our calories are coming from sugary beverages and calorie-dense, nutrient-poor foods, it is understandable why we find many obese patients with micronutrient deficiencies prior to weight loss surgery. It is therefore important to screen for these and to treat their nutritional deficiencies prior to surgery to help to prevent major or fatal nutritional complications that may occur in the long-term after bariatric surgery.

4. Surgical origins for micronutrient deficiencies

4.1 Roux-en-Y gastric bypass

Roux-en-Y gastric bypass (RYGB) is the most commonly performed bariatric surgery in North America and remains the major surgical option for individuals with medically-complicated obesity. The divided RYGB combines restriction of food intake, due to the small size of the gastric pouch and constriction at the gastrojejunal anastomosis, with malabsorption induced by bypass of the duodenum and variable lengths of jejunum (see Figure 1). A small proximal stomach pouch is created with a stapler device and is connected to distally transected jejunum. The remnant stomach and proximally transected jejunum is then reattached in a Y-shaped configuration to the distal small intestine. Malabsorption of both fat and nitrogen has been identified in studies of the Roux-en-Y reconstruction (29). Malabsorption was corrected by providing oral, exogenous pancreatic enzymes. The RYGB bypasses native stomach that secretes intrinsic factor which is required for vitamin B12 absorption, as well as proximal small intestine which is required for absorption of copper, iron, and thiamine. The length of small intestine between the gastrojejunostomy and the jejunojejunostomy is not exposed to bile, thus limiting absorption of fat soluble vitamins due to absence of micelle formation. Reduced vitamin D levels due to malabsorption induce inadequate calcium absorption and utilization.

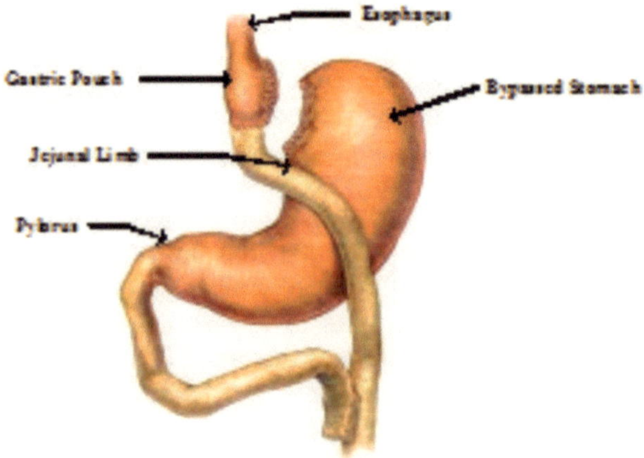

Fig. 1. Roux-en-y gastric bypass. The orientation of the gastro-jejunal anastomosis can be different depending upon whether it is formed during an open or laparoscopic surgery. The location of the jejuno-jejunal anastomosis alters the length of the common channel, which extends from the jejuno-jejunostomy to the ileocecal valve. (Adapted with permission from 31)

There are multiple studies of micronutrient deficiencies after RYGB. A major study of 493 patients after laparoscopic RYGB revealed deficiencies of vitamin A (11%), vitamin C (34.6%), vitamin D (7%), thiamine (18.3%), riboflavin (13.6%), vitamin B6 (17.6%), and vitamin B12 (3.6%) at 1 year after surgery (30). The results must be considered with regards to the body's reserves for different vitamins (18 days for thiamine and 3 to 5 years for vitamin B12 and vitamin E).

4.2 Adjustable gastric banding

Laparoscopic adjustable gastric banding (LAGB) is an effective strategy for the surgical treatment of morbidly obese patients and is the most common bariatric procedure in Europe and Australia. Restriction is created by placing a silicone band around the fundus of the stomach, approximately 4 cm distal to the gastroesophageal junction. The level of gastric constriction by the band can be adjusted by addition or removal of saline through a subcutaneous port placed above the abdominal musculature (see Figure 2). Since the introduction of the modern adjustable gastric band in 1994, this procedure has continued to gain momentum as a therapeutic alternative to RYGB. Since LAGB is a restrictive procedure, nutritional deficiencies are not expected post-operatively. However, recent reports of micronutrient deficiencies are now emerging. A study of LAGB in adolescents revealed vitamin D deficiency as the second most common micronutrient deficiency (after iron deficiency anemia) within the first two years after surgery (32).

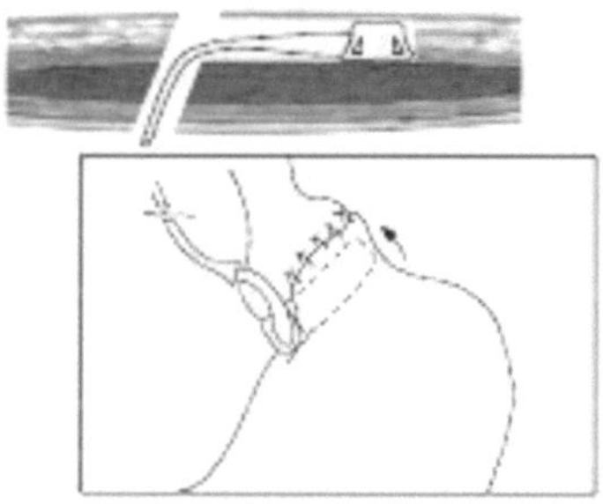

Fig. 2. Gastric Adjustable Band. As shown in the lower half of this drawing, the band is placed laparoscopically around the upper part of the stomach, approximately 4 cm below the gastroesophageal junction. As shown in the upper half of this drawing, the access port in placed subcutaneously on top of the abdominal musculature. The ring or band is connected to the access port by tubing and its volume can be adjusted by accessing the port in order to add or remove sterile saline (Adapted with permission from Allergan, Inc. from http://www.allergan.com/assets/pdf/lapband_dfu.pdf).

4.3 Vertical sleeve gastrectomy

Sleeve gastrectomy (SG), or gastric sleeve, is a surgical weight-loss procedure in which the stomach is reduced to about 15% of its original size by surgical removal of a large portion of the stomach along the greater curvature. Despite being described as a solely restrictive procedure, micronutrient deficiencies post operatively are common. A recently published study from the Netherlands showed that 21% patients were Vitamin D deficient within one year of having a SG (33). This deficiency occurred despite daily multi-vitamin supplementation. Bone loss and bone remodeling also occurs following SG in as little as one year. Significant bone mass loss and remodeling were recorded in a study using bone densitometry and bone remodeling markers (34). Despite the presence of micronutrient deficiencies induced by SG, studies show that fewer nutrient deficiencies occur after SG as compared to RYGB (35). However, SG is often combined with the duodenal switch procedure as described in section 4.4.

4.4 Biliopancreatic diversion

Biliopancreatic diversion (BPD), or the Scopinaro procedure, is the original weight loss surgery. This procedure is now rarely performed because of problems with severe malnutrition and severe early complications, including death (36, 37). BPD is the hallmark of a malabsorptive procedure that produces substantial and sustained weight loss, but the malabsorption of fat and protein is paralleled by malabsorption of fat soluble and water soluble vitamins, minerals, and trace elements.

This operation has been replaced by malabsorptive procedures that obtain a "physiological" biliopancreatic diversion, through formation of a jejuno-enteric anastomosis ≤120 cm from the ileocecal valve (i.e. by preparation of a long Roux limb or by preparation of a long biliopancreatic limb). Malabsorption induced by a short common channel in part involves inadequate micelle formation, with subsequent development of steatorrhea.

By comparison, in the duodenal switch procedure, the duodenum is transected 5 cm distal to the pylorus; the distal duodenal segment (stump) is then oversewn. Small intestine is transected approximately 1/3 of its length to the ileocecal valve. The distal transected segment is used in the production of an anastomosis to proximal duodenum and the proximal transected segment is used in the production of an entero-enteric anastomosis (which is 75 to 100 cm proximal to the ileocecal valve).

In comparison to RYGB, low serum levels of zinc and copper are more common in individuals after biliopancreatic diversion (38). A randomized trial of RYGB compared to duodenal switch revealed increased deficiencies of thiamine, vitamin A, and vitamin D in the first year after duodenal switch (107).

5. Medical origins for micronutrient deficiencies

5.1 Preoperative deficiencies

Major micronutrients that have been examined preoperatively include vitamin D (vitamin D deficiency is reported in 25% to 96% of morbidly obese individuals) (39-42) and thiamine (15% prevalence of low preoperative thiamine levels among 437 consecutive obese patients) (43). Obesity was identified as a risk factor, in a preoperative surgical population, for finding low plasma ascorbic acid concentrations (44). In preoperative obese patients in Israel, common micronutrient deficiencies included iron (35%), folic acid (24%), and vitamin B12 (3.6%) with high levels of parathyroid hormone identified in 39% of patients (45). A high prevalence of vitamin A deficiency in obese, preoperative patients has been described (46), but daily supplementation with 5,000 IU of retinol acetate (ester derivative of Vitamin A) did not fully resolve vitamin A deficiency 6 months after RYGB.

5.2 Weight loss supplements and programs

Special dietary programs and dietary supplements, which are commonly utilized by morbidly obese individuals, have been associated with development of micronutrient deficiency (47, 48). Starvation, which has been previously suggested as a treatment for obesity, can also contribute to the development of thiamine deficiency.

5.3 Pharmacological agents

Pharmacologic agents can result in micronutrient depletion through multiple mechanisms. Excretion of urinary zinc is enhanced by diuretics, such as hydrochlorothiazide (49, 50).

A second proposed mechanism involves molecular mimicry. The prototype drug for this proposed mechanism is conversion of metronidazole to an analog of thiamine, an inhibitor of thiamine pyrophosphokinase (51).

Thiamine deficiency induced by parenteral feedings (52) may be caused by consumption induced by a high glucose load or may be induced by development of sepsis (53), especially in patients being treated for postoperative complications. More severe beriberi is associated with the development of lactic acidosis and "fulminant beriberi" may be related to thiamine depletion induced by a high glucose load in patients receiving total parenteral nutrition (54).

Alcohol consumption appears to be a toxic origin for depletion of multiple micronutrients, including B vitamins (55), folate (due to a weak antifolate effect) (56), and zinc and selenium (57).

5.4 Small intestinal bacterial overgrowth

Small intestinal bacterial overgrowth is another potential explanation for the development of micronutrient deficiencies. After Roux-en-Y gastric bypass, there is relative achlorhydria of the gastric pouch, which may permit upper gut bacterial overgrowth. As another potential origin for small bowel bacterial overgrowth, it has been suggested that small intestinal bacterial overgrowth in patients with diabetes mellitus is related to the presence of a gut motility disorder (58). In support of this mechanism, the prevalence of small intestinal bacterial overgrowth is higher in diabetic patients who have evidence for autonomic neuropathy (59). In a preliminary study, we have previously noted upper gut bacterial overgrowth among patients who have undergone an adjustable gastric band, perhaps induced by stasis in the proximal gastric pouch (60).

In our previous study, postoperative thiamine deficiency after RYGB was associated with small intestinal bacterial overgrowth (31). Consumption of micronutrients by small intestinal bacteria has been reported but is not fully understood. There are multiple studies of the effect of bacteria on vitamin B12 and thiamine. A major observation in this field has been that bacteria secrete thiaminases, which can cleave thiamine (61-63). Staphylococcus aureus produces a thiaminase type II that is regulated at both the transcriptional as well as the enzymatic level. Thiaminase type II catalyzes the cleavage (deamination) of thiamine.

6. Deficiencies of micronutrients

6.1 Water soluble vitamins

The biochemical roles of water-soluble vitamins and their associated deficiency disorders are shown in Table 2. There is only minor storage in the body of most water-soluble vitamins.

VITAMIN	DEFICIENCY STATE	SYMPTOMS
Thiamine (Vitamin B1)	Beriberi	See Table 3
Riboflavin (Vitamin B2)	Ariboflavinosis	Anemia, Stomatitis, Glossitis, Dermatitis
Niacin (Vitamin B3)	Pellagra	Diarrhea, Dermititis, Ataxia, Confusion
Folic Acid	Folate deficiency anemia	Weakness, Anorexia, Weight Loss
Pyridoxine (Vitamin B6)		Dermititis, Confusion, Neuropathy
Cobalamin (Vitamin B12)	Pernicious Anemia	Depression, Ataxia, Parasthesias
Ascorbic Acid (Vitamin C)	Scurvy	Malaise, Myalgias, Petechia, Gum Disease

Table 2. Water soluble vitamins and their deficiencies

6.1.1 Thiamine

Thiamine or vitamin B1 deficiency is a major nutritional complication following RYGB (31). Thiamine deficiency or beriberi was originally described in individuals with multi-organ involvement, including cardiac, gastrointestinal or neuropsychiatric symptoms that corrected with "beriberi factor" or thiamine (see Table 3)). We have described after RYGB the presence of thiamine deficiency that does not correct with oral thiamine. "Bariatric beriberi" is associated with small intestinal bacterial overgrowth and antibiotic therapy may be required to correct thiamine deficiency.

Among the major clinical presentations of beriberi, patients with neuropsychiatric beriberi may have auditory and visual hallucinations, or aggressive behavior. Wernicke's disease presents with confusion (impairment of memory or altered mental state), nystagmus, ataxia, and ophthalmoplegia. Patients with high output cardiovascular disease (wet beriberi) have been reported to have tachycardia, respiratory distress, or lower extremity edema, with right ventricular dilation and lactic acidosis. Patients with neurological (dry beriberi) present with numbness or muscle weakness, pain of lower greater than upper extremities, or convulsions. Gastrointestinal beriberi induces delayed emptying of the stomach. After gastric bypass surgery, common symptoms include nausea and emesis in patients who may have megajejunum and constipation in patients who may have megacolon. A recent case study supports the notion that thiamine deficiency can induce both a sensory ataxia and optic neuropathy (64), a symptom complex more commonly believed to suggest copper deficiency.

Only a small percentage of total body thiamine is present in whole blood. Measurement of erythrocyte transketolase activity is an alternative approach for determination of thiamine deficiency (65). This bioassay is based upon binding of the catalytic activity of the enzyme transketolase to thiamine pyrophosphate. Due to the seriousness of thiamine deficiency, recent European guidelines suggest that after bariatric surgery, patients should have follow-up evaluation of their thiamine status for at least 6 months and receive parenteral thiamine supplementation (66).

A standard therapy for thiamine deficiency is thiamine HCl 100 mg taken orally twice daily. In patients who do not respond to oral thiamine, the presence of small intestinal bacterial overgrowth must be considered. Acute psychosis and Wernicke's encephalopathy are medical emergencies. These conditions require hospitalization with supportive care and a minimum of 250 mg of thiamine given daily intramuscular or intravenously (infused over 3 to 4 hours to reduce the risk of an anaphylactoid reaction) for at least 3 to 5 days (67). Most patients report symptomatic improvement within several days after the first parenteral dose of thiamine HCl. An autopsy is recommending for those individuals who have died from suspected Wernicke encephalopathy (66).

BERIBERI SUBTYPE	SYMPTOMS AND FINDINGS
Neuropsychiatric	Hallucinations; Aggressive Behavior; Confusion; Nystagmus; Ataxia; Ophthalmoplegia
Neurologic (Dry beriberi)	Numbness; Muscle Weakness and Pain of Lower>Upper Extremities; Convulsions; Exaggerated Tendon Reflexes
High Output Cardiac (Wet beriberi)	Tachycardia; Bradycardia; Respiratory Distress; Leg Edema; Right Ventricular Dilation; L-Lactic Acidosis
Gastroenterologic	Nausea; Vomiting; Slow Gastric Emptying; Megajejunum; Constipation; Megacolon

Table 3. Clinical features of beriberi

6.1.2 Riboflavin

Riboflavin or vitamin B2 is present in the flavocoenzymes, flavin adenine dinucleotide and flavin mononucleotide. Flavocoenzymes are a major participant in a number of reactions important in metabolic pathways and in the proper functioning of glutathione peroxidase (required for metabolism of hydroperoxides) and glutathione reductase (generates reduced glutathione from oxidized glutathione). Biochemical but not clinical riboflavin deficiency has been reported after bariatric surgery (30). Clinical symptoms of riboflavin deficiency include sore throat, stomatitis, anemia, and a scaly dermatitis. It has been suggested that riboflavin deficiency may play a role in the development of migraine-like headaches. The standard treatment for riboflavin deficiency is 5-10 mg daily of oral riboflavin.

Since the reliability of the serum assay for vitamin B2 is uncertain, a clinical improvement in a potential symptom during supplementation with oral riboflavin may support the diagnosis of a deficiency state.

6.1.3 Niacin

Nicotonic acid or vitamin B3 is converted into both nicotinamide, a component of nicotinamide adenine dinucleotide (involved in catabolic reactions), and nicotinamide adenine dinucleotide phosphate (involved in anabolic reactions). Clinical deficiency of niacin has not been reported after bariatric surgery, although it has likely been present in patients with multiple B vitamin deficiencies. It is difficult to diagnose niacin deficiency by laboratory studies, but the diagnosis is supported by low plasma niacin. Deficiency of niacin is termed pellagra, which includes neurologic, dermatologic, and gastrointestinal involvement. Patients may present with headaches, ataxia or myoclonus, anxiety-depression, delusions or hallucinations, painful, scaly dermititis, and a malabsorptive disorder or diarrhea with colitis. The initial treatment of pellagra is initiation of oral niacin 100-500 mg, three times daily (this may induce flushing). Symptomatic improvement during niacin supplementation could support a diagnosis of niacin deficiency.

6.1.4 Folate

In studies of patients with small intestinal bacterial overgrowth, a high serum folate level is an identified and validated marker for bacterial overgrowth (68). Folate levels in patients after RYGB must therefore be considered in the context of a patient's risk for development of small intestinal bacterial overgrowth. In patients who have folate deficiency after bariatric surgery, the potential for another small intestinal malabsorptive disorder, including celiac sprue, should be considered. Patients with folate deficiency are generally detected in this patient population in individuals with a normocytic, mixed anemia with an increased red cell distribution width. Symptoms of folate deficiency include weakness, anorexia, and weight loss. Treatment of folate deficiency begins with oral folic acid, 1 to 5 mg daily.

6.1.5 Vitamin B6

The active form of vitamin B6 is pyridoxal phosphate. A clinical diagnosis of vitamin B6 deficiency has not been widely recognized after bariatric surgery. Patients with vitamin B6 deficiency can present with dermatitis, confusion, anemia and neurologic symptoms. Peripheral neuropathy has also been reported with vitamin B6 deficiency (69). Treatment can be started with oral vitamin B6 at 30 mg daily; a post-therapy increased level of pyridoxal phosphate is then consistent with repletion of vitamin B6.

6.1.6 Vitamin B12

Vitamin B12 deficiency is a well-described nutritional deficiency after bariatric surgery and is likely multifactorial in origin (30). RYGB results in the exclusion of the majority of parietal cell mass, which is a site of R factor and intrinsic factor production. Relative achlorhydria after bariatric surgery prevents oral cyanocobalamin from being deconjugated from pteryl groups, before cyanocobalamin absorption.

Because of vitamin B12 storage in the body, development of vitamin B12 deficiency may become clinically relevant 3 to 5 years after bariatric surgery. Methyl malonic acid blood levels will increase when vitamin B12 stores are depleted (70). A low normal blood level of vitamin B12 can indicate the presence of deficiency. Clinical manifestations of vitamin B12 deficiency include the multiple presentations of pernicious anemia or the development of peripheral neuropathy. In treatment of vitamin B12 deficiency, daily oral cobalamin is considered less effective than the intra-muscular preparation. Treatments for Vitamin B12 deficiency include: i. oral vitamin B12 (cyanocobalamin) 350 to 500 mcg per day, ii. intramuscular vitamin B12 1,000 mcg every month or 3,000 mcg every 6 months, iii. nasal (500 mcg once weekly), or iv. sublingual (500 mcg, once daily) preparation.

6.1.7 Vitamin C

Biochemical evidence for vitamin C or ascorbic acid deficiency is common after bariatric surgery (44). Ascorbic acid deficiency is suggested by clinical symptoms. In our clinical practice, bariatric patients present with fatigue or complaint of arthralgias. Early reported symptoms include malaise, myalgias, and petechia, with progression to gum disease (scurvy). Standard treatment for a patient with vitamin C deficiency is oral ascorbic acid 200 mg daily.

6.2 Fat soluble vitamins

Signs and symptoms of the fat soluble vitamin (A, D, E, and K) deficiency are summarized in Table 4.

VITAMIN	SYMPTOMS
A	Nyctalopia, Blindness
D	Arthralgias, Myalgias, Fasciculations
E	Anemia, Dysarthria, Ataxia, Myopathy
K	Bleeding Disorder

Table 4. Fat soluble vitamins and their deficiencies

6.2.1 Vitamin A

Vitamin A complex includes retinols, beta-carotenes, and carotenoids, and there is approximately a 1 year supply stored in human liver. When ingested in high doses, excessive doses of vitamin A may cause headache, vomiting, diplopia, alopecia, dryness of the mucous membranes, bone abnormalities, and liver damage. Signs of toxicity usually appear with sustained daily intakes exceeding 15,000 IU. As alternative therapy, signs of toxicity have not been observed while receiving beta-carotene, a previtamin A analogue.

Vitamin A deficiency after bariatric surgery is most commonly seen in patients who have undergone a biliopancreatic diversion, duodenal switch, or extended Roux-en-Y gastric bypass. In these procedures, the mechanism of deficiency is most likely related to fat soluble vitamin malabsorption induced by bile acid deficiency. In addition, individuals with zinc deficiency have impaired protein synthesis that may alter retinol transport from the liver to other organs. Manifestations of vitamin A deficiency in a bariatric patient include nocturnal visual difficulty, dry skin, dry hair, and pruritus. Other potential manifestations include decreased visual acuity and reduced resistance to infections. Treatment of vitamin A deficiency includes supplemental vitamin A, 10,000 IU daily by mouth (with co-therapy of any existing iron deficiency since vitamin A deficiency may persist in the presence of iron deficiency).

6.2.2 Vitamin D

Vitamin D deficiency after RYGB induces metabolic bone disease (71). Vitamin D deficiency activates a metabolic cascade resulting in decreased calcium absorption and insufficient calcium availability. This cascade induces subsequently hypocalcemia, secondary hyperparathyroidism, and development of osteoporosis and osteomalacia (72-74). Patients will see their physician for symptoms of bony pain, back pain, or aching of the limbs (75).

There is a high frequency of and serious nature of metabolic bone disease after RYGB including bone biopsy-proven osteomalacia with marrow fibrosis (76). Symptoms may be present for as long as 2 to 5 years prior to evaluation.

Studies of patients after RYGB demonstrate that maintenance of normal serum calcium involves increasing bony release of calcium and decreasing urinary calcium secretion. After RYGB, a high prevalence of bone resorption and hyperparathyroidism may exist independent of intake of calcium and Vitamin D status (77, 78). This raises a concern that the present recommendations for daily calcium and vitamin D supplementation may not be protective after RYGB, especially in female patients. Commonly, in postoperative follow up after RYGB, patients will still have evidence for inadequate blood levels of vitamin D despite vitamin D oral supplements.

For monitoring, 24-hour urinary calcium determination and a serum alkaline phosphatase level every 6 to 12 months is commonly suggested. However, urine calcium secretion can be altered by concomitant use of diuretics. If urinary calcium excretion is low and the serum alkaline phosphatase activity is increased, alkaline phosphatase should be fractionated. If the alkaline phosphatase is of bone origin, then a serum parathyroid level should be measured. An increase in serum parathyroid level supports supplementation with additional vitamin D and calcium. It is important to obtain a total 25-hydroxy vitamin D level every 12 months or earlier if a patient has a low 24-hour urinary calcium excretion. Low vitamin D levels require consideration of several explanations, including bile salt deficiency, rapid weight loss phase, and small intestinal bacterial overgrowth (which may interfere with vitamin D absorption).

To try to prevent vitamin D deficiency and thus secondary metabolic bone disease, post-operative RYGB patients should receive at least 1.2 grams daily of elemental calcium and 800 international units (IU) of vitamin D daily. In those patients with low serum levels of 25-hydroxy vitamin D, 50,000 IU of vitamin D (ergocalciferol) taken orally once per week for six to eight weeks is prescribed with a recheck of the 25-hydroxy Vitamin D level after eight weeks to confirm repletion (79). The reported dose for treatment of rickets is at least 600,000 IU, which has been given as rapidly as 150,000 IU, taken four times daily during 1 day of treatment. In treatment of osteomalacia, significant improvement in patients' clinical symptoms, functional status, biochemical indices and bone mineral density has been reported after treatment with a combination of ergocalciferol (100,000 IU daily) and calcium carbonate (1 to 2.5 g daily).

6.2.3 Vitamin E

Vitamin E consists of tocopherols and tocotrienols. This fat-soluble vitamin is located in cell membranes, and it may be active in preventing lipid peroxidation. Most adults tolerate doses of vitamin E up to 1000 mg/day (0.67 mg of vitamin E is 1 IU) without gross signs or biochemical evidence of toxicity (80).

Deficiency of vitamin E should be considered in bariatric patients who have visual symptoms (retinopathy), non-specific neurological symptoms (ataxia, dysarthria, muscle weakness due to myopathy, or ptosis), or hemolytic anemia. Treatment of vitamin E deficiency should include oral vitamin E 800 to 1200 IU daily.

6.2.4 Vitamin K

Vitamin K describes a group of compounds which contain the 2-methyl-1,4-naphthoquinone moiety. These compounds are essential for the formation of prothrombin, and five factors (factors VII, IX, and X, and proteins C and S) involved in regulation of blood clotting. Vitamin K is moderately (40 to 70%) well absorbed from the jejunum and ileum (81).

Absorption of vitamin K depends on the normal flow of bile and pancreatic secretion, and its absorption is enhanced by dietary fat. The total body pool of vitamin K is small. Most of the daily requirements for vitamin K is provided through biosynthesis by the intestinal flora. Deficiency of vitamin K leads to increase risk of bleeding disorders.

Vitamin K deficiency is rare after bariatric surgery. There is a report of 5 babies with intracranial hemorrhage whose mothers had undergone bariatric surgery (82), suggesting vitamin K deficiency. Replacement of vitamin K can be accomplished with an oral form (2.5 to 25 mg daily) or with parenteral delivery of vitamin K (5-15 mg, intramuscularly or subcutaneously).

6.3 Essential minerals

Most studies of essential minerals after bariatric surgery involve iron and calcium. It is not presently known whether long-term deficiencies occur with other minerals after bariatric surgery.

6.3.1 Iron

Development of anemia after bariatric surgery is common and the origins for anemia are complex. Many patients after bariatric surgery require iron supplementation for treatment of anemia. Several potential mechanisms may explain iron malabsorption after bariatric surgery, including relative achlorhydria (acid may improve absorption of non-heme iron from plant sources by oxidation of Fe^{2+} to the better-absorbed Fe^{3+} cation) and bypass of proximal small intestine (the major location for iron absorption). Identification of iron deficiency in a bariatric patient requires consideration of other potential gastrointestinal origins for the development of iron deficiency anemia. Routine treatment of iron deficiency includes use of an iron/vitamin C complex or 150 to 200 mg/day of oral elemental iron in any preparation (gluconate/sulfate/fumarate). Parenteral iron is occasionally needed in those patients who have a poor response to oral iron therapy, especially in premenopausal women with heavy menstrual bleeding (83).

It is not commonly known that iron supplementation has risks. Iron supplementation for whatever purpose should be monitored, since electron transfer from transition metals such as iron to oxygen-containing molecules can initiate free radical reactions. Large doses of unnecessary iron supplements could induce an acquired iron overload disorder.

6.3.2 Calcium

Vitamin D deficiency and calcium malabsorption can occur simultaneously. Vitamin D deficiency activates a metabolic cascade resulting in hypocalcemia and secondary hyperparathyroidism. Steatorrhea due to malabsorption induces calcium malabsorption through the interaction of dietary calcium with intraluminal triglycerides.

Isolated serum calcium measurement is not an adequate marker of calcium metabolism. Patients may present with complaints of bony pain, back pain, or aching of the limbs. Bariatric surgery patients can maintain normal serum calcium by decreasing urinary calcium secretion. Urine calcium secretion can however be altered by concomitant use of diuretics. Treatment of calcium deficiency requires minimally oral calcium of ≥ 1.2 grams daily and concomitant correction of vitamin D deficiency.

6.3.3 Iodine

There are no reports of iodine deficiency after bariatric surgery. Weight loss after bariatric surgery is associated with resolution of subclinical hypothyroidism (84).

6.4 Trace elements

Trace elements function as co-factors for antioxidant enzymes or proteins. Trace elements in supplements provide a relatively narrow range of safety between deficiency and toxicity. Because of their ability to donate or accept electrons, transition metals have potential antioxidant properties.

6.4.1 Zinc

Zinc is important in the bioactivity of hundreds of mammalian proteins and is a co-factor in cytosolic superoxide dismutase. Zinc may reduce the formation of the highly toxic hydroxyradical (OH^-) from H_2O_2 produced through the antagonism of redox-active transition metals, such as iron and copper (85). There are reports of biochemical zinc deficiency after bariatric surgery (86). However, clinical zinc deficiency in bariatric patients has not been well studied. Symptoms of zinc deficiency can include a dermatological eruption, alopecia, glossitis, hypoalbuminemia and nail dystrophy. Initial treatment of zinc deficiency is with oral zinc gluconate, 50 mg, taken every other day.

6.4.2 Copper

Copper is a co-factor in cytosolic superoxide dismutase as well as cytochrome oxidase. Animal studies support a linkage in the absorption of copper and zinc (most likely in the stomach and upper small intestine), but a recent study using a human cell line suggests that a different copper transport protein is active in copper absorption in humans (87). Ingestion of fructose appears to reduce the biological activity of copper, as demonstrated by decreasing the activity of superoxide dismutase in erythrocytes (88).

Copper deficiency may result from the use of liquid vitamin supplements that do not contain copper. The occurrence of decreased serum copper levels has been reported through case reports involving bariatric patients, generally >10 years after RYGB (89). Copper deficiency in susceptible individuals can induce anemia and neutropenia, or pancytopenia (90, 91). There have also been, in the past several years, reports of RYGP patients who have developed a myelopathy-like disorder with spastic gait and sensory ataxia associated with low serum copper levels (92). The clinical and neuroimaging findings in these patients are similar to the findings identified in patients with vitamin B12 deficiency. Similar symptoms associated with low serum copper have been reported in individuals with Celiac sprue (93). This condition has been termed by Dr. Kumar "human swayback", which is an unfortunate description since research workers studying swayback in lambs have been reported to develop multiple sclerosis, raising the question of an infectious etiology (94). Unfortunately, copper supplements given to patients with low serum copper levels and symptoms of myeloneuropathy do not appear to lead to a significant improvement in their neurologic symptoms (95). Further work is needed to better understand the origin for and the treatment for this rare neurologic complication.

Optic neuropathy has been reported to occur in patients after bariatric surgery in association with low serum copper levels (96). However, copper infusion therapy had no effect on the optic neuropathy. From this report, it is therefore unclear whether the damage was irreversible or whether other micronutrient deficiencies may have been involved in the optic neuropathy.

Treatment of copper deficiency can begin with oral copper gluconate, 2 to 4 mg, taken every other day. Higher daily oral doses involving use of 6 mg copper have been reported to be required in some patients (97). Correction of copper deficiency in individual patients may necessitate intravenous infusions of copper chloride (98).

6.4.3 Selenium

Selenium is a trace element that is known to be essential for activation of glutathione peroxidase, a key enzyme in the body's defense against oxygen-derived free radicals. Selenium supplementation, alone and in combination with other micronutrients, has been extensively studied. Selenium deficiency induces a cardiomyopathy in those regions of the world in which selenium levels in the soil are low, as in China. There is a case report of a patient presenting with a severe cardiomyopathy 9 months after biliopancreatic diversion (99). Treatment of selenium deficiency begins with sodium selenite, 100 micrograms daily taken orally.

6.4.4 Chromium

It is not known whether chromium is a required cofactor in humans. Chromium deficiency has not been reported after bariatric surgery. The potential role of chromium in human nutrition is based on observations from patients receiving total parenteral nutrition. Case reports have discussed, in patients with total parenteral nutrition, development of an abnormal intravenous glucose tolerance test, weight loss, and peripheral neuropathy associated with decreased blood chromium levels (100).

6.4.5 Manganese

Manganese is an important cofactor in inducible mitochondrial superoxide dismutase. Manganese deficiency has not been reported after bariatric surgery. Deficiency of manganese in animal models inhibits collagen deposition during wound healing and induces skeletal deformation.

7. Symptoms and findings of micronutrient deficiencies

7.1 Anemia

This is the most commonly recognized and treatable nutrient deficiency after bariatric surgery (101, 102). Patients with normal hemoglobin levels can have low ferritin levels after RYGB, supporting the addition of iron supplementation at that time. Iron deficiency anemia can be monitored by checking hemoglobin, hematocrit, and mean corpuscular volume as part of a complete blood count. Routine treatment of iron deficiency includes treatment with an iron/vitamin C complex or with 150 to 200 mg/day of oral elemental iron in any preparation (gluconate/sulfate/fumarate). If there is an incomplete response to oral iron therapy and vitamin B12 and an evaluation by a gastrointestinal specialist has not provided a specific diagnosis, one must then consider additional micronutrient deficiencies and other origins for anemia. Other nutritional origins of anemia must be excluded by examining levels of folate, zinc, copper, and vitamins A and E (see Table 5).

As mentioned above, a gastrointestinal specialist should be consulted when anemia does not correct with iron and vitamin B12 supplementation, in order to exclude blood (i.e. iron) loss from a colon source, a stomal ulcer, a duodenal ulcer, or antritis. Blood loss from the gastric remnant can at times be addressed by a double balloon enteroscopy. The lengths of the Roux limb and the pancreaticobiliary limb may preclude direct endoscopic visualization of the duodenum and bypassed stomach. If one needs to visualize the "bypassed" stomach and duodenum, this can be accomplished by intraoperative endoscopy performed through a laparoscopically-assisted gastrotomy, which will allow insertion of an endoscope directly into the bypassed stomach.

7.2 Neurologic symptoms

Neurologic complaints are reported by about 1% of post-operative patients in surveys, but are described by 5% of patients in prospective studies (103). A main determination is whether the neurologic complaint is indeed related to a post-operative disorder. Patients present most commonly with peripheral neuropathy after RYGB (104). Micronutrient deficiencies involving vitamin B12 and copper are reported in bariatric surgery patients who have been seen for neurologic symptoms (105). Reported neurologic emergencies include Wernicke's disease and Guillain-Barre syndrome.

In patients with neurologic symptoms, blood levels of vitamin B12, vitamin B2, vitamin B6, vitamin E, copper, thiamine, and niacin should be obtained (see Table 5). Physicians must remember that patients may expect to have neurological symptoms after RYGB (and therefore may not report their symptoms) and patients may believe that neurologic symptoms are related to their history of diabetes mellitus.

It is not clear whether the routine use of chewable multivitamins containing minerals after bariatric surgery prevent neurologic disorders. It is not known whether neurologic symptoms can be consistently reversed by treatment of specific micronutrient deficiencies. There are only anecdotal reports of the use of micronutrient infusions for the treatment of neurologic symptoms (a typical intravenous infusion would include, mixed in 5% dextrose in aqueous solution, a standard injectable multivitamin formulation [several are commercially available] with a mixture of trace elements, such as Multitrace 5 concentrate, and both 100 mg thiamine hydrochloride and 1 mg folic acid). Revision of bariatric surgery in order to reduce the length of bypassed small intestine has been reported to be of clinical benefit in a patient with neurologic symptoms (105). Physicians should be cautious, should encourage strongly the use of supplemental multivitamins, and should routinely screen all patients for neurologic symptoms during their postoperative visits.

SYMPTOM	LABORATORY TESTING
Anemia	Ferritin; Vitamin B12; Folate; Zinc; Copper; Vitamins A; Vitamin E
Neurologic Symptoms	Vitamin B12; Vitamin E; Copper; Thiamine; Vitamin B2; Vitamin B6; Plasma Niacin
Visual Symptoms	Vitamin A; Vitamin E; Whole blood thiamine; Copper
Bleeding Disorder	Complete Blood Count; Prothrombin Time
Skin Disorders	Vitamin A; Vitamins B2; Vitamin B6; Zinc; Plasma Niacin
Edema	Selenium; Plasma Niacin; Whole Blood Thiamine

Table 5. Laboratory testing after bariatric surgery

7.3 Visual disorders

Manifestations of vitamin A deficiency include nocturnal visual difficulty and decreased visual acuity. Vitamin E deficiency can induce visual symptoms related to retinopathy. Patients with thiamine deficiency can present with complaints of difficulty focusing their vision or persistent blurred vision; on physical examination, nystagmus is often identified. Optic neuropathy has been reported in patients with deficiencies of copper and thiamine. In laboratory evaluation, one should consider obtaining serum levels of vitamin A, vitamin E, copper and whole blood thiamine (see Table 5).

7.4 Skin disorders

Symptoms of zinc deficiency include a dermatological eruption, but it is unclear whether this occurs after bariatric surgery. Manifestations of vitamin A deficiency include xerosis and pruritus. Essential fatty acid deficiency, niacin deficiency, and riboflavin deficiency can cause a scaly dermititis. The two essential fatty acids, linoleic acid and linolenic acid, are both present in flaxseed oil, soybean oil, and canola oil. One can consider ordering serum levels of vitamin B2, vitamin A, zinc, and plasma niacin (see Table 5).

7.5 Edema

Underlying heart failure is a major concern when a bariatric patient presents with edema. Patients with thiamine deficiency can develop high output cardiovascular disease (wet beriberi) and may present with tachycardia, bradycardia, respiratory distress, lower extremity edema, right > left ventricular dilation, and lactic acidosis. Selenium deficiency is another known cause of heart failure. Evaluation of edema could include determination of serum selenium, plasma niacin, and whole blood thiamine levels (see Table 5).

In considering other medical conditions, edema could be caused by obstructive sleep apnea. Edema can develop in patients with hypoalbuminemia. An underlying hepatic disorder, potentially the end result of steatohepatitis, should be considered. Other origins of hypoalbuminemia include an inflammatory process and small intestinal bacterial overgrowth. There is a serious syndrome of post-operative diarrhea associated with hypoalbuminenia and diffuse edema. This disorder may be induced by severe protein-calorie malnutrition due to a physiological biliopancreatic diversion, such as an extended (distal) Roux-en-Y gastric bypass or a duodenal switch. In addition, it has been reported that this syndrome improves with antibiotic therapy (106) supporting the role of small intestinal bacterial overgrowth. Finally, niacin deficiency can induce a diarrheal illness or colitis that may be responsible for development of hypoalbuminemia as an origin for peripheral edema.

8. Conclusions

There is an increasing prevalence of obesity in developed countries. Dietary intake may be both an origin for obesity as well as an origin for the development of micronutrient deficiencies. Since dietary and activity programs fail to produce sufficient weight loss in most obese individuals, bariatric surgery will continue to be the major therapeutic options for patients with medically-complicated obesity. Many patients after bariatric surgery will develop micronutrient deficiencies despite suggestions for the use of ongoing vitamin and mineral supplementation. Common micronutrient deficiencies after bariatric surgery include deficiencies of iron, vitamin B12, thiamine, and vitamin D. The risks of micronutrient deficiencies are highest in those individuals who have undergone a malabsorptive surgical procedure. Other origins for micronutrient deficiencies include the utilization of pharmacological agents or dietary supplements, and the presence of upper gut or small intestinal bacterial overgrowth. Micronutrient deficiencies must be considered when patients develop specific symptom complexes. It is not yet known whether an ongoing survey of symptoms or a regularly scheduled determination of blood levels of micronutrients will prove to be the best detection method to screen bariatric patients for micronutrient deficiencies.

9. References

[1] Ogden, CL, Carroll, MD. Prevalence of overweight, obesity, and extreme obesity among adults: United States, Trends 1960-1962 through 2007-2008. Accessed online: http://www.cdc.gov/NCHS/data/hestat/obesity_adult_07_08/obesity_adult_07_08.pdf

[2] Diabetes Prevention Program Research Group. (2002). Reduction in the incidence of type 2 diabetes with lifestyle intervention or metformin. *NEJM*, 346, 6, pp. 393–403

[3] Look AHEAD Research Group. (2007). Reduction in weight and cardiovascular disease risk factors in individuals with type 2 diabetes: one-year results of the look AHEAD trial. *Diabetes Care*, 30, 6, pp. 1374–83

[4] Xanthakos, SA. (2009). Nutritional deficiencies in obesity and after bariatric surgery. *Pediatr Clin North Am*, 56, 5, pp. 1105-1121

[5] Kant, AK, Graubard, BI, Kumanyika, SK. (2007). Trends in black-white differentials in dietary intakes of U.S. Adults, 1971-2002. *Am J Prev Med*, 32, 4, pp. 264-72

[6] Frazao, E, Allshouse, J. (2000). Strategies for intervention: commentary and debate. Symposium: sugar and fat-from genes to culture. American Society for Nutritional Sciences. *J Nutr*, 133, pp. 844-47
[7] Neilson, SJ, Popkin, BM. (2003). Patterns and trends in food portion sizes, 1977-1998. *JAMA*, 289, pp. 450-53
[8] Shahar, D, Shai, I, Vardi, H, Shahar, A, Fraser, D. (2005). Diet and eating habits in high and low socieconomic groups. *Nutrition*, 21, pp. 559-66
[9] Drewnowski, A, Pecter, SE. (2004). Poverty and Obesity: The Role of Energy Density and Energy Costs. *Am J Clin Nutr*, 79, pp. 6-16
[10] Drewnowski, A. (2004). Obesity and the food environment: Dietary energy density and diet costs. *Am J Prev Med*, 27, Suppl 3, pp. S154-S162
[11] Tanumihardjo, SA, Anderson, C, Kaufer-Horwitz, M, Bode, L, Emenaker, NJ, Haqq, AM, Satia, JA, Silver, HJ, Stadler, DD. (2007). Poverty, obesity, and malnutrition: an international perspective recognizing the paradox. *J Amer Diet Assoc*, 107, pp. 1966-72
[12] Olson, CM. (1999). Nutrition and Health Outcomes Associated with Food Insecurity and Hunger. *J Nutr*, 129, Suppl 2S, pp. S521-S524
[13] Aasheim, ET, Hofso, D, Hjelmesath, J, Birkeland, KI, Bohmer, T. (2008). Vitamin Status in morbidly obese patients: a cross-sectional study. *Am J Clin Nutr*, 87, pp. 362-69
[14] Flancbaum, L, Belsley, S, Drake, V, et al. (2006). Preoperative nutritional status of paient undergoing Roux-en-Y gastric bypass for morbid obesity. *J Gastrointestinal Surgery*, 10, pp. 1033-37
[15] Kaidar-Person, O, Person, B, Szomstein, S, Rosenthal, RJ. (2008). Nutritional deficiencies in morbidly obese patients: a new form of malnutrition? *Obes Surg*, 18, pp. 870-76
[16] Garcia, OP, Long, KZ, Rosado, JL. (2009). Impact of micronutrient deficiencies on obesity. *Nutrition Rev*, 67, 10, pp. 559-72
[17] Kimmons, JE, Michels Blanck, H, Tohill, BC, Zhang, J, Khan, LK. (2006). Associations between body mass index and the prevalence of low micronutrient levels among US adults. *Med Gen Med*, 8, 4, p. 59
[18] Burke, LE, Wang, J, Sevick, MA. (2011). Self-monitoring in weight loss: a systematic review of the literature. *J Am Diet Assoc*, 111, pp. 92-102
[19] Wing, RR. (1998). Behavioral approaches to the treatment of obesity. In: *Handbook of Obesity*, Bray, GA, Bouchard, C, James, WPT, eds. pp. 855-77, Marcel Dekker, New York, NY
[20] Baker, RC, Kirschenbaum, DS. (1993). Self-monitoring may be necessary for successful weight control. *Behav Ther*, 24, pp. 377-9429]
[21] Burke, LE, Elci, OU, Wang, J, et al. (2009). Self-monitoring in behavioral weight loss treatment: SMART trial short-term results. *Obesity*, 17, Suppl 2, p. S273
[22] Burke, LE, Styn, MA, Glanz, K, et al. (2009). SMART trial: A randomized clinical trial of self-monitoring in behavioral weight management design and baseline findings. *Contemp Clin Trials*, 30, pp. 540-51
[23] National Center for Health Statistics. Accessed online:
National Health and Nutrition Examination Survey 2011.
[24] US Department of Agriculture, Agricultural Research Service, Beltsville Human Nutrition Research Center, Food Surveys Research Group. (2011). *MyPyramid*

Intakes and Snacking Patterns of U.S. Adults: What We Eat in America, NHANES 2007-2008. Food Surveys Research Group Dietary Data Brief No. 5. Accessed online: http://ars.usda.gov/Services/docs.htm?docid=19476.

[25] Kimmons, J, Gillespie, C, Seymour, J, Serdula, M, Michels Blanck, H. (2009). Fruit and vegetable intake among adolescents and adults in the United States: percentage meeting individualized recommendations. *Medscape J Med,* 11, 1, p. 26 Accessed online: http://www.ncbi.nlm.nih.gov/pmc/articles/PMC2654704/?report=printable

[26] Ogden, CL, Kit, BK, Carroll, MD, Park, S. (2011). Consumption of sugar drinks in the United States, 2005–2008. NCHS data brief, no 71. National Center for Health Statistics, Hyattsville, MD.

[27] Malik, VS, Schulze, MB, Hu, FB. (2006). Intake of sugar-sweetened beverages and weight gain: a systematic review. *Am J Clin Nutr,* 84, 2, pp. 274–88

[28] Vartanian, LR, Schwartz, MB, Brownell, KD. (2007). Effects of soft drink consumption on nutrition and health: A systematic review and meta-analysis. *Am J Public Health,* 97, 4, pp. 667–75

[29] Bradley, EL III, Isaacs, JT, Mazo, JD, Hersh, T, Chey, WY. (1977). Pathophysiology and significance of malabsorption after Roux-en-Y reconstruction. *Surgery,* 81, pp. 684-91

[30] Clements, RH, Katasani, VG, Palepu, R, Leeth, RR, Leath, TD, Roy, BP, Vickers, SM. (2006). Incidence of vitamin deficiency after laparoscopic Roux-en-Y gastric bypass in a university hospital setting. *Am Surg,* 72, 12, pp. 1196-202

[31] Lakhani, SV, Shah, HN, Alexander, K, Finelli, FC, Kirkpatrick, JR, Koch, TR. (2008). Small intestinal bacterial overgrowth and thiamine deficiency after Roux-en-Y gastric bypass surgery in obese patients. *Nutrition Res,* 28, 5, pp. 293-98

[32] Nadler, EP, Youn, HA, Ren, CJ, et al. (2008). An update on 73 US obese pediatric patients treated with laparoscopic adjustable gastric banding: comorbidity resolution and compliance data. *J Pediatr Surg,* 43, 1, pp. 131-6

Aarts, EO, Janssen, IM, Berends, FJ. (2011). The gastric sleeve: losing weight as fast as micronutrients? *Obes Surg,* 21, 2, pp. 207-1176]

[34] Nogués, X, Goday, A, Peña, MJ, et al. (2010). Bone mass loss after sleeve gastrectomy: a prospective comparative study with gastric bypass. *Cir Esp,* 88, 2, pp. 103-9

[35] Gehrer, S, Kern, B, Peters, T, et al. (2010). Fewer nutrient deficiencies after laparoscopic sleeve gastrectomy (LSG) than after laparoscopic Roux-Y-gastric bypass (LRYGB)-a prospective study. *Obes Surg,* 20, 4, pp. 447-53

Bajardi, G, Latteri, M, Ricevuto, G, Mastrandrea, G, Florena, M. (1992). Biliopancreatic diversion: early complications. *Obes Surg,* 2, 2, pp. 177-8038]

[37] de Luis, DA, Pacheco, D, Izaola, O, Terroba, MC, Cuellar, L, Martin, T. (2008). Clinical results and nutritional consequences of biliopancreatic diversion: three years of follow-up. *Ann Nutr Metab,* 53, pp. 234-9

Balsa, JA, Botella-Carretero, JI, Gómez-Martín, JM, et al. (2011). Copper and zinc serum levels after derivative bariatric surgery: differences between Roux-en-Y Gastric bypass and biliopancreatic diversion. *Obes Surg,* 21, 6, pp. 744-50

[39] Ernst, B, Thurnheer, M, Schmid, SM, Schultes, B. (2009). Evidence for the necessity to systematically assess micronutrient status prior to bariatric surgery. *Obes Surg,* 19, 1, pp. 66-73

[40] Buffington, C, Walker, B, Cowan, GS Jr, Scruggs, D. (1993). Vitamin D deficiency in the morbidly obese. *Obes Surg*, 3, 4, pp. 421-24

[41] Moizé, V, Deulofeu, R, Torres, F, de Osaba, JM, Vidal, J. (2011). Nutritional intake and prevalence of nutritional deficiencies prior to surgery in a Spanish morbidly obese population. *Obes Surg*, 21, 9, pp. 1382-8

[42] Ducloux, R, Nobecourt, E, Chevallier, JM, Ducloux, H, Elian, N, Altman, JJ. (2011).Vitamin D deficiency before bariatric surgery: should supplement intake be routinely prescribed? *Obes Surg*, 21, 5, pp. 556-60

[43] Carrodeguas, L, Kaidar-Person, O, Szomstein, S, Antozzi, P, Rosenthal, R. (2005). Preoperative thiamine deficiency in obese population undergoing laparoscopic bariatric surgery. *Surg Obes Relat Dis*, 1, 6, pp. 517-22

[44] Riess, KP, Farnen, JP, Lambert, PJ, Mathiason, MA, Kothari, SN. (2009). Ascorbic acid deficiency in bariatric surgical population. *Surg Obes Relat Dis*, 5, 1, pp. 81-6

[45] Schweiger, C, Weiss, R, Berry, E, et al. (2010). Nutritional deficiencies in bariatric surgery candidates. *Obes Surg*, 20, 2, pp. 193-7

[46] Pereira, S, Saboya, C, Chaves, G, et al. (2009). Class III obesity and its relationship with the nutritional status of vitamin A in pre- and postoperative gastric bypass. *Obes Surg*, 19, 6, pp. 738-44

[47] Sechi, GP, Serra, A, Pirastru, MI, Sotgui, S, Rosati, G. (2002). Wernicke's encephalopathy in a woman on slimming diet. *Neurology*, 58, pp. 1697-98

[48] Sechi, GP. (2010). Dietary supplements and the risk of Wernicke's encephalopathy. *Clin Pharmacol Ther*, 88, p. 164

[49] Pak, CY, Ruskin, B, Diller, E. (1972). Enhancement of renal excretion of zinc by hydrochlorothiazide. *Clin Chim Acta*, 39,2, pp. 511-7

[50] Reyes, AJ, Olhaberry, JV, Leary, WP, Lockett, CJ, Van Der Byl, K. (1983). Urinary zinc excretion, diuretics, zinc deficiency and some side-effects of diuretics. *SA Medical Journal*, 64, pp. 936-41

[51] Alston, TA, Abeles, RH. (1987). Enzymatic conversion of the antibiotic metronidazole to an analog of thiamine. *Arch Biochem Biophys*, 257, 2, pp. 357-62

[52] Francini-Pesenti, F, Brocadello, F, Manara, R, Santelli, L, Laroni, A, Caregaro, L. (2009). Wernicke's syndrome during parenteral feeding: not an unusual complication. *Nutrition*, 25, 2, pp. 142-6

[53] Donnino, MW, Carney, E, Cocchi, MN, et al. (2010). Thiamine deficiency in critically ill patients with sepsis. *J Crit Care*, 25, 4, pp. 576-81

[54] Kitamura, K, Yamaguchi, T, Tanaka, H, Hashimoto, S, Yang, M, Takahashi, T. (1996). TPN-induced fulminant beriberi: a report on our experience and a review of the literature. *Surg Today Jpn J Surg*, 26, pp. 769-76

[55] Dastur, DK, Santhadevi, N, Quadros, EV, et al. (1976). The B-vitamins in malnutrition with alcoholism: A model of intervitamin relationships. *Br J Nutr*, 36, pp. 143-59

[56] Lindenbaum, J, Roman, MJ. (1980). Nutritional anemia in alcoholism. *Am J Clin Nutr*, 33, 12, pp. 2727-35

[57] Gonzalez-Reimers, E, Martin-Gonzalez, MC, Aleman-Valls, MR, et al. (2009). Relative and combined effects of chronic alcohol consumption and HCV infection on serum zinc, copper, and selenium. *Biol Trace Elem Res*, 132, pp. 75-84

[58] Bures, J, Cyrany, J, Kohoutova, D, et al. (2010). Small intestinal bacterial overgrowth syndrome. *World J Gastroenterol*, 16, 24, pp. 2978-90

[59] Ojetti, V, Pitocco, D, Scarpellini, E, et al. (2009). Small bowel bacterial overgrowth and type 1 diabetes. *Eur Rev Med Pharmacol Sci*, 13, 6, pp. 419-23

[60] Bal, B, Finelli, FC, Shope, TR, Koch, TR. (2010). Association between the adjustable gastric band and upper gut bacterial overgrowth. *Am J Gastroenterol*, 105, Suppl 1, p. S83

[61] Begum, A, Drebes, J, Perbandt, M, Wrenger, C, Betzel, C. (2011). Purification, crystallization and preliminary X-ray diffraction analysis of the thiaminase type II from Staphylococcus aureus. *Acta Crystallogr Sect F: Struct Biol Cryst Commun*, 67, Pt 1, pp. 51-3

[62] Toms, AV, Haas, AL, Park, JH, Begley, TP, Ealick, SE. (2005). Structural characterization of the regulatory proteins TenA and TenI from Bacillus subtilis and identification of TenA as a thiaminase II. *Biochemistry*, 44, 7, pp. 2319-29

[63] Muller, IB, Bergmann, B, Groves, MR, et al. (2009). The vitamin B1 metabolism of Staphylococcus aureus is controlled at enzymatic and transcriptional levels. *PLoS One*, 4, 11, p. e7656

[64] Spinazzi, M, Angelini, C, Patrini, C. (2010). Subacute sensory ataxia and optic neuropathy with thiamine deficiency. *Nat Rev Neurol*, 6, pp. 288-293

[65] Herve, C, Beyne, P, Letteron, P, Delacoux, E. (1995). Comparison of erythrocyte transketolase activity with thiamine and thiamine phosphate ester levels in chronic alcoholic patients. *Clin Chim Acta*, 234, pp. 91-100

[66] Galvin, R, Brathen, G, Ivashynka, A, et al. (2010). EFNS guidelines for diagnosis, therapy and prevention of Wernicke encephalopathy. *Eur J Neurol*, 17, 12, pp: 1408-18

[67] Thomson, AD, Marshall, EJ. (2006). The treatment of patients at risk of developing Wernicke's encephalopathy in the community. *Alcohol Alcohol*, 41, pp. 159-67

[68] Camilo, E, Zimmerman, J, Mason, JB, et al. (1996). Folate synthesized by bacteria in the human upper small intestine is assimilated by the host. *Gastroenterology*, 110, 4, pp. 991-8

[69] Moriwaki, K, Kanno, Y, Nakamoto, H, Okada, H, Suzuki, H. (2000). Vitamin B6 deficiency in elderly patients on chronic peritoneal dialysis. *Adv Perit Dial*, 16, pp. 308-12

[70] Herrmann, W, Obeid, R. (2008). Causes and early diagnosis of vitamin B12 deficiency. *Dtsch Arztebl Int*, 105, 40, pp. 680-5

[71] Collazo-Clavell, ML, Jimenez, A, Hodgson, SF, Sarr, MG. (2004). Osteomalacia after Roux-en-Y gastric bypass. *Endocr Pract*, 10, 3, pp. 195-198

[72] Johnson, JM, Maher, JW, Samuel, I. (2005). Effects of gastric bypass procedures on bone mineral density, calcium, parathyroid hormone, and vitamin D. *J Gastrointest Surg*, 9, 8, pp. 1106-10

[73] Johnson, JM, Maher, JW, DeMaria, EJ, Downs, RW, Wolfe, LG, Kellum, JM. (2006). The long-term effects of gastric bypass of vitamin D metabolism. *Ann Surg*, 243, 5, pp. 701-4

[74] El-Kadre, LJ, Rocha, PRS, de Almeida Tinoco, AC, Tinoco, RC. (2004). Calcium metabolism in pre- and postmenopausal morbidly obese women at baseline and after laparoscopic Roux-en-y gastric bypass. *Obes Surg*, 14, 8, pp. 1062-1066

[75] Holick, MF. (2006). High prevalence of vitamin D inadequacy and implications for health. *Mayo Clin Proc*, 81, 3, pp. 353-73

[76] Al-Shoha, A, Qui, S, Palnitkar, S, et al. (2009). Osteomalacia with bone marrow fibrosis due to severe vitamin D deficiency after a gastrointestinal bypass operation for severe obesity. *Endocr Pract*, 15, 6, pp. 528–33
[77] Valderas, JP, Velasco, S, Solari, S, et al. (2009). Increase of bone resorption and the parathyroid hormone in postmenopausal women in the long-term after Roux-en-Y gastric bypass. *Obes Surg*, 19, 8, pp. 1132-8
[78] Signori, C, Zalesin, KC, Franklin, B, et al. (2010). Effect of gastric bypass on vitamin D and secondary hyperparathyroidism. *Obes Surg*, 20, 7, pp. 949-52
[79] Dawson-Hughes, B, Heaney, RP, Holick, MF, Lips, P, Meunier, PJ, Vieth, R. (2005). Estimates of optimal vitamin D status. *Osteoporos Int*, 16, pp. 713–716
[80] Bendich, A, Machlin, LJ. (1988). Safety of oral intake of vitamin E. *Am J Clin Nutr*, 48, pp. 612-61993]
[81] Shearer, MJ, McBurney, A, Barkhan, P. (1974). Studies on the absorption and metabolism of phylloquine (vitamin K) in man. *Vit Horm*, 32, pp. 513-514
[82] Eerdekens, A, Debeer, A, Van Hoey, G, et al. (2010). Maternal bariatric surgery: Adverse outcomes in neonates. *Eur J Pediatr*, 169, 2, pp. 191-6
[83] Varma, S, Baz, W, Badine, E, et al. (2008). Need for parenteral iron therapy after bariatric surgery. *Surg Obes Relat Dis*, 4, 6, pp. 715-719
[84] Chikunguwo, S, Brethauer, S, Nirujogi, V, et al. (2007). Influence of obesity and surgical weight loss on thyroid hormone levels. *Surg Obes Relat Dis*, 3, 6, pp. 631-5
[85] Powell, SR. (2000). The antioxidant properties of zinc. *J Nutr*, 130, pp. 1447S-1454S
[86] Sallé, A, Demarsy, D, Poirier, AL, et al. (2010). Zinc deficiency: A frequent and underestimated complication after bariatric surgery. *Obes Surg*, 20, 12, pp. 1660-70
[87] Zimnicka, AM, Ivy, K, Kaplan, JH. (2011). Acquisition of dietary copper: a role for anion transporters in intestinal apical copper uptake. *Am J Physiol Cell Physiol*, 300, 3, pp. C588-99
[88] Reiser, S, Smith, JC Jr., Mertz, W, et al. (1985). Indices of copper status in humans consuming a typical American diet containing either fructose or starch. *Am J Clin Nutr*, 42, pp. 242-51
[89] Kumar, N, Ahlskog, JE, Gross, JB Jr. (2004). Acquired hypocupremia after gastric surgery. *Clin Gastroenterol Hepatol*, 2, pp. 1074-79
[90] Todd, LM, Godber, IM, Gunn, IR. (2004). Iatrogenic copper deficiency causing anaemia and neutropenia. *Ann Clin Biochem*, 41, pp. 414-416
[91] Fuhrman, MP, Herrmann, V, Masidonski, P, Eby, C. (2000). Pancytopenia after removal of copper from total parenteral nutrition. *J Parenter Enteral Nutr*, 24, 6, pp. 361-6
[92] Kumar, N. (2006). Copper deficiency myelopathy (human swayback). *Mayo Clinic Proc*, 81, pp. 1371-84
[93] Goodman, BP, Mistry, DH, Pasha, SF, et al. (2009). Copper deficiency myeloneuropathy due to occult celiac disease. *Neurologist*, 15, 6, pp. 355-6
[94] Dean, G, McDougall, EI, Elian, M. (1985). Multiple sclerosis in research workers studying swayback in lambs: an updated report. *J Neurol Neurosurg Psychiatry*, 48, pp. 859-65
[95] Kelkar, P, Chang, S, Muley, SA. (2008). Response to oral supplementation in copper deficiency myeloneuropathy. *J Clin Neuromuscular Dis*, 10, 1, pp. 1-3

[96] Naismith, RT, Shepherd, JB, Weihl, CC, Tutlam, NT, Cross, AH. (2009). Acute and bilateral blindness due to optic neuropathy associated with copper deficiency. *Arch Neurol*, 66, 8, pp. 1025-7

[97] Prodan, CI, Bottomley, SS, Holland, NR, et al. (2006). Relapsing hypocupraemic myelopathy requiring high-dose oral copper replacement. *J Neurol Neurosurg Psychiatry*, 77, pp. 1092-3

[98] Hoffman, HN 2nd, Phyliky, RL, Fleming, CR. (1988). Zinc-induced copper deficiency. *Gastroenterology*, 94, 2, pp. 508-12

[99] Boldery, R, Fielding, G, Rafter, T, Pascoe, AL, Scalia, GM. (2007). Nutritional deficiency of selenium secondary to weight loss (bariatric) surgery associated with life-threatening cardiomyopathy. *Heart Lung Circ*, 16, 2, pp. 123-6

[100] Jeejeebhoy, KN, Chu, RC, Marliss, EB, Greenberg, GR, Bruce-Robertson, A. (1977). Chromium deficiency, glucose intolerance, and neuropathy reversed by chromium supplementation, in a patient receiving long-term total parenteral nutrition. *Am J Clin Nutr*, 30, 4, pp. 531-8

[101] Marinella, MA. (2008). Anemia following Roux-en-Y surgery for morbid obesity: a review. *South Med J*, 101, pp. 1024-31

[102] Von Drygalski, A, Andris, DA. (2009). Anemia after bariatric surgery: more than just iron deficiency. *Nutr Clin Pract*, 24, pp. 217-26

[103] Koffman, BM, Greenfield, LJ, Ali, II, Pirzada, NA. (2006). Neurologic complications after surgery for obesity. *Muscle Nerve*, 33, pp. 166-76

[104] Thaisetthawatkul, P, Collazo-Clavel, ML, Sarr, MG, Norell, JE, Dyck, PJB. (2004). A controlled study of peripheral neuropathy after bariatric surgery. *Neurology*, 63, pp. 1462-70

[105] Juhasz-Pocsine, K, Rudnicki, SA, Archer, RL. (2007). Neurologic complications of gastric bypass surgery for morbid obesity. *Neurology*, 68, 21, pp. 1843-50

[106] Machado, JD, Campos, CS, Lopes Dah Silva, C, et al. (2008). Intestinal bacterial overgrowth after Roux-en-Y gastric bypass. *Obes Surg*, 18, 1, pp. 139-43

[107] Aasheim, ET, Björkman, S, Søvik, TT, et al. (2009). Vitamin status after bariatric surgery: a randomized study of gastric bypass and duodenal switch. *Am J Clin Nutr*, 90, 1, pp. 15-22

11

Foot Drop as a Complication of Weight Loss After Bariatric Surgery – Is It Preventable?

Frank J. M. Weyns[1], Frauke Beckers[2],
Linda Vanormelingen[3], Marjan Vandersteen[3] and Erik Niville[4]
[1]*Department of Neurosurgery, Ziekenhuis Oost-Limburg, Genk (B),*
[2]*School of Life Sciences, Universiteit Hasselt,*
[3]*Department of Basic Medical Science, Universiteit Hasselt,*
[4]*Department of Abdominal Surgery, Ziekenhuis Oost-Limburg, Genk (B),*
Belgium

1. Introduction

Peroneal neuropathy, causing foot drop, is a common mononeuropathy accounting for approximately 15 % of all the mononeuropathies in adults. (A. Cruz-Martinez, et al. 2000, E. Shahar , et al., 2007) A relationship between peroneal nerve palsy and weight loss has been well documented over the last decades. (D.G. Sherman, et al., 1977, K.A. Sotaniemi ,1984, E. Streib, 1993, I. Aprile et al., 2000, M.J.H. Harrison, 1984) During World War II, foot drop was frequently observed in prisoners of war. Prolonged sitting as well as weight loss were speculated to be the cause of foot drop. (F. Kaminsky. 1947, D. Denny-Brown, 1947) In the sixties, foot drop was also related to cancer. Paraneoplastic phenomena were thought to be the cause of this neurological condition, however all patients with foot drop had significant weight loss due to the primary disease. (D.I. Rubin, et al.,1998) In severe diabetes (with weight loss) also many patients developed peripheral nerve problems. Here, 'diabetic neuropathy' was thought to be the main reason for this condition. During the last decade many reports of foot drop due to starvation or weight loss were published. (A. Cruz-Martinez, et al. 2000, E. Shahar , et al., 2007, D.G. Sherman, et al., 1977, K.A. Sotaniemi ,1984, E. Streib, 1993, I. Aprile et al., 2000, D.I. Rubin, et al., 1998, P.J. Koehler, et al., 1997, I. Lutte, et al., 1997) It became clear that substantial weight loss itself could cause foot drop. Further study of the pathogenesis of this condition is required.

2. Material and methods

In our institution 160 patients were operated for persisting foot drop between January 1995 and December 2005. In all cases an L5 radiculopathy was excluded and a peroneal neuropathy -with a conduction block at the fibular head- was demonstrated by electromyography. When selected, all patients were interviewed to detect the possible cause of their neurological condition. The different pathophysiological conditions are summarized in figure 1. Weight loss (>10% of body weight) was found in 43.5 % of the patients, the reasons being dieting, bariatric surgery, severe illness (pneumonia, cancer, diabetes,…), psychiatric disorder, etc.

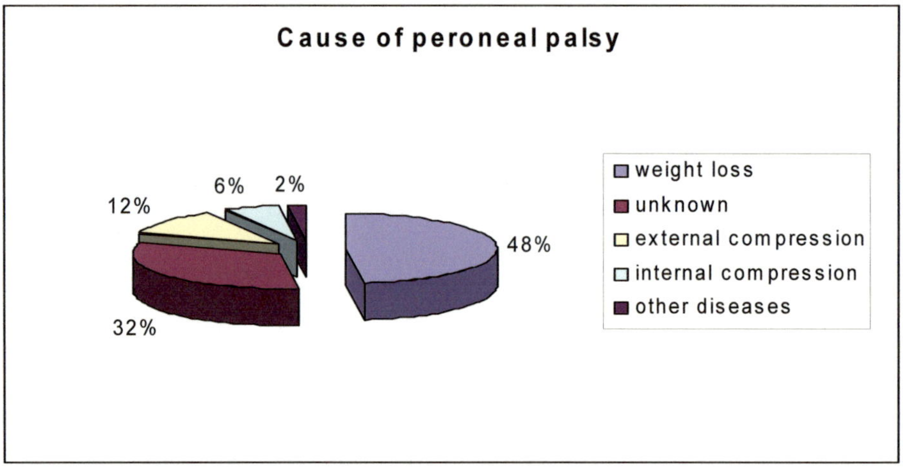

Fig. 1. Cause of peroneal palsy in 160 operated patients: 77 pts with weight loss, 51 pts with unknown cause, 19 pts with external compression (due to positioning), 10 pts with internal compression (fibular fracture, haematoma, cystic lesions) and 3 patients with other diseases (rheumatoid arthritis, diabetes and later diagnosed amyotrophic lateral sclerosis (ALS))

The patients with foot drop following bariatric surgery were compared to a matched control group of patients who did not develop foot drop after bariatric surgery. This control group consisted of patients who all underwent a gastric banding procedure for obesity. Both study groups were statistically similar for sex, age and total weight loss. Statistical analysis was performed using the method of logistic regression and the Chi-square test.

3. Results

Between January 1995 and December 2005, 160 patients were operated for persisting foot drop (Figure 2 and 3). Of these 160 patients, 43,5% (78 patients) developed their pathology after a period of serious weight loss (>10% of their body weight). There were many reasons for this weight loss: dieting, bariatric surgery, severe illness (pneumonia, cancer, diabetes,…), psychiatric disorder, etc. The influence of weight loss on the development of foot drop is clearly demonstrated in this population. This matter will be described in a separate article. In these analyses we noted that the weight loss occurred in a very short period. For all 78 patients maximal weight loss was observed within 18 months (varying from two weeks to 18 months with a mean time interval of 4 months).

Nine patients developed foot drop after bariatric surgery. These patients are listed in table 1. The mean weight loss for these patients was 45 kg (38.3 % of their initial body weight), ranging from 20 kg to 74 kg. This weight reduction took place during a mean period of 8.6 months (ranging from 1 month to 18 months). We compared this patient group with a control group of patients who underwent bariatric surgery (gastric banding) but did not develop peroneal neuropathy. Our control group consists of ten patients, listed in table 2. The mean weight loss in these patients was 43.8 kg (38.5 % of their initial body weight), ranging from 23 kg to 98 kg. The weight reduction took place during a mean period of 21.7 months (ranging from 10 months to 36 months).

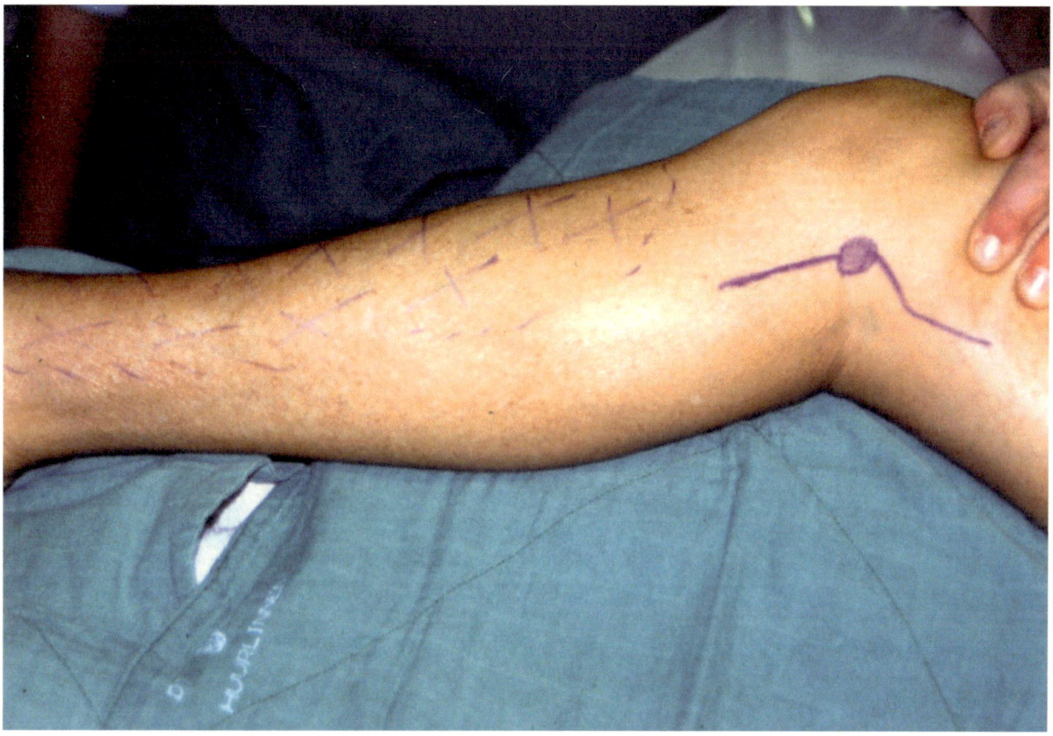

Fig. 2. Incision for peroneal nerve decompression. Dotted line shows the region of sensory deficit.

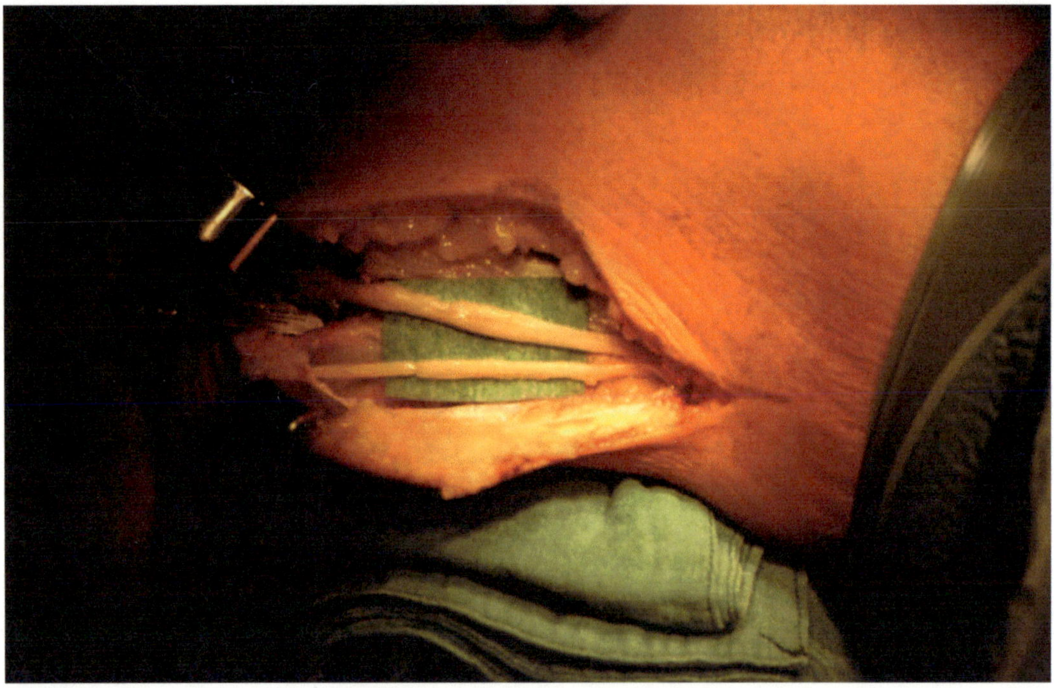

Fig. 3. Peroperative view after decompression of the peroneal nerve with internal neurolysis of the two branches: superficial and deep peroneal nerve.

Using the Chi-square test, we found statistically significant differences in the amount of weight loss between the two study groups ($p<0.0457$). Using the method of logistic regression, we can conclude that weight loss in a short period of time is associated with a higher risk for developing foot drop (Odds ratio = 0.822 with 95% reliability interval between 0.678 and 0.996). The nerve palsy was resolved by neurolysis of the peroneal nerve at the fibular head in all cases.

patient	age	sex	type of surgery	weight loss kg (%)	time period (months)
1	39	M	gastric banding	50(33%)	18
2	46	F	bypass	20(20%)	7
3	27	F	gastric banding	28(29%)	9
4	48	F	gastric banding	64(46%)	12
5	45	M	bypass	74(53%)	7
6	45	F	bypass	64(50%)	6
7	22	F	bypass	42(38%)	5
8	30	F	gastric banding	30(37%)	6
9	40	F	gastric banding	34(39%)	7

Table 1. Nine patients developed foot drop after bariatric surgery

patient	age	sex	type of surgery	weight loss kg (%)	time period (months)
1	37	F	gastric banding	39(39%)	36
2	27	F	gastric banding	29(30%)	18
3	50	F	gastric banding	98(58%)	36
4	44	F	gastric banding	33(39%)	18
5	54	F	gastric banding	29(24%)	12
6	19	F	gastric banding	50(38%)	24
7	57	F	gastric banding	39(42%)	21
8	30	F	gastric banding	41(42%)	30
9	49	M	gastric banding	47(37%)	12
10	46	M	gastric banding	39(36%)	10

Table 2. Ten control patients without peroneal palsy.

4. Discussion

Peroneal nerve palsy is a common mononeuropathy accounting for approximately 15 % of all the mononeuropathies in adults.(A. Cruz-Martinez, et al. 2000, E. Shahar , et al., 2007) As early as 1876, it was recognized that some patients with chronic disease, developed peroneal nerve palsies.(13,14) While weight loss may have played a role, the neuropathy was generally ascribed to a toxin or infectious agent. In 1929 Woltman was the first author to report the association of massive weight reduction to the existence of foot drop. In 1947 Kaminsky as well as Denny-Brown reported several cases of peroneal nerve palsy in prisoners of war (up to 10 % of prisoners) and attributed this neurological condition to the prolonged dietary restriction. Later peroneal nerve palsy was correlated to cancer.(D.I. Rubin DI, et al., 1998) In a population of more than 400, 000 patients (in which more than 8000 newly diagnosed cases of cancer), Koehler et al. found a relative risk of 8,6 to develop peroneal nerve palsy compared with patients without cancer.(P.J. Koehler, et al., 1997) A paraneoplastic factor or neurotoxicity due to the use of different antineoplastic drugs were considered to cause this syndrome. (P.J. Koehler, et al., 1997) Here as well, malnutrition and secondary weight loss were mentioned as side-phenomena.

Over the last decades, the correlation between weight loss and peroneal neuropathy was well documented. (A. Cruz-Martinez, et al. 2000, D.G. Sherman, et al 1977, K.A. Sotaniemi ,1984, E. Streib, 1993, I. Aprile et al., 2000, M.J.H. Harrison, 1984) In 1977 Sherman et al. described this correlation in 7 patients after excessive weight loss. In their study weight reduction was the only obvious common feature to all their patients. Cruz-Martinez et al. (2000) demonstrated a peroneal neuropathy due to excessive weight loss in 20% of 150 patients with peroneal symptoms. There were many reasons for this weight loss: dieting, bariatric surgery, psychiatric disorders and other severe diseases like cancer, diabetes, acute pneumonia, etc.(E. Shahar , et al., 2007, M.J.H. Harrison, 1984, D. Denny-Brown, 1947, D.I. Rubin DI, et al., 1998, B.E. Sprofkin, 1958, E.W. Massey, J.M. Massey, 1987, G.D. Scott, 1979) Until now the exact way in which weight loss causes nerve palsy, is still unknown. We consider it due to a compression syndrome caused by nerve oedema as it is known in diabetic neuropathy. This intraneural oedema, caused by metabolic changes can cause nerve dysfunction especially at risk areas (anatomical tunnel regions). Electromyographic studies in all our patients confirmed peroneal nerve palsy with a conduction block at the fibular head. For this reason, we operated upon all patients with persisting foot drop longer than 3 weeks. Up until now, there are controversies upon the optimal therapy for this specific condition. In literature, there are no large studies comparing the conservative and the surgical treatment of peroneal neuropathy in this condition. Recovery after conservative treatment varies strongly from study to study and most of these studies deal with only small groups of patients. (A. Cruz-Martinez, et al. 2000, E. Shahar , et al., 2007, D.G. Sherman, et al. 1977, K.A. Sotaniemi ,1984, E. Streib, 1993, D.I. Rubin DI, et al., 1998, E.W. Massey, J.M. Massey, 1987)

We were also able to demonstrate a statistically significant correlation between weight loss and peroneal neuropathy. In addition we illustrated the short time interval in which the weight loss occurred (2 weeks to 18 months with an average of 4 months). These findings are described in a separate article. To investigate the importance of the period in which patients develop their weight loss, especially in a population of bariatric surgery patients, a comparison was made between a subgroup of our peroneal nerve palsy patients and a matched control group of patients who were submitted for bariatric surgery (gastric banding) but did not develop peroneal neuropathy. Of the 160 patients who were treated surgically for persisting peroneal nerve palsy, 9 patients developed foot drop after obesity surgery (table 2). The mean weight loss for these patients was 45 kg (38.3 % of their initial body weight). The weight reduction took place during a mean period of 8.6 months. Our control group consisted of 10 patients(table 2). The mean weight loss for these patients was 42.6 kg (37.4 % of their initial body weight). The weight reduction took place during a mean period of 21.7 months.

In contrast to earlier studies (eg. Waldström et al., 1991), we demonstrated that important weight loss is correlated with a higher risk to develop foot drop and that the time period in which the weight loss is achieved is important. A rapid reduction of body weight is correlated with a higher risk to develop foot drop. A slow weight reduction is recommended to avoid such disabling disease.

5. References

Aprile I, Padua L, Padua R et al. Peroneal mononeuropathy: predisposing factors and clinical and neurological relationships. Neurol Sci 2000; 21: 367-371

Cruz-Martinez A, Arpa J, Palau F. Peroneal neuropathy after weight loss. J Periph Nerv Syst 2000; 5: 101-105

Denny-Brown D. Neurological conditions resulting from prolonged and severe dietary restriction. Medicine 1947; 26: 41-113

Harrison M J H. Peroneal neuropathy during weight reduction. J Neurol Neurosurg Psych 1984; 47: 1260

Kaminsky F. Peroneal palsy by crossing the legs. JAMA 1947; 134: 206

Koehler PJ, Busher M, Rozeman CAM et al. Peroneal nerve neuropathy in cancer patients: a paraneoplastic syndrome? J Neurol 1997; 244: 328-332.

Lutte I, Rhys C, Hubert C et al. Peroneal nerve palsy in anorexia nervosa. Arch Neurol Belg 1997; 97: 251-254

Massey EW, Massey JM. Peroneal palsy in depressed patients. Weight loss, psychomotor retardation predispose patients to this condition. Psychosomatics 1987; 28: 93-94.

Rubin DI, Kimmel DW, Cascino TL. Outcome of peroneal neuropathies in patients with systemic malignant disease. Cancer 1998; 83: 1602-1606.

Scott G D. Anorexia nervosa presenting as foot drop. J Neurol Neurosurg Psych 1979; 55: 58-60

Shahar E, Landau E, Genizi J. Adolescence peroneal neuropathy associated with rapid marked weight reduction: case report and literature review. Eur J Paediatr Neurol 2007; 11: 50-54

Sherman DG, Easton JD. Dieting and peroneal nerve palsy. JAMA 1977; 238: 230-231.

Sotaniemi KA. Slimmer's paralysis - peroneal neuropathy during weight reduction J Neurol Neurosurg Psych 1984; 47: 564-566.

Sprofkin B E. Peroneal paralysis. A hazard of weight reduction. Arch Intern Med 1958; 102: 82-87

Streib E. Weight loss and foot drop. Iowa Med 1993; 83: 224-225

Wadström C, Backman L, Persson HE et al. The effect of excessive weight reduction on peripheral and central nervous functions. A study in obese patients treated by gastric banding. Eur J Surg 1991; 157: 39-44.

Woltman H W. Crossing of the legs as a factor in the of peroneal palsy. J Am Med Assoc 1929; 93/ 670-672

12

Diabetes Improvement Following Bariatric and Metabolic Surgery

Rodolfo Lahsen, Marcos Berry and Patricio Lamoza
Clinica Las Condes,
Chile

1. Introduction

Obesity rates are increasing worldwide. Free fatty acids derived from visceral adipose tissue impair insulin sensitivity and β-cell function (lipo-toxicity), leading to the metabolic syndrome and type 2 diabetes.

Weight loss is the cornerstone for diabetes prevention and treatment, thus lifestyle and eventually pharmacological interventions that achieve significant weight loss are widely accepted. Nevertheless, long-term compliance to diet and exercise as well as safety and efficacy concerns regarding obesity drugs limit their benefits in real world. Moreover, weight gain is a common and undesirable side-effect of several oral antidiabetic drugs and insulins.

Bariatric surgery has demonstrated to be an effective and safe treatment option for type 2 diabetic patients who are severely obese, what is linked to weight loss and other mechanisms. Considering weight loss-independent mechanisms for diabetes improvement, investigators in several countries have started mostly metabolic than bariatric procedures for mildly obese or even overweight patients, focused on diabetes rather than obesity, and their early results have been encouraging.

1.1 Obesity and type 2 diabetes

Obesity is and its related metabolic disorders are increasing worldwide, especially in developing countries in western hemisphere (Ford & Mokdad, 2008). In most cases, an increase in body mass index (BMI) reflects an underlying increase in body fat that leads to diabetes, hypertension and dyslipidaemia (Bays, 2009), cardiovascular risk factors that are associated with increased mortality (Berrington et al, 2010).

Cardiometabolic risk increases not only with BMI, but waist circumference as well (National Institutes of Health [NIH], 1998). Waist circumference correlates tightly with visceral adipose tissue, and currently is a widely accepted assessment of the accumulation of intraabdominal or visceral adiposity (Despres et al, 2001).

Visceral adipose tissue is more likely to be related to insulin resistance than subcutaneous adipose tissue (Banerji et al, 1997, as cited in Zinman, 2006). Visceral obesity-derived cardiometabolic risk factors are frequently linked to insulin resistance and tend to cluster, what is clinically recognised as the metabolic syndrome (Alberti et al, 2009).

These factors follow a common and progressive course, so the prevalence of metabolic syndrome is 10 to 15% in normoglycaemic individuals, 44 to 64% in prediabetic, and 78 to 84% in type 2 diabetic patients (Isomaa et al, 2001). In other words, the more hyperglycaemic, the more dysmetabolic the individual will be.

Metabolic and ultimately cardiovascular complications of visceral obesity are summarised in Figure 1.

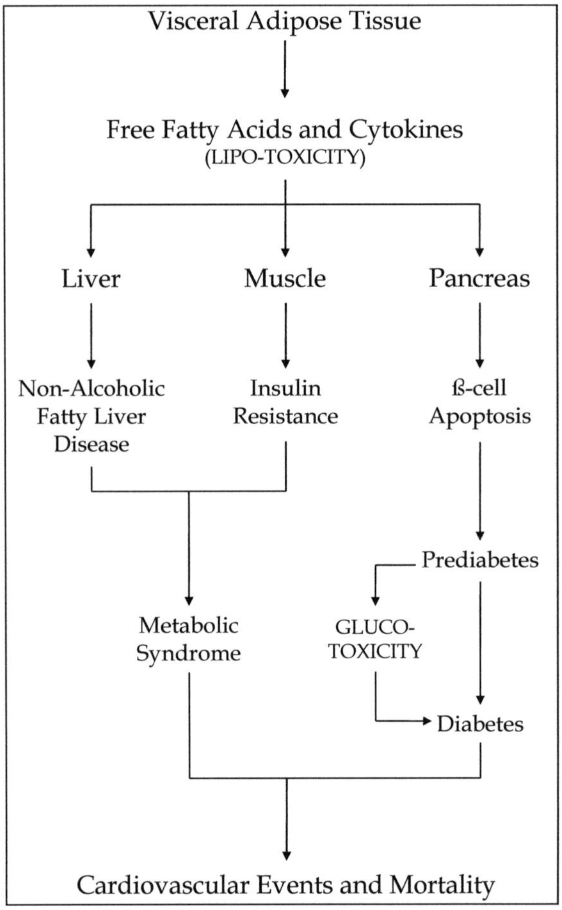

Fig. 1. Cardiometabolic risk derived from visceral obesity.

Visceral adipose tissue shows a high lipolytic activity, releasing free fatty acids (FFAs) to portal and then systemic circulation (Wajchenberg, 2000). FFAs, as well as cytokines and tumor necrosis factor-α (TNF-α), both derived from visceral adipose tissue, impair insulin action at target cells in liver and muscle, causing a postbinding defect that blocks tyrosine kinase activity,1 uncoupling insulin signal transduction (Le Roith & Zick, 2001). Insulin resistance is a key factor for the development of non-alcoholic fatty liver disease (NAFLD), and atherogenic dyslipidaemia.

Insulin resistance is followed by pancreatic β-cell compensation and hyperinsulinaemia, due to fuel and neurohormonal signals derived from fat, liver, intestine, and brain (Prentki,

2006). Hyperinsulinaemia stimulates sodium reabsortion at kidneys, as well as sympathetic nervous system activity, leading to vasoconstriction and enhanced cardiac output, increasing blood pressure (Reaven et al, 1996). In addition, hyperinsulinaemia exerts anti-lipolytic and lipogenic actions, thus maintaining and increasing visceral adipose tissue (Wajchenberg, 2000).

Nevertheless, while FFAs are one of the β-cell compensation signals, they can cause ultimately β-cell apoptosis, leading to prediabetic states and type 2 diabetes (Bell, 2003; Kasuga, 2006). Prediabetes (impaired fasting glucose and/or impaired glucose tolerance), in other words, slightly elevated plasma glucose levels, accelerates pancreatic failure through gluco-toxicity.

1.2 Weight loss in diabetes prevention and treatment

Weight loss is the cornerstone for diabetes prevention and treatment, thus lifestyle and eventually pharmacological interventions that achieve significant weight loss are widely accepted.

1.2.1 Lifestyle intervention in diabetes prevention

Modest weight loss, as part of a comprehensive intervention in lifestyle, has demonstrated significant reductions in the incidence of diabetes in high risk populations. In the Finnish Diabetes Prevention Study the intervention group showed a greater lose of weight when compared with a control group (weight reduction >5% in 43 versus 13% of the subjects, respectively), with a risk of type 2 diabetes reduced by 58% at 3.2 years (Tuomilehto et al, 2001). In the American Diabetes Prevention Program, the average weight loss in the lifestyle intervention group was 5.6 kg compared with 0.1 kg in the placebo group, with a risk of type 2 diabetes reduced by 58% at 2.8 years (Diabetes Prevention Program [DPP] Research Group, 2002). In the Indian Diabetes Prevention Programme, the lifestyle modification group reduced their risk of type 2 diabetes by 28.5% at 2.5 years compared with the control group, without loosing weight (Ramachandran et al, 2006).

1.2.2 Pharmacologic Interventions in diabetes prevention

Weight loss and antidiabetic drugs have been tested in the prevention of type 2 diabetes. Orlistat, a gastrointestinal lipase inhibitor used in the treatment of overweight and obesity, showed a 37.3% reduction in diabetes incidence at 4 years in obese subjects (Torgerson et al, 2004). Acarbose, an enteric α-glycosidase inhibitor used in the treatment of type 2 diabetes, reduced diabetes incidence by 25% at 3.3 years in subjects with impaired glucose tolerance (Chiasson et al, 2002). Another antidiabetic drug, metformin, which enhances insulin sensitivity at liver and muscle tissues, showed a 31% reduction in diabetes incidence at 2.8 years (DPP Research Group, 2002).

Two effective obesity drugs, rimonabant and sibutramine, have been recently withdrawn in several countries because long-term safety concerns.

1.2.3 Lifestyle intervention in diabetes treatment

One-year results of the ongoing Look-AHEAD clinical trial, which is intended to assess whether intensive lifestyle intervention decreases major cardiovascular events in type 2 diabetic subjects, showed a significant weight reduction with lifestyle intervention when compared with a control group (-8.6 vs. -0.7%, respectively). Diabetes control and other cardiovascular disease risk factors were also improved, with reduced medicine use (Pi-Sunyer et al, 2007).

Long-term compliance to diet and exercise could be a major issue in clinical practice. In addition, weight gain is a common and undesirable side-effect of several oral antidiabetic drugs and insulins (Turner et al, 1998; Kahn et al, 2006).

2. Diabetes improvement following weight loss surgery

Currently accepted indications for bariatric surgery are BMI ≥40 kg/m^2 or BMI ≥35 kg/m^2 when comorbidities are associated (NIH, 1998). Bariatric surgery has demonstrated significant weight reduction, and improvement on cardiometabolic risk factors such as type 2 diabetes mellitus, dyslipidaemia, and hypertension, in severely obese patients. Moreover, this procedures are associated with 29% decreased overall mortality at 15-year follow-up (Sjostrom et al, 2007). Because the improvement observed not only in excess weight reduction, but in cardiometabolic risk factors as well, these procedures have been recently recognised as "bariatric and metabolic". Principal mechanisms leading to diabetes and metabolic improvement following bariatric and metabolic procedures are summarised in Table 1.

MECHANISM	CLINICAL BENEFIT
Decreased Lipo-toxicity (weight loss)	Improved metabolic syndrome
Decreased ghrelin and increased PYY	Decreased appetite and increased satiety
Enhanced incretin effect	Improved diabetes control

Table 1. Main mechanisms for diabetes and metabolic improvement following surgery.

2.1 Decreased lipo-toxicity

Diabetes remission, defined as fasting plasma glucose <126 mg/dL (7.0 mmol/L) without hypoglycaemic therapy, occurs in 72 and 36% at two an ten years respectively in surgical patients, compared with 21 and 13% in conventionally treated subjects. On the other hand, diabetes incidence in non-diabetics is 1 and 8% at two and ten years respectively in the surgical group compared with 8 and 24% in the control group (Sjostrom et al, 2004, as cited in Dixon et al, 2011).

Undoubtedly, such metabolic benefit is closely related to weight loss because a marked reduction in FFA-derived lipo-toxicity. Lipo-toxicity impairs insulin action at target tissues and increases pancreatic β-cell apoptosis. One randomised controlled trial that compared laparoscopic adjustable gastric banding (LAGB), a pure restrictive technique, versus comprehensive medical therapy for obese type 2 diabetic individuals showed a significant 5.5-fold higher remission at two years in the surgical group (Dixon et al, 2008). In this regard, procedures that achieve weight loss and decrease lipo-toxicity should be viewed as "metabolic".

2.2 Weight loss-independent mechanisms for diabetes control

Bypass or malabsortive procedures appear to result in greater metabolic benefit than restrictive ones, and a common observation is that diabetes remission is achieved within days to weeks of undergoing surgery, before significant weight loss has occurred (Pories et al, 1995). These facts lead to conclude that additional and, at some extent, weight loss-independent mechanisms are involved. These mechanisms, thus more metabolic than bariatric, could be summarised as reduced caloric intake and enhanced incretin effect (Lahsen & Berry, 2010).

2.2.1 Reduced caloric intake

Gastrointestinal hormones and peptides involved in the regulation of energy homeostasis may be modified following bariatric surgery. Roux-en-Y Gastric Bypass (RYGB) and Sleeve Gastrectomy (SG) increase peptide YY (PYY) (Morinigo et al, 2006) and reduce ghrelin levels (Cummings et al, 2002, Karamanakos et al, 2008). PYY is an appetite suppressant peptide secreted by distal ileum and colon, whereas ghrelin is an orexigenic hormone secreted by gastric fundus. Thus, post surgery changes in gut-derived hormones result in decreased appetite and increased satiety, which enhance patients' compliance to lifestyle intervention guidance.

2.2.2 Incretin effect

Food intake is followed by the release of several intestinal peptides, some of which increase insulin levels. The increase in insulin secretion is higher after oral or enteral glucose ingestion when compared to intravenous administration, what is called the incretin effect. Glucagon-like peptide-1 (GLP-1) and glucose-dependent insulinotropic peptide (GIP) are the two most studied peptides, being GLP-1 probably the most important in terms of carbohydrate homeostasis. GLP-1 secretion from L-cells at the ileum rises after a meal and enhances insulin biosynthesis and release by pancreatic β-cells, decreases glucagon release by pancreatic α-cells, improves glucose uptake and glycogen synthesis in liver and peripheral tissues, slows gastric emptying, and decreases appetite and increases satiety at central nervous system. GIP is released from K-cells in duodenum, and stimulates post-meal insulin secretion and promotes β-cell mass expansion (Drucker, 2003). Type 2 diabetes is associated with a reduced or lost incretin effect that contributes with impaired insulin secretion (Toft-Nielsen et al, 2001). Bariatric surgery, especially RYGB, significantly enhances GLP-1 levels and activity in severely obese subjects with or without diabetes (Laferrere et al, 2007).

3. Metabolic surgery in non-severely obese type 2 diabetics

Theoretically, it could be plausible the design of surgical techniques focused mainly on weight loss, caloric intake, or incretin effect, depending on patients' individual needs and careful clinical judgment.

3.1 Duodenal-Jejunal bypass and the Hindgut and Foregut hypothesis

Experimental studies were performed in non-obese diabetic rats, who underwent duodenal-jejunal bypass (DJB), a stomach-preserving RYGB that excludes proximal intestine, or gastrojejunostomy (GJ), which creates a shortcut for ingested nutrients without bypassing intestine (Rubino et al, 2006). No differences in body weight, food intake, or nutrient absorption were observed between surgical groups, however DJB-treated rats improved their oral glucose tolerance. When GJ rats were reoperated to exclude proximal intestine a marked improvement in oral glucose tolerance was observed and, conversely, restoration of duodenal passage in DJB rats impaired oral glucose tolerance. In this study, Rubino demonstrated that bypassing proximal intestine directly ameliorates diabetes by weight loss-independent mechanisms.

At some extent, two theories are born. The "hindgut hypothesis", is explained by the rapid nutrient delivery to distal intestine that enhance the secretion of GLP-1, PYY, and oxyntomodulin, which are involved in the reduction of food intake and gastrointestinal motility, and improvement in glucose homeostasis. The second theory, the "foregut hypothesis" or duodenal exclusion, clearly demonstrates that duodenum and proximal jejunum bypass of nutrients plays a major role in diabetes resolution.

3.2 Rationale for metabolic surgery in diabetic patients with BMI <35 kg/m^2

The American Diabetes Association established for first time in 2009 that bariatric procedures should be considered for diabetic adults with BMI ≥35 kg/m^2 when diabetes is poor controlled with lifestyle and pharmacologic therapy. American Diabetes Association does not recommend surgery in patients with BMI <35 kg/m^2 outside a research protocol (American Diabetes Association, 2009). Nevertheless, and as observed in landmark diabetes clinical trials, most type 2 diabetic individuals are overweight or mildly obese, with a BMI close to 30 kg/m^2, below the cut-off for eligibility in current guidelines, disregarding the presence of a visceral pattern of obesity (Lahsen & Berry, 2010). Precisely, type 2 diabetic individuals having the metabolic syndrome have a very high risk of cardiovascular complications (Isomaa et al, 2001). Table 2 summarises the criteria followed by the authors to consider bariatric and metabolic surgery in type 2 diabetic subjects.

BODY MASS INDEX (kg/m^2)	OBSERVATIONS
≥ 35	Consider surgery
< 35	Consider surgery when metabolic syndrome is present
< 30	Consider surgery only as part of a Clinical Research Protocol

Table 2. Selection criteria for bariatric and metabolic surgery in type 2 diabetes.

In recent years, several groups performing both established and novel surgical procedures in type 2 subjects with BMI <35 kg/m^2 have shown encouraging metabolic results. It must be noted that these procedures should be performed as part of a clinical research protocol with local ethical approval.

3.3 Clinical results of metabolic surgery

Our group started a clinical research protocol assessing DJB in early 2008, and 19 non-obese (BMI <30 kg/m^2) type 2 diabetic patients underwent surgery by late 2010. Our preliminary metabolic results are encouraging, however surgical technique modifications have been done due to concerns regarding gastroparesis, a previously reported surgery-derived adverse effect on gastric emptying. This issue was handled performing a non-restrictive SG, turning DJB into a modified duodenal switch, a well known procedure with proven benefits on glucose metabolism. The authors have seen better results, less morbidity (no gastroparesis) and a better metabolic control with diabetes remission in near 75% of the cases, what was presented at the XIV Latin American Diabetes Association Congress held in Santiago, Chile, in november 2010 (Table 3).

Variable	Pre-Surgery	Post-Surgery	P*
BMI, kg/m^2	27.7	25.3	<0.001
Fasting plasma glucose, mg/dL (mmol/L)	163 (9.1)	131 (7.3)	0.01
HbA1c, %	8.3	6.7	<0.001
Patients with HbA1c <7%, %	26.3	73.60	0.05**
Pharmacologic treatment (n)			
None	0	6	
Oral monotherapy	2	9	
Oral combination therapy	15	3	
Insulin	2	1	

* T test; ** Fisher test.

Table 3. Clinical results of Modified Duodenal-Jejunal Bypass in 19 non-obese type 2 diabetic patients.

But, Why to perform "the most aggressive" surgery in non-obese patients? What about their weight loss? To answer the first question it must be considered the almost pure hormonal effect that is achieved in this subset of patients, where weight loss is not the "common factor" observed in restrictive and malabsortive bariatric procedures. Answering the second question requires considering that obese patients with different degree of severity who undergo the same surgery lose almost the same excess weight proportion, what can be explained as an "accommodation" of the caloric intake to the metabolism "real requirements". Our patients, with BMI between 25 and 30 kg/m^2, experienced a moderated lose of weight during the first 12 weeks after surgery, recovering later their inicial weight or maintaining BMI close to 25 kg/m^2, with no excessive weight loss. This fact was also noted by Scopinaro, who performed a novel surgical procedure in type 2 diabetic individuals with BMI <35 kg/m^2, achieving metabolic control and moderated weight loss (Scopinaro et al, 2007).

3.4 Novel metabolic procedures

Clinical researchers worldwide are performing novel surgical and endoscopic procedures and assessing their metabolic and surgical long-term efficacy and safety.

3.4.1 Sleeve gastrectomy

While SG is considered a pure restrictive technique, it is noteworthy that weight loss-mediated decrease in lipo-toxicity is metabolic *per se*, and SG reduces ghrelin, increases peptide YY, and increases GLP-1 (Peterli et al, 2009), so SG must be viewed as metabolic surgery as well. We have assessed clinical and metabolic results in obese patients with easily controlled or recently diagnosed diabetes, which underwent SG with promising results: remission of the disease, no medication longer required, and very low morbidity rates.

3.4.2 Endobarrier®

One of the non invasive metabolic procedures currently under investigation is the "Endobarrier®", a polypropylene sleeve endoscopically installed, anchored to the pylorus, that extends until the first portion of the jejunum. Its mechanism of action is the isolation of the food from the pancreatic enzymes and bile. This device has to be removed at 12 month, while an acceptable glycaemic control has been observed, and early results in obese patients also shows a moderated weight loss.

4. Current and future indications for metabolic surgery

Current obesity guidelines consider surgery when type 2 diabetes is associated with BMI ≥35 kg/m^2, however diabetes guidelines have incorporated surgical options very recently. In 2009 the American Diabetes Association established that bariatric surgery should be considered for diabetic adults with BMI ≥35 kg/m^2 if metabolic control is difficult to achieve with lifestyle and pharmacological therapy. In March 2011 the International Diabetes Federation released a position paper which considers with some restrictions bariatric surgery for type 2 diabetic patients with BMI ≥30 kg/m^2, and historically, for first time includes bariatric surgery in a diabetes treatment algorithm.

Probably future guidelines will consider not only BMI but also waist circumference and other elements of the metabolic syndrome as well as the presence and extent of diabetic chronic complications, patients' preference and quality of life.

5. Conclusions

Bariatric surgery has demonstrated to be an effective and safe therapy for obesity in subjects with BMI ≥40 kg/m^2, and in type 2 diabetic patients with BMI ≥35 kg/m^2.

The major factor involved in metabolic improvement after surgery is weight loss, which decreases lipo-toxicity. Any procedure that achieves weight loss must be recognised as metabolic.

There are weight loss-independent mechanisms for metabolic improvement that can be summarised as decreased appetite and increased satiety, due to post surgical changes in ghrelin and PYY, and enhanced β-cell function, due to an increased incretin effect.

Novel surgical techniques have been developed in recent years, aimed to correct dysmetabolism through weight loss-independent mechanisms in type 2 diabetic patients who are mildly obese or even overweight, with promissory early results.

Nowadays, these procedures have been part of clinical investigation protocols approved by each local ethics committee.

Future indications for metabolic procedures will consider other factors than BMI.

6. References

Alberti, KGMM.; Eckel, RH.; Grundy, SM.; Zimmet, PZ.; Cleeman, JI.; Donato, KA.; Fruchart, JC.; James, WPT.; Loria, CM.; Smith, SC. (2009) Harmonizing the Metabolic Syndrome. A Joint Interim Statement of the International Diabetes Federation Task Force on Epidemiology and Prevention; National Heart, Lung, and Blood Institute; American Heart Association; World Heart Federation; International Atherosclerosis Society; and International Association for the Study of Obesity. *Circulation*, Vol.120, No.16, (October 2009), pp. 1640-1645.

American Diabetes Association. (2009) Standards of medical care in diabetes - 2009. *Diabetes Care*, Vol.32, Supplement No.1, (January 2009), pp. S13-S61.

Bays, HE. (2009) "Sick Fat", Metabolic Disease, and Atherosclerosis. *The American Journal of Medicine*, Vol.122, No.1A, (January 2009), pp. S26-S37.

Bell, D. (2003) β-Cell Rejuvenation with Thiazolidinediones. *The American Journal of Medicine*, Vol.115, No.8A, (December 2003), pp. 20S-23S.

Berrington, A.; Hartge, P.; Cerhan, JR.; Flint, AJ.; Hannan, L.; Maclnnis, RJ.; Moore, SC.; Tobias, GS.; Anton-Culver, H.; Freeman, LB.; Beeson, WL.; Clipp, SL.; English, DR.; Folsom, AR.; Freedman, M.; Giles, G.; Hakansson, N.; Henderson, KD.; Hoffman-Bolton, J.; Hoppin, JA.; Koenig, KL.; Lee, IM.; Linet, MS.; Park, Y.; Pocobelli, G.; Schatzkin, A.; Sesso, HD.; Weiderpass, E.; Willcox, BJ.; Wolk, A.; Zeleniuch-Jacquotte, A.; Willett, W., & Thun, MJ. (2010) Body-Mass Index and Mortality among 1.46 Million White Adults. *The New England Journal of Medicine*, Vol.363, No.23, (December 2010), pp. 2211-2219.

Chiasson, JL.; Josse, RG.; Gomis, R.; Hanefeld, M.; Karasik, A.; Laakso, M., for the STOP-NIDDM Trial Research Group. (2002) Acarbose for prevention of type 2 diabetes mellitus: the STOP-NIDDM randomised trial. *The Lancet*, Vol.359, No.9323, (June 2002), pp. 2072-2077.

Cummings, DE.; Weigle, DS.; Frayo, S.; Breen, PA.; Ma, MK.; Dellinger, EP., & Purnell, JQ. (2002)Plasma Ghrelin levels after Diet-Induced Weight Loss or Gastric Bypass Surgery. *The New England Journal of Medicine*, Vol.346, No.6, (May 2002), pp. 1623-1630.

Despres, JP.; Lemieux, I., & Prud'homme, D. (2001) Treatment of obesity: need to focus on high risk abdominally obese patients. *British Medical Journal*, Vol.322, No.7288, (March 2001), pp. 716-720.

Diabetes Prevention Program Research Group. (2002) Reduction in the Incidence of Type 2 Diabetes with Lifestyle Intervention or Metformin. *The New England Journal of Medicine*, Vol.346, No.6, (February 2002), pp. 393-403.

Dixon, JB.; O'Brien, PE.; Playfair, J.; Chapman, L.; Schachter, LM.; Skinner, S.; Proietto, J.; bailey, M., & Anderson, M. (2008) Adjustable Gastric Banding and Conventional Therapy for Type 2 Diabetes: a Randomized Controlled Trial. *The Journal of the American Medical Association*, Vol.299, No.3, (January 2008), pp. 316-323.

Dixon, JB.; Zimmet, P.; Alberti, KG., & Rubino, F., on behalf of the International Diabetes Federation Taskforce on Epidemiology and Prevention. (2011) Bariatric surgery: an IDF statement for obese Type 2 diabetes. *Diabetic Medicine*, Vol.28, No.6, (June 2011), pp. 628-642.

Drucker, DJ. (2003) Enhancing Incretin Action for the Treatment of Type 2 Diabetes. *Diabetes Care*, Vol.26, No.10, (October 2003), pp. 2929-2940.

Ford, ES. & Mokdad, AH. (2008) Epidemiology of obesity in the western hemisphere. *The Journal of Clinical Endocrinology & Metabolism,* Vol.93, No.11, (November 2008), pp. S1-S8.

Isomaa, B.; Almgren, P.; Tuomi, T.; Forsen, B.; Lahti, K.; Nissen, M.; Taskinen, MR., & Groop, L. (2001) Cardiovascular Morbidity and Mortality Associated With the Metabolic Syndrome. *Diabetes Care,* Vol.24, No.4, (April 2001), pp. 683-689.

Kahn, SE.; Haffner, SM.; Heise, MA.; Herman, WH.; Holman, RR.; Jones, NP.; Kravitz, BG.; Lachin, JM.; O'Neill, MC.; Zinman, B., & Viberti, G., for the ADOPT Study Group. (2006) Glycemic Durability of Rosiglitazone, Metformin, or Glyburide Monotherapy. *The New England Journal of Medicine,* Vol.355, No.23 (December 2006), pp. 2427-2443.

Karamanakos, SN.; Vanegas, K.; Kalfarentzos, F., & Alexandrides, TK. (2008) Weight loss, appetite suppression, and changes in fasting plasma ghrelin and peptide YY levels after Roux-en-Y gastric bypass and sleeve gastrectomy. A prospective, double-blind study. *Annals of Surgery,* Vol.247, No.3 , (March 2008), pp. 401-407.

Kasuga, M. (2006) Insulin resistance and pancreatic β cell failure. *The Journal of Clinical Investigation,* Vol.116, No.7, (July 2006), pp. 1756-1760.

Laferrere, B.; Heshka, S.; Wang, K.; Khan, Y.; McGinty, J.; Teixeira, J.; Hart, AB., & Olivan, B. (2007) Incretin Levels and Effect Are Markedly Enhanced 1 Month After Roux-en-Y Gastric Bypass Surgery in Obese Patients With Type 2 Diabetes. *Diabetes Care,* Vol.30, No.7, (July 2007), pp. 1709-1716.

Lahsen, R., & Berry, M. (2010) Surgical Interventions to Correct Metabolic Disorders. *The British Journal of Diabetes & Vascular Disease,* Vol.10, No.3, (June 2010), pp. 143-147.

Le Roith, D., & Zick, Y. (2001) Recent Advances in Our Understanding of Insulin Action and Insulin resistance. *Diabetes Care,* Vol.24, No.3 (March 2001), pp. 588-597.

Morinigo, R.; Moize, R.; Musri, M.; Lacy, AM.; Navarro, S.; Marin, JL.; Delgado, S.; Casamitjana, R., & Vidal, J. (2006) Glucagon-Like Peptide-1, Peptide YY, Hunger, and Satiety after Gastric Bypass Surgery in Morbidly Obese Subjects. *The Journal of Clinical Endocrinology & Metabolism,* Vol.91, No.5, (May 2006), pp. 1735-1740.

National Institutes of Health. National Heart, Lung, and Blood Institute in cooperation with The National Institute of Diabetes and Digestive and Kidney Diseases. (1998) Clinical Guidelines on the Identification, Evaluation, and Treatment of overweight and Obesity in Adults. The Evidence Report. NIH Publication No. 98-4083, (September 1998).

Peterli, R.; Wolnerhanssen, B.; Peters, T.; Devaux, N.; Kern, B.; Christoffel-Courtin, C.; Drewe, J.; von Flue, M., & Beglinger, C. (2009) Improvement in Glucose Metabolism After Bariatric Surgery: Comparison of Laparoscopic Roux-en-Y Gastric Bypass and Laparoscopic Sleeve Gastrectomy. *Annals of Surgery,* Vol.250, No.2 , (August 2009), pp. 234-241.

Pi-Sunyer, X.; Blackburn, G.; Brancati, FL.; Bray, GA.; Bright, R.; Clark, JM.; Curtis, JM.; Espeland, MA.; Foreyt, JP.; Graves, K.; Haffner, SM.; Harrison, B.; Hill, JO.; Horton, ES.; Jakicic, J.; Jeffery, RW.; Johnson, KC.; Kahn, S.; Kelley, DE.; Kitabchi, AE.; Knowler, WC.; Lewis, CE.; Maschak-Carey, BJ.; Montgomery, B.; Nathan, DM.; Patricio, J.; Peters, A.; Redmon, B.; Reeves, RS.; Ryan, DH.; Safford, M.; Van Dorsten, B.; Wadden, TA.; Wagenknecht, L.; Wesche-Thobaben, J.; Wing, RR., & Yanovski, SZ., for the Look-AHEAD Research Group. (2007) Reduction in Weight and Cardiovascular Disease Risk Factors in Individuals with Type 2 Diabetes. One-year results of the Look-AHEAD trial. *Diabetes Care*, Vol.30, No.6, (June 2007), pp. 1374-1383.

Pories, WJ.; Swanson, MS.; MacDonald, KG.; Long, SB.; Morris, PG.; Brown, BM.; Barakat, HA.; deRamon, RA.; Israel, G.; Dolezal, JM., & Dohm, L. (1995) Who Would Have Thought it? An Operation Proves to Be the Most Effective Therapy for Adult-Onset Diabetes Mellitus. *Annals of Surgery*, Vol.222, No.3, (September 1995), pp. 339-352.

Prentki, M., & Nolan, CJ. (2006) Islet β cell failure in type 2 diabetes. *The Journal of Clinical Investigation*, Vol.116, No.7 (July 2006), pp. 1802-1812.

Ramachandran, A.; Snehalatha, C.; Mary, S.; Mukesh, B.; Bhaskar, AD., & Vijay, V., for the Indian Diabetes Prevention Programme (IDPP). (2006) The Indian Diabetes Prevention Programme shows that lifestyle modification and metformin prevent type 2 diabetes in Asian Indian subjects with impaired glucose tolerance (IDPP-1). *Diabetologia*, Vol.49, No.2, (February 2006), pp. 289-297.

Reaven, GM.; Lithell, H., & Landsberg, L. (1996) Hypertension and Associated Metabolic Abnormalities - The Role of Insulin Resistance and the Sympathoadrenal System. *The New England Journal of Medicine*, Vol.334, No.6, (February 1996), pp. 374-381.

Rubino, F.; Forgione, A.; Cummings, DE.; Vix, M.; Gnuli, D.; Mingrone, G.; Castagneto, M., & Marescaux, J. (2006) The Mechanism of Diabetes Control After Gastrointestinal Bypass Surgery Reveals a Role of the Proximal Small Intestine in the Pathophysiology of Type 2 Diabetes. *Annals of Surgery*, Vol.244, No.5 , (November 2006), pp. 741-749.

Scopinaro, N.; Papadia, F.; Marinari, G.; Camerini, G., & Adami, G. (2007) Long-Term Control of Type 2 Diabetes Mellitus and the Other Major Components of the Metabolic Syndrome after Biliopancreatic Diversion in Patients with BMI <35 kg/m^2. *Obesity Surgery*, Vol.17, No.2, (February 2007), pp. 185-192.

Sjostrom, L.; Narbro, K.; Sjostrom, CD.; Karason, K.; Larsson, B.; Wedel, H.; Lystig, T.; Sullivan, M.; Bouchard, C.; Carlsson, B.; Bengtsson, C.; Dahlgren, S.; Gummesson, A.; Jacobson, P.; Karlsson, J.; Lindroos, AK.; Lonroth, H.; Naslund, I.; Olbers, T.; Stenlof, K.; Torgerson, J.; Agren, G., & LMS Carlsson, for the Swedish Obese Subjects Study. (2007) Effects of Bariatric Surgery on Mortality in Swedish Obese Subjects. *The New England Journal of Medicine*, Vol.357, No.8, (August 2007), pp. 741-752.

Toft-Nielsen, MB.; Damholt, MB.; Madsbad, S.; Hilsted LM.; Hughes, TE.; Michelsen, BK., & Holst, JJ. (2001) Determinants of the Impaired Secretion of Glucagon-Like Peptide-1 in Type 2 Diabetic Patients. *The Journal of Clinical Endocrinology & Metabolism*, Vol.86, No.8, (August 2001), pp. 3717-3723.

Torgerson, JS.; Hauptman, J.; Boldrin, MN., & Sjostrom, L. (2004) Xenical in the Prevention of Diabetes in Obese Subjects (XENDOS) Study. *Diabetes Care*, Vol.27, No.1, (January 2004), pp. 155-161.

Tuomilehto, J.; Lindstrom, J.; Eriksson, JG.; Valle, TT.; Hamalainen, H.; Ilanne-Parikka, P.; Keinanen-Kiukaanniemi, S.; Laakso, M.; Louheranta, A.; Rastas, M.; Salminen, V., & Uusitupa, M., for the Finnish Diabetes Prevention Study Group. (2001) Prevention of Type 2 Diabetes Mellitus by Changes in Lifestyle among Subjects with Impaired Glucose Tolerance. *The New England Journal of Medicine*, Vol.344, No.18, (May 2001), pp. 1343-1350.

Turner, RC.; Holman, RR.; Stratton, IM.; Cull, CA.; Matthews, DR.; Manley, SE.; Frighi, V.; Wright, D.; Neil, A.; Kohner, E.; McElroy, H.; Fox, C., & Hadden, D., for the United Kingdom Prospective Diabetes Study (UKPDS) Group. (1998) Effect of intensive blood-glucose control with metformin on complications in overweight patients with type 2 diabetes (UKPDS 34). *The Lancet*, Vol.352, No.9131, (September 1998), pp. 854-865.

Wajchenberg, BL. (2000) Subcutaneous and Visceral adipose Tissue: Their Relation to the Metabolic Syndrome. *Endocrine Reviews*, Vol.21, No.6, (December 2000), pp. 697-738.

Zinman, B. (2006) Type 2 Diabetes Mellitus: Magnitude of the Problem and Failure to Achieve Glycemic Control. *Endocrinology and Metabolism Clinics of North America*, Vol.35, Supplement 1, (December 2006), pp. 3-5.

13

Bariatric Surgery on Obese Type 2 Diabetes Patients

Junichirou Mori, Yoshihiko Sato and Mitsuhisa Komatsu
Shinshu University, Japan

1. Introduction

Amidst a worldwide epidemic of diabetes, the World Health Organization estimates that 346 million people have diabetes and an estimated 3.4 million people died from consequences of high blood sugar in 2004[1]. Over time, diabetes can damage the heart, blood vessels, eyes, kidneys, and nerves. Especially diabetes increases the risk of heart disease and stroke.

Obesity carries with it significant risks of diabetes. Improvement in obesity is attendant with improvements in this ailment[2][3], and obese people consequently have been treated through pharmacotherapy, and intervention in life habits, including diet and exercise. Even with such treatment, however, it is very difficult to have satisfactory body weight loss. In the last few years, many studies have performed to compare intensive glucose control therapy with standard therapy. Most of the results show that body weight did not change with both intensive glucose control therapy and standard therapy[4][5]. Moreover, many patients who are initially successful at weight loss then go on to rebound[6]. Thus, promoting weight loss is a major issue in treatment, especially in severely obese patients. Recently, there has been an increase in patients with a BMI > 35 undergoing bariatric surgery and there has been a notable increase in studies describing effect of bariatric surgery on type 2 diabetes patients[6].

2. Effect of bariatric surgery on obesity and diabetes

Although an average of 55.9% loss in excess body weight was observed in bariatric surgery[6], the extent of operation-induced weight loss varies depending on the surgical method[7]. While loss in body weight from intervention in life habits is insufficient, it was 46.2% for gastric binding and 59.5% for gastric bypass, respectively, thus showing that bariatric surgery leads to more efficient weight-loss results[6]. However, although bariatric surgery generally leads to a great improvement in diabetes[8] (Table 1), there is a gradation of results depending on the procedure[9]. Additionally for type 2 diabetes patients, studies on gastric bypass have shown that improvements in fasting plasma glucose and insulin sensitivity are evident prior to weight loss[10][11]. These kinds of changes are not observed in gastric binding[6][12]. From these results, apart from improvements in insulin sensitivity induced through weight loss, gastric bypass is also thought to improve glucose metabolism.

	Total (n)	Gastric Binding (n)	Gastric Bypass (n)
Absolute Weight Loss (Kg)	-41.9 (266)	-26.0 (56)	-50.54 (129)
BMI Decrease (kg/m2)	-14.0 (306)	-9.1 (56)	-18.0 (166)
Excess Loss (%)	-57.3 (267)	-41.0 (83)	-65.7 (184)
Fasting Insulin (pmol/L)	-123.9 (160)	-49.5 (56)	-153.7 (90)
HbA1c (%)	-2.4 (171)	-1.2 (83)	-3.0 (88)
Fasting Glucose (mmol/L)	-4.0 (296)	-3.2 (56)	-3.4 (164)
BMI: body mass index			

Table 1. Efficacy for Improvement in Diabetes-Related Outcomes for Diabetic and Glucose-Intolerant Patients [8].

Incretin	Secretion	Function	Change after bariatric surgery
GLP-1	Distal ileum , Colon	Increase insulin release Slowing gastric emptying Controlling Glucagon secretion Induce satiety by working on the central nervous system	Increase
Ghrelin	Stomach	Stimulate appetite Increasing activity in the stomach Suppression of insulin secretion Increase growth hormone secretion	Decrease (Roux-en-Y Gastric Bypass)

Table 2. Summary of Intestin.

3. Effects of bariatric surgery on intestine hormone

One hypothesis to explain this phenomenon is the influence of gastrointestinal hormones. Glucagon-like peptide-1 (GLP-1), an intestinal hormone secreted from the distal ileum and colon in response to nutrient ingestion[9]. GLP-1 acts on the beta cells to increase the level of cyclic AMP, leading to replenishment of the readily releasable pool of insulin granules during glucose-stimulated insulin secretion[13]. Not only improving beta-cell function, GLP-1 is also involved in the proliferation and regeneration of pancreatic β-cells[14][15]. Outside pancreatic effects, GLP-1 decreases dietary intake by slowing gastric emptying[16], controlling secretion of gastric acid[17] and glucagon[18], and induce satiety by working on the central nervous system[19][20]). There have been numerous studies detailing a post-operative increase in GLP-1 secretion from gastric bypass, and this increase occurs prior to post-gastric bypass weight loss[21-24]. Studies show that the post-gastric bypass GLP-1 level is significantly higher when compared to the post-gastric binding GLP-1 level[25][26]. When considering the effect of GLP-1, it is possible that the increase in endogenous GLP-1 secretion plays an important role in the improvement of glucose metabolism by the gastric bypass surgery.

Although ghrelin is similar to GLP-1 in that it is related to the appetite, it is actually an appetite-stimulating hormone[27-29]. It is likely that the appetite stimulating from ghrelin is due to its increasing activity in the stomach[28][30] and suppressing of insulin secretion[30]. Ghrelin levels increase in dietary restriction-induced weight loss and when there is a negative energy balance, and conversely, decrease when eating or in the case of the obese[31)32)]. However in the case of the obese, ghrelin levels become unchanged even when eating, and therefore, ghrelin level is a potential factor in obesity[33)]. There are many reports demonstrating that fasting ghrelin levels decrease after Roux-en-Y Gastric Bypass compared to pre-operation[34)35)]. It has been reported that decrease in ghrelin levels occurs immediately following surgery and lasts for more than a year[36) 37)]. Through Roux-en-Y Gastric Bypass, food bypasses the distal stomach in which ghrelin is released, and this may account for the post-bypass decrease in ghrelin levels[34)].

4. Incretin-therapy on type 2 diabetes patients

Recently GLP-1 analog/receptor agonists and GLP-1 degradation inhibitors are in clinical use. The beneficial points of these antidiabetes agents are glucose-dependent insulinotropism which may be reduced the risk of hypoglycemia[38)]. Liraglutide is a GLP-1 analog with 97% sequence identity to human hormone. The mean reduction in HbA1c by liraglutide (1.8mg) was 1.14%[39)]. In addition to effective glucose lowering, liraglutide produced beneficial effects on body weight. The mean reduction in body weight after 16weeks treatment of 1.8mg liraglutide was 3.6kg and was sustained thoughout the 52 week study[39)]. These results support the hypothesis that the bariatric surgery leads to a great improvement of diabetes not only by the reduction of the storage capacity of the stomach but also by the change in intestinal hormone.

5. Clinical application of bariatric surgery in Asia

As previously stated, there are reports that bariatric surgery leads to dramatic improvement in type 2 diabetes compared to pharmacotherapy and lifestyle intervention-based treatment. Will bariatric surgery replace conventional medication and/or life style intervention-based treatment in Asia? At present, however, most of these reports are not necessarily targeting regular subjects, given the subjects' extremely high average BMI of 47.9 kg/m^2 and relatively young average age of 40.2 years old[6)].

Obesity in the Asian population is much less than in Western populations. The Ministry of Health, Labour and Welfare, Japan reported that only 3.7% of the population is obese (BMI>30)[40)]. The rate of obesity in diabetes is reported to be similar to that in the rest of the Japanese population[41)], and at present bariatric surgery has only a limited application in Japan. To increase the application of bariatric surgery in Asia, there is a need for a high-evidence level cohort study based on previous research that varies by age and obesity level in order to further the discussion on whether bariatric surgery should be given precedence over conventional medication and life style intervention-based treatment in patients with a BMI > 35.

6. Summary

Recently, in certain countries, there has been an increase in obese patients undergoing bariatric surgery which leads to more efficient weight-loss results. Bariatric surgery is an effective treatment option for severely obese patients for whom weight loss has been problematic with conventional pharmacotherapy and/or life style intervention-based treatment. Gastric bypass has been shown not only to decrease body weight but to have an effect on incretin (Table2). Change in incretin, especially GLP-1, could support the improvement in body weight. GLP-1 also has beneficially affect on pancreatic β-cells function, proliferation and regeneration. Thus even if diabetes did not cure by bariatric surgery, change in incretin have beneficially effect on diabetes. Therefore to choose the operative procedure of bariatric surgery, especially on patients who have basic disease, it is necessary to think about dynamic state of incretin.

7. References

[1] World Health Organization: Diabetes. Fact sheet No312, Geneva, 2011

[2] Pi-Sunyer X, Blackburn G, Yonavski SZ et al: Reduction in weight and cardiovascular disease risk factors in individuals with type 2 Diabetes: one-year results of the look AHEAD trial. Diabetes Care 30: 1374-1383, 2007

[3] Espeland MA, Bray GA, Wing R et al: Describing patterns of weight changes using principal components analysis: results from the Action for Health in Diabetes (Look AHEAD) research group. Ann Epidemiol 19: 701-710, 2009

[4] Patel A, MacMahon S, Travert F et al: Intensive blood glucose control and vascular outcomes in patients with type 2 diabetes. N Engl J Med 358: 2560-2572, 2008

[5] Gerstein HC, Miller ME, Friedewald WT et al: Long-term effects of intensive glucose lowering on cardiovascular outcomes. N Engl J Med 364: 818-828, 2011

[6] Buchwald H, Estok R, Sledge I et al: Weight and type 2 Diabetes after bariatric surgery: systematic review and meta-analysis. Am J Med 122: 248-256, 2009

[7] Garb J, Welch G, Zagarins S, Kuhn J, Romanelli J: Bariatric surgery for the treatment of morbid obesity: a meta-analysis of weight loss outcomes for laparoscopic adjustable gastric banding and laparoscopic gastric bypass. Obes Surg 19: 1447-1455, 2009

[8] Buchwald H, Avidor Y, Schoelles K et al: Bariatric surgery: a systematic review and meta-analysis. JAMA 292: 1724-1737, 2004

[9] Pournaras DJ, LeRoux CW: The effect of bariatric surgery on gut hormones that alter appetite: Diabetes Metab. 35: 508-512, 2009

[10] Bose M, Teixeira J, Laferrère B et al: Weight loss and incretin responsiveness improve glucose control independently after gastric bypass surgery. J Diabetes 2: 47-55, 2009

[11] Bikman BT, Zheng D, Dohm GL et al: Mechanism for improved insulin sensitivity after gastric bypass surgery. J Clin Endocrinol Metab 93: 4656-4663, 2008

[12] VincentRP, leRouxCW: Changes in gut hormones after bariatric surgery. Clin Endocrinol 69: 173-179, 2008

[13] Yajima H, Komatsu M, Shermerhorn T et al: cAMP enhances insulin secretion by an action on the ATP-sensitive K+ channel-independent pathway of glucose signaling in rat pancreatic islets. Diabetes 48:1006-1012, 1999

[14] Holst JJ: The physiology of glucagon-like peptide 1.Physiol Rev 87: 1409-1439, 2007

[15] Buteau J, Roduit R, Susini S, Prentki M: Glucagon-like peptide-1 promotes DNA synthesis, activates phosphatidylinositol 3-kinase and increases transcription factor pancreatic and duodenal homeobox gene 1 (PDX-1) DNA binding activity in beta (INS-1)-cells. Diabetologia 42: 856-864, 1999

[16] Edholm T, Degerblad M, Schmidt PT, Hellström PM et al: Differential incretin effects of GIP and GLP-1 on gastric emptying, appetite and insulin-glucose homeostasis. Neurogastroenterol Motil 22:1191-1200, 2010

[17] Nauck MA, Niedereichholz U, Schmiegel WH et al: Glucagon-like peptide 1 inhibition of gastric emptying outweighs its insulinotropic effects in healthy humans. Am J Physil 273: E981-E988, 1997
[18] Asmar M, Bache M, Knop FK, Madsbad S, Holst JJ: Do the actions of glucagon-like peptide-1 on gastric emptying, appetite, and food intake involve release of amylin in humans? J Clin Endocrinol Metab 95: 2367-2375, 2010.
[19] MaX, BruningJ, AshcroftFM: Glucagon-like peptide 1 stimulates hypothalamic proopiomelanocortin neurons. J Neurosci 27: 7125-7129, 2007
[20] Pannacciulli N, Le DS, Krakoff J et al: Postprandial glucagon-like peptide-1 (GLP-1) response is positively associated with changes in neuronal activity of brain areas implicated in satiety and food intake regulation in humans. NeuroImage 35: 511-517, 2007
[21] MacDonald PE, El-Kholy W, Wheeler MB et al: The multiple actions of GLP-1 on the process of glucose-stimulated insulin secretion. Diabetes 51: S434-S442, 2002
[22] Goldfine AB, Mun EC, Patti ME et al: Patients with neuroglycopenia after gastric bypass surgery have exaggerated incretin and insulin secretory responses to a mixed meal. J Clin Endocrinol Metab 92: 4678-4685, 2007
[23] LeRoux CW, Aylwin SJ, Bloom SR et al: Gut hormone profiles following bariatric surgery favor an anorectic state, facilitate weight loss, and improve metabolic parameters. Ann Surg 243: 108-114, 2006
[24] Morínigo R, Moizé V, Vidal J et al: Glucagon-like peptide-1, peptide YY, hunger, and satiety after gastric bypass surgery in morbidly obese subjects. J Clin Endocrinol Metab 91: 1735-1740, 2006
[25] Korner J, Bessler M, Inabnet W, Taveras C, Holst JJ: Exaggerated glucagon-like peptide-1 and blunted glucose-dependent insulinotropic peptide secretion are associated with Roux-en-Y gastric bypass but not adjustable gastric banding. Surg Obes Relat Dis 3: 597-601, 2007
[26] Rodieux F, Giusti V, D'Alessio DA, Suter M, Tappy L: Effects of gastric bypass and gastric banding on glucose kinetics and gut hormone release. Obesity (Silver Spring) 16: 298-305, 2008
[27] Murphy KG, Bloom SR: Gut hormones and the regulation of energy homeostasis. Nature 444: 854-859, 2006
[28] Cummings DE, Overduin J: Gastrointestinal regulation of food intake. J Clin Invest 117: 13-23, 2007
[29] Nakazato M, Murakami N, Date Y, Kojima M, Matsuo H, Kangawa K, Matsukura S: A role for ghrelin in the central regulation of feeding. Nature 409:194-198, 2001
[30] Zwirska-Korczala K, Konturek SJ, Brzozowski T et al: Basal and postprandial plasma levels of PYY, ghrelin, cholecystokinin, gastrin and insulin in women with moderate and morbid obesity and metabolic syndrome. J Physiol Pharmacol 58:13-35, 2007
[31] HansenTK, Dall R, Jørgensen JO et al: Weight loss increases circulating levels of ghrelin in human obesity. Clin Endocrinol 56: 203-206, 2002
[32] Cummings DE, Foster-Schubert KE, Overduin J: Ghrelin and energy balance: focus on current controversies. Curr Drug Targes 6: 153-169, 2005
[33] English PJ, Ghatei MA, Malik IA, Bloom SR, Wilding JP: Food fails to suppress ghrelin levels in obese humans. J Clin Endocrinol Metab 87: 2984, 2002

[34] Lin E, Gletsu N, Smith CD et al: The effects of gastric surgery on systemic ghrelin levels in the morbidly obese. Arch Surg 139: 780-784, 2004

[35] N. A. Tritos, E. Mun, A. Bertkau, R. Grayson, E. Maratos-Flier, and A. Goldfine: Serum ghrelin levels in response to glucose load in obese subjects post-gastric bypass surgery. Obes Res 11: 919-924, 2003

[36] Leonetti F, Silecchia G, DiMario U et al: Different plasma ghrelin levels after laparoscopic gastric bypass and adjustable gastric banding in morbid obese subjects. J Clin Endocrinol Metab 88: 4227-4231, 2003

[37] LeRoux CW, Welbourn R, Olber T et al: Gut hormones as mediators of a:etite and weight loss after Roux-en-Y gastric bypass. Ann Surg. 246: 780-785, 2007

[38] Ross SA and Ekoe JM: incretin agents in type 2 diabetes. Can Fam Physician56(7): 639-648, 2010

[39] Garber A, Henry R, Ratner R, Garcia-Hernandez PA Rodriguez-Pattzi H, Olvera-Alvarez I: Liraglutide versus glimepiride monotherapy for type 2 diabetes (LEAD-3 Mono): a randomized, 52-week, phase III, duble-blind, parallel-treatment trial. Lancet 373(9662): 473-481. 2008

[40] Ministry of Health, Labour and Welfare, Japan: Outline of the diabetes mellitus field study 2002. Tokyo, 2004

[41] Sone H, Mizuno S, Fujii H, Yoshimura Y, Yamasaki Y, Ishibashi S, Katayama S, Saito Y, Ito H, Ohashi Y, Akanuma Y, Yamada N: Is the diagnosis of metabolic syndrome useful for predicting cardiovascular disease in Asian diabetic patients? Analysis from the Japan Diabetes Complications Study. Diabetes Care. 28:1463-1471, 2005

14

Bariatric and Metabolic Surgery for Asians

Kazunori Kasama, Yosuke Seki and Tsuyoshi Yamaguchi
Yotsuya Medical Cube, Weight Loss and Metabolic Surgery Center, Japan

1. Introduction

Over the past few decades, there has been a dramatic increase in the prevalence of obesity in many countries. The World Health Organization (WHO) estimates that more than 1 billion adults worldwide are overweight; of these, at least 300 millions are obese. (1) Obesity is associated with multiple chronic diseases, including type 2 diabetes, hypertension, coronary heart disease, stroke and several cancers.(2)

Definitions of overweight (BMI >25) and obesity (BMI>30) are based essentially on criteria derived from studies that involved populations of European origin. The validity of these criteria in Asian populations has yet to be determined. It has been suggested that the associations of BMI with body composition and health outcomes may differ between Asian and European populations. Studies have shown that for a given BMI, Asians generally have a higher percentage of body fat than do Europeans. Asian populations have also been shown to have elevated risks of type 2 diabetes, hypertension, and hyperlipidemia at a relatively low level of BMI.(3)

2. Obesity in Asia

In most Asian countries, the prevalence of overweight and obesity have increased many times over in the past few decades, and the magnitude varies between countries (4,5,6). Southeast Asia and the Western Pacific region are currently facing an epidemic of diseases associated with obesity such as diabetes and CVD. India has the highest number of people with diabetes in the world and China occupies the second position (7).

Table 1 (8) shows the prevalence of overweightness and obesity in Asian countries in comparison with the United States. Many Asian countries have rates which are not very different from that of the U.S.

The highest rate of obesity in Asia is in Thailand(9) and the lowest is in India (6) followed by Philippines (10). China, which once had the leanest of populations, is now rapidly catching up with the West in terms of prevalence of overweight and obesity which had occurred in a remarkably short time (11,12)

The obesity pandemic was restricted to developed, high-income countries until a few decades ago, but recently it has penetrated even the poorest of nations. Asia has undergone considerable socioeconomic transition in the last three decades, which has resulted in increased availability of food, better transport facilities and better health care facilities. The changing trend was seen first in urban populations and in recent years, with improving socioeconomic scenarios in rural areas, the changes were seen even among the urbanizing rural populations. The recent epidemiological data among urban and semi urban southern Indian populations illustrates the changing scenario (13). In addition, reduced physical activity at work due to mechanization, improved motorized transport and preferences for viewing television and video games to outdoor games during leisure time, have resulted in positive energy balance in most Asian countries (14).

	Survey year	Prevalence of overweight adults (%)	Prevalence of obese adult (%)
United States	2007-2008	34.0	0.2
India	1998-1999	10.0	2.2
Malaysia	1996-1997	16.6	4.4
Philippines	1998	16.9	3.3
Taiwan	1993–1996	21.1	4.0
Japan	2001	23.0	3.0
Singapore	1998	24.4	6.0
China	1999-2000	25.0	4.0
Hong Kong	1996-1997	25.1	3.8
South Korea	2001	27.4	3.2

Table 1. Comparison of prevalence of adult obesity in Asian countries versus the United States.

In parallel with the increase in adult obesity, obesity in children is also increasing. Childhood obesity has reached more than 25% in many developing countries. The etiological factors for childhood obesity include genetic, metabolic, and behavioral components. An imbalanced energy intake versus energy expenditure due to consumption of energy dense food and increase in sedentary habits has mainly contributed to increases in childhood obesity, both in developed and developing countries (15).

Asian populations generally have a lower BMI than many other ethnic groups, but the association between BMI and glucose intolerance is as strong as in any other population (16). The risk of diabetes (odds ratio) was significant for urban Indian populations with a BMI of >23kg/m2 (17). This has been confirmed by studies from other parts of India (18), by studies in migrant Indians and in other Asian populations (19). According to WHO recommendations, a BMI of 18.5–22kg/m2 is considered healthy for Asian populations (20). Insulin resistance is one of the major etiological factors for diabetes and the risk association between obesity and diabetes is mediated through insulin resistance.

Many Asian populations have a higher total and central adiposity for a given body weight when compared to matched Caucasian populations. A higher prevalence of metabolic syndrome in south Asians is mostly attributed to the higher prevalence of central adiposity.

The IDF criteria for metabolic syndrome recommends use of ethnic specific thresholds for waist circumference, which includes ≥ 90 cm in men, and ≥ 80 cm in women of Asian origin (21). The Japanese population is an exception.

It has also been noted that for a given BMI, Asians have higher body fat percentage compared with Caucasians (22,23). Higher insulin resistance and an increased risk of diabetes may be partially attributed to this feature. The differences in anthropometric characteristics are evident even in Asian children who are shown to have higher body fat percentage at lower levels of body weight (24,25) and also a tendency for abdominal obesity (26).

In the cohorts of East Asians(27), including Chinese, Japanese, and South Koreans, the lowest risk of death was seen among persons with a BMI in the range of 22.6 to 27.5. The risk was elevated among persons with BMI levels either higher or lower than that range – by a factor of up to 1.5 among those with a BMI of more than 35.0 and by a factor of 2.8 among those with a BMI of 15.0 or less. A similar U-shaped association was seen between BMI and the risks of death from cancer, cardiovascular diseases and other causes.

A WHO expert consultation concluded in 2004 that Asians generally have a higher percentage of body fat than Caucasian people of the same age, sex, and BMI. Also, the proportion of Asians with risk factors for type 2 diabetes and cardiovascular disease is substantial even below the existing WHO BMI cut-off point of 25 kg/m2. Thus, WHO cut-off points did not provide an adequate basis for taking action on risks related to overweight and obesity in many populations in Asia. The WHO recommended for many Asian populations additional trigger points for public health action, which were identified as 23 kg/m2 or higher, representing increased risk, and 27·5 kg/m2 or higher, as representing high risk. The suggested categories are as follows: less than 18·5 kg/m2 underweight; 18·5–23 kg/m2 increasing but acceptable risk; 23–27·5 kg/m2 increased risk; and 27·5 kg/m2 or higher high risk. (3)

3. Diabetes in Asia

Type 2 diabetes is now a global health priority.(28) The International Diabetes Federation has predicted that the number of individuals with diabetes will increase from 240 million in 2007 to 380 million in 2025, with 80% of the disease burden in low- and middle-income countries.(29) More than 60% of the world's population with diabetes will come from Asia, because it remains the world's most populous region. The number of individuals with diabetes and impaired glucose tolerance (IGT) in each Asian country will increase substantially in coming decades (Table 2).(30)

	Diabetes		Impaired Glucose Tolerance	
Country	2007	2025	2007	2025
India	40850	69882	35906	56228
China	39809	59270	64323	79058
Japan	6978	7171	12891	12704
Bangladesh	3848	7416	6819	10647
Korea	3074	4163	3224	4240
Total Asia	113536	179742	157067	213218

All values are in thousands

Table 2. Top 5 Countries in Asia With the Highest Number of Persons With Type 2 Diabetes and Impaired Glucose Tolerance in the Age Group 20 to 79 Years in 2007 and Projected Data in 2025 (30)

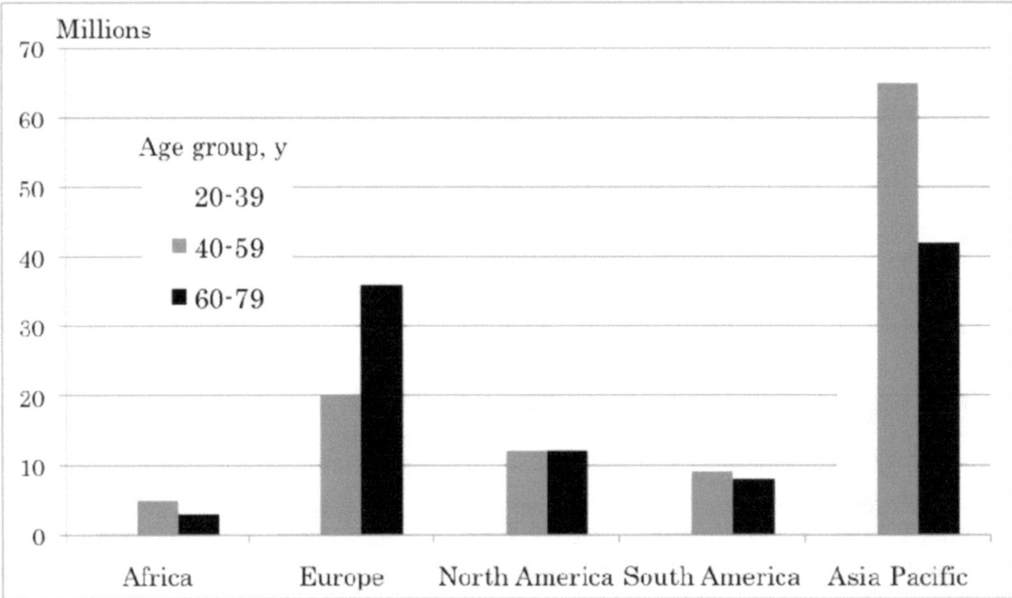

Fig. 1. Number of persons with diabetes in different age group (30)

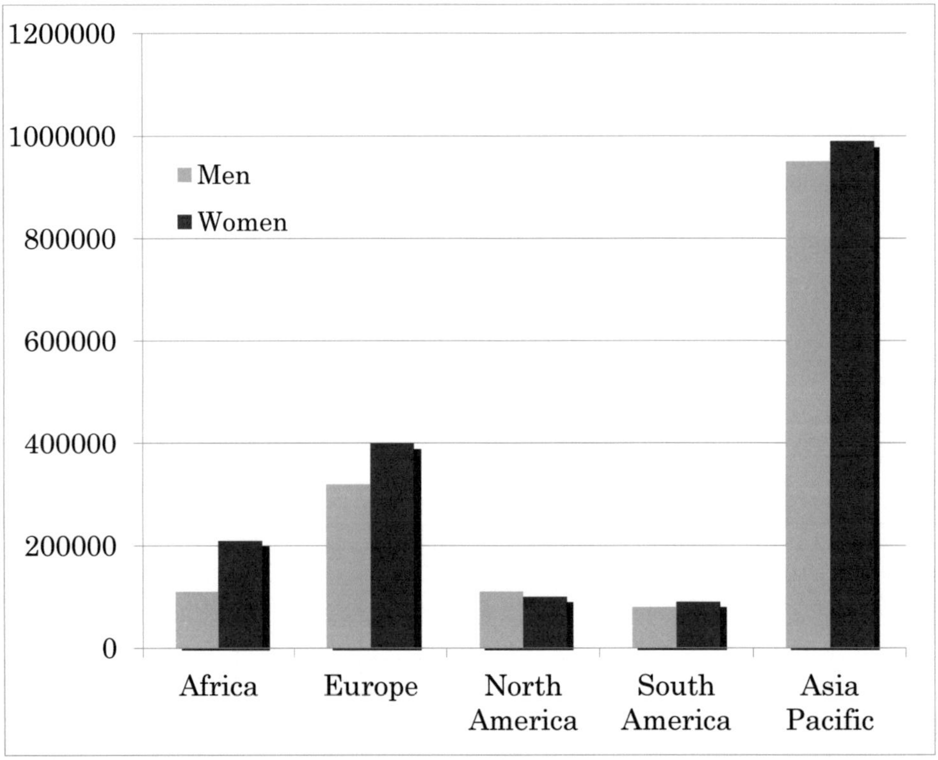

Deaths attributable to diabetes , Age 20~79 years.

Fig. 2. Number of Deaths Attributable to Diabetes in Different Regions of the World in 2007 (30)

Unlike in the West, where older populations are most affected, the burden of diabetes in Asian countries is disproportionately high in young to middle-aged adults. (Figure 1) And also the number of deaths attributable to diabetes in Asian Pacific region is extremely high.(Figure 2) (30)

Amid this global epidemic of diabetes, Asian countries undergoing economic and nutritional transitions have experienced a particularly notable increase.(30) In China, the prevalence of diabetes increased from 1% in 1980 to 5.5% in 2001(31), with much higher rates in urban areas such as Shanghai(32). Nearly 10% of Chinese adults residing in affluent regions such as Hong Kong and Taiwan have diabetes (33). Among individuals with diabetes, two-thirds in mainland China and one-half in Hong Kong and Taiwan remain undiagnosed.

In urban Indian adults, diabetes prevalence increased from 3% in the early 1970s to 12% in 2000, with a narrowing rural-urban gradient (34). In 2006, the rate of type 2 diabetes in rural south India was 9.2%, compared with an increase from 13.9% in 2000 to 18.6% in 2006 in urban south India. (35)

Asians have lower rates of overweightness and obesity than their Western counterparts, using conventional definitions. Despite lower BMI, some Asian countries have similar or even higher prevalence of diabetes than Western countries.(36) These data confirm that the risk of type 2 diabetes starts at a lower BMI for Asians than for Europeans.(37)

Asian populations, especially those of South Asian descent, are more prone to abdominal obesity and low muscle mass with increased insulin resistance compared with their Western counterparts. (38,39,40,41,42,43,44) Thus, waist circumference reflecting central obesity is a useful measure of obesity-related risk of type 2 diabetes, especially in individuals with normal BMI values. (38,45)

Data suggest that the increased risk of type 2 diabetes in Asian populations may be attributed to increased abdominal and visceral adiposity for a given BMI.(46)

In Asian populations, the amount of visceral fat (including mesenteric fat) and fatty liver was significantly associated with subclinical atherosclerosis.(47) In addition, increased waist circumference has been associated with substantially increased risk of developing diabetes (48,49) as well as increased risk of cardiovascular and all-cause mortality, independent of BMI.(50,51,52,53)

In the 1980s, Japanese researchers first revealed that reduced early insulin response was an independent predictor for diabetes.(54) Fukushima et al (55) found that at all stages of glucose intolerance, Japanese individuals had reduced early and late phases of insulin responses. In Japanese men with normal glucose tolerance, even a small increase in BMI produced a decrease in beta cell function disproportionate to that in insulin sensitivity. (56) In a sample of Chinese patients with type 2 diabetes, 50% were of normal weight, with low BMI correlating with low levels of fasting plasma C-peptide and high glycated hemoglobin levels.(57) In a prospective survey of Japanese Americans, visceral fat area and reduced incremental insulin response were independent predictors for diabetes. (58) Taken together, in some Asian populations, inadequate beta cell response to increasing insulin resistance results in a loss of glycemic control and increased risk of diabetes, even with relatively little weight gain.

Among lean, healthy individuals matched for age, BMI, waist circumference, birth weight, and current diet, Asians had higher levels of postprandial glycemia and lower insulin sensitivity than Caucasians in response to a 75-g carbohydrate load.(59) These findings raise the possibility that Asians are more genetically susceptible to insulin resistance and diabetes than Caucasians.

Asian patients with diabetes continue to exhibit high risk for renal complications. (60) In observational studies as well as clinical trials, Asian patients with diabetes were more likely to develop end stage renal disease (ESRD) than their Caucasian counterparts. In a 25-year prospective survey, 60% of young Japanese patients with type 2 diabetes diagnosed before age 35 became blind or had developed ESRD at a mean age of 50. (61)

4. Bariatric and metabolic surgery in Asia

The history of bariatric surgery started when Taiwan adopted the JI bypass as the first bariatric surgery in Asia in the 1970s. (62) The first gastric partitioning was performed at Taiwan in 1981. (63) The first gastric bypass was introduced into Japan in 1982 and the VBG into Singapore in 1987. (64,65)

With the development of laparoscopic surgery, bariatric surgery has entered the realm of minimally invasive surgery. Laparoscopic VBG (LVBG) was successfully performed in Taiwan in 1998 and emerged as an alternative to the conventional VBG. (66) After the success of laparoscopic adjustable gastric banding (LAGB) in Europe and Australia, Asian countries also started to perform LAGB since 1999, first in Singapore.(13) Further, laparoscopic Roux-en-Y gastric bypass (LRYGBP) was also introduced into Taiwan in 2000(67) and subsequently proven to be a more effective but complicated bariatric operation than LVBG.(68) LRYGBP has also been developed in Japan 2002 and other Asian countries. (69). Laparoscopic Sleeve Gastrectomy was introduced into South Korea in 2002 (70)

Asian Pacific Bariatric Surgery Group (APBSG), which was founded in 2004 and officially changed its name to Asian Pacific Metabolic and Bariatric Surgery Society (APMBSS) in 2008, held a consensus meeting in 2005 and modified the indication for bariatric surgery for Asian.

Consensus in Asia-Pacific 2005 (63)

1. Obese patients with a BMI >37
2. Obese patients with a BMI >32 and the presence of diabetes or two significant obesity-related co-morbidities.
3. Have been unable to lose or maintain weight loss using dietary or medical measures.
4. Age of patient >18 years and <65 years. Under special circumstance and in consultation with a pediatrician, bariatric surgery may be used on children under 18.

Because bariatric surgery currently is the most effective treatment for type 2 diabetes, APBSG not only modified the indications for bariatric surgery but also emphasized its role in diabetic treatment. It was the first bariatric guideline of the world to mention a focus especially on diabetes.

In the national report session at the 2nd congress of the International Federation for Surgery of Obesity and Metabolic Disorders Asian Pacific Chapter (IFSO-APC), which was held in Hokkaido, Japan, in 2011, the representatives of Asian countries reported on their respective situations. According to the session reports, more than 5,500 cases of bariatric and metabolic surgery were performed in Asia 2010. India had 3000 cases followed by Taiwan (Figure 3).

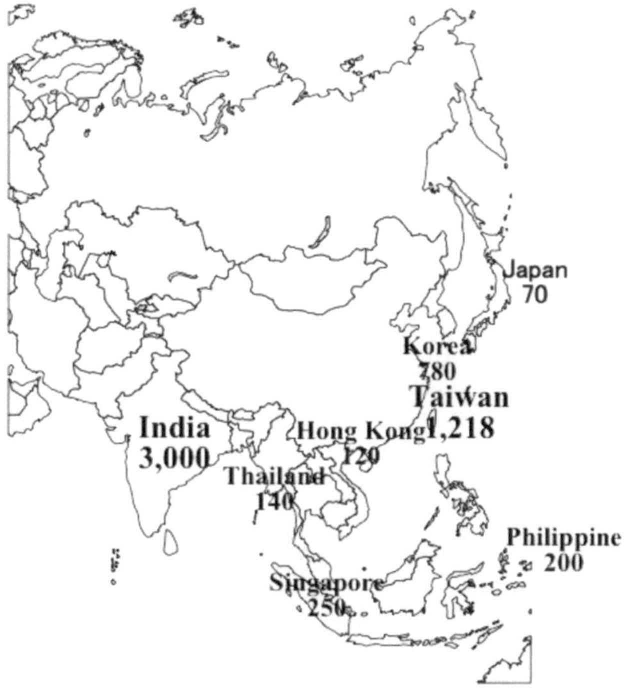

Fig. 3. Bariatric and Metabolic Surgery Cases in 2010 (IFSO-APC 2011 National Report)

Laparoscopic Gastric bypass still formed the majority of the procedures and LSG was rapidly increasing.

A systematic review of bariatric surgery in Asia with citation of 160 papers from Asia was also reported IFSO-APC 2011 by Seki Y, et al. The report summarized as Table3.

		Asian (Seki et al)	All
RYGBP	%EWL	74.8%	61.6% a
	Mortality	0%	0.5% in Open, 0.2% in laparoscopic
LAGB	%EWL	59.1%	45.5% a
	Mortality	0.07%	0.1%
LSG	%EWL	67.9%	55.4% b
	Mortality	0.32%	0.19%

a) Buchwald et al. (n=22094, pre-OP mean BMI 46.9 kg/m2),
b) Brethauer et al. (n=2570, pre-OP mean BMI 51.2 kg/m2)
RYGBP: Roux en Y Gastric Bypass, LAGB: Laparoscopic Adjustable Gastric Banding, LSG: Laparoscopic Sleeve Gastrectomy

Table 3. Systemic review results of bariatric surgery for Asians.

From the current evidence, including 14 studies and 4,257 patients, bariatric surgery for Asians is an effective weight loss procedure although long-term data are limited. The postoperative mortality rates have been acceptably low.

Regarding the anti-diabetic effect of bariatric surgery for Caucasians, LRYGB and LSG showed similar results. (71) But for East Asians, a prospective randomized control study for type 2 diabetes patients by Lee WJ et al.(72) suggested different results. Gastric bypass was far superior to LSG on remission of diabetes and metabolic disorders. Duodenal exclusion would play significant role in remission of type 2 diabetes for East Asian populations. Limitation of remission of diabetes after LSG was also reported (73). Patients with fasting C-peptide over 6ng/ml could have a very good remission of diabetes and patients with c-peptide less than 3ng/ml could only have 14% of remission rate of diabetes after LSG. The problem is that a majority of East Asian diabetes patients are more prone to having a beta cell dysfunction than Caucasians and with fasting C-peptide less than 3 ng/ml (74). These results provide us with data showing that Asians, at least East Asians including Taiwanese, Chinese, South Korean and Japanese, have a higher rate of remission from type 2 diabetes after bypass surgery than with LSG.

4. IFSO-APC consensus statement 2011

According to the ethnicity of Asians, the IFSO-Asian Pacific chapter (APC) consensus statement was established in 2011. Forty four bariatric experts from the Asia Pacific and other regions were chosen to have voting privileges for the IFSO-APC consensus at 2nd IFSO APC congress on 24th February 2011 in Rusutsu, Hokkaido, Japan. All voting delegates represented their respective societies or countries. The IFSO-APC consensus based upon the antecedent statements and guidelines regarding bariatric and metabolic surgery, especially in the Asian Pacific region, including the National Institute of Health (NIH) statements (75), Obesity Surgery Society of India (OSSI), Japan Society for Surgery of Obesity (JSSO), Asian Consensus Meeting on Metabolic Surgery (ACMOMS)(76), Obesity Surgery Society of Australia and New Zealand (OSSANZ), APMBSS(63), Diabetes Surgery Summit (DSS)(77) and Asian Diabetes Surgery Summit (ADSS). Before voting on the consensus, representatives from each society presented their statements or guidelines. These statements and guidelines were used to establish the consensus of the IFSO-APC. A computerized audience-response voting system was used to analyze agreement or disagreement with the wording of the consensus.

"Consensus" was established with the agreement of over 75% of delegates and a "Viewpoint" was recognized with an agreement between 66% and 75%.

Results: Ninety five percent of the delegates agreed with the necessity of establishment of the IFSO-APC consensus statement, and 98% agreed with the necessity of new indicators for Asian patients.

IFSO-APC Consensus statements 2011

- Bariatric surgery should be considered for the treatment of obesity for acceptable Asian candidates with BMI > 35 regardless of the existence of co-morbidities
- **Agree 75% Consensus**

- Bariatric/ GI metabolic surgery should be considered for the treatment of T2DM or metabolic syndrome for patients who are inadequately controlled by lifestyle alternations or medical treatment for acceptable Asian candidates with BMI > 30
- **Agree 76.7% Consensus**
- The surgical approach may be considered as a non-primary alternative to treat inadequately controlled T2DM or metabolic syndrome for suitable Asian candidates with BMI > 27.5.
- **Agree 67.5% Viewpoints**
- Any surgery for T2DM or metabolic syndrome for Asian patients with a BMI < 27.5 should be strictly performed only under clinical study protocols with the informed consent of the patient and prior approval from an ethics committee.
- **Agree 88.1% Consensus**
- Any surgery for T2DM or metabolic syndrome for Asian patients with a **BMI < 27.5** should be strictly performed only under clinical study protocols with the informed consent of the patient and prior approval from the ethics committee.
- **Agree 88.1% Consensus**
- IFSO-APC generally recommends the procedures below for Bariatric and GI metabolic surgery for Asians, currently
- Gastric bypass, Sleeve gastrectomy, Gastric banding, BPD/DS
- **Agree 95.3% Consensus**
- Although novel GI surgical procedures show promising results for Asians other than the four mentioned previously, currently these should be used only in the context of IRB approval.
- **Agree 97.6% Consensus**
- Clinical study should be organized by highly experienced bariatric surgeons, with experience in over **100** cases of bariatric surgery
- **Agree 80% Consensus**

And another three sentences were agreed to by a majority of the voting delegates to form IFSO-APC consensus statements.

Furthermore, an International Diabetes Federation (IDF) position statement in 2011 March (78) also concluded surgery should be considered as an alternative treatment option in Asian patients with a BMI between 27.5 and 32.5 kg/m2 when diabetes cannot be adequately controlled by an optimal medical regimen, especially in the presence of other major cardiovascular disease risk factors.

These results indicate the progress of the Asian region differs from other regions and that it will play significant role in progression of metabolic surgery not only in Asia but also all over the world.

5. References

[1] Abelson P, Kennedy D. The obesity epidemic. Science 2004;304:1413.
[2] Aekplakorn W, Bunnag P, Woodward M, et al. A risk score for predicting incident diabetes in the Thai population. Diabetes Care. 2006; 29(8):1872- 1877.
[3] Ann Intern Med. 1991 Dec 15;115(12):956-61.

[4] Balkau B, Deanfield JE, Despres JP, et al. Inter- national Day for the Evaluation of Abdominal Obesity (IDEA): a study of waist circumference, cardio- vascular disease, and diabetes mellitus in 168,000 primary care patients in 63 countries. Circulation. 2007; 116(17):1942-1951.
[5] Boyko EJ, Fujimoto WY, Leonetti DL, Newell-Morris L. Visceral adiposity and risk of type 2 diabetes: a prospective study among Japanese Americans. Diabetes Care. 2000;23(4):465-471.
[6] Buchwald H, Avidor Y, Braunwald E et al. A systematic review and meta-analysis. JAMA 2004; 13: 1724-37.
[7] Chan WB, Tong PCY, Chow CC, et al. The associations of body mass index, C peptide and metabolic status in Chinese type 2 diabetic patients. Diabet Med. 2004;21(4):349-353.
[8] Chen KM, Lee WJ, Lai HS et al. Fifteen years' experience with gastric partitioning for obesity treatment. J Formos Med Assoc 1998; 97: 381-6.
[9] Cheung BM, Wat NM, Man YB, et al. Development of diabetes in Chinese with the metabolic syndrome: a 6-year prospective study. Diabetes Care. 2007; 30(6):1430-1436.
[10] Cho NH, Jang HC, Choi SH, et al. Abnormal liver function test predicts type 2 diabetes: a community- based prospective study. Diabetes Care. 2007; 30(10):2566-2568.
[11] Deurenberg P, Deurenberg-Yap M, Guricci S. Asians are different from Caucasians and from each other in their body mass index/body fat per cent relationship. Obes Rev. 2002; 3(3):141-146.
[12] Dixon JB, Zimmet P, Alberti KG et al. Bariatric surgery: an IDF statement for obese Type 2 diabetes. Diabet Med. 2011 Jun;28(6):628-42
[13] Fukushima M, Usami M, Ikeda M, et al. Insulin secretion and insulin sensitivity at different stages of glucose tolerance: a cross-sectional study of Japanese type 2 diabetes. Metabolism. 2004;53(7): 831-835.
[14] Funakoshi S, Fujimoto S, Hamasaki A et al. Analysis of factors influencing pancreatic beta-cell function in Japanese patients with type 2 diabetes: association with body mass index and duration of diabetes exposure. Diabetes Res Clin Pract. 2008 Dec;82(3):353-8.
[15] Gu D, Reynolds K, Duan X, et al; InterASIA Collaborative Group. Prevalence of diabetes and impaired fasting glucose in the Chinese adult population: International Collaborative Study of Cardiovascular Disease in Asia (InterASIA). Diabetologia. 2003; 46(9):1190-1198.
[16] Haslam DW, James WP. Obesity. Lancet 2005;366:1197-209.
[17] Huxley R, James WP, Barzi F, et al; Obesity in Asia Collaboration. Ethnic comparisons of the cross- sectional relationships between measures of body size with diabetes and hypertension. Obes Rev. 2008; 9(suppl 1):53-61.
[18] International Diabetes Federation, Diabetes Atlas, 4th edition, 2009.
[19] International Diabetes Federation. Diabetes Atlas. 3rd ed. Brussels, Belgium: International Diabetes Federation; 2006.
[20] J. Parizkova, M.-K. Chin, M. Chia, and J. Yang, "An international perspective on obesity, health and physical activity: current trends and challenges in China and Asia," Journal of Exercise Science and Fitness, vol. 5, no. 1, pp. 7–23, 2007.

[21] J.C.N. Chan, V. Malik, W. Jia, et al, Diabetes in Asia: Epidemiology, Risk Factors, and Pathophysiology, JAMA 301: 20, 2129–2140 2009
[22] Jia WP, Pang C, Chen L, et al. Epidemiological characteristics of diabetes mellitus and impaired glucose regulation in a Chinese adult population: the Shanghai Diabetes Studies, a cross-sectional 3-year follow-up study in Shanghai urban communities. Diabetologia. 2007; 50(2):286-292.
[23] K. G. M. M. Alberti, P. Zimmet, and J. Shaw, "Metabolic syndrome—a new world-wide definition. A consensus statement from the International Diabetes Federation," Diabetic Medicine, vol. 23, no. 5, pp. 469–480, 2006.
[24] K. M. Flegal, M. D. Carroll, C. L. Ogden, and L. R. Curtin, "Prevalence and trends in obesity among US adults, 1999- 2008," Journal of the American Medical Association, vol. 303, no. 3, pp. 235–241, 2010.
[25] K.H. Yoon, J.H. Lee, J.W. Kim et al., "Epidemic obesity and type 2 diabetes in Asia," The Lancet, vol. 368, no. 9548, pp. 1681–1688, 2006.
[26] Kadowaki T, Miyake Y, Hagura R, et al. Risk factors for worsening to diabetes in subjects with impaired glucose tolerance. Diabetologia. 1984;26 (1):44-49.
[27] Karter AJ, Ferrara A, Liu J, Moffet H, Ackerson L, Selby J. Ethnic disparities in diabetic complications in an insured population. JAMA. 2002;287(19): 2519-2527.
[28] Kasama K, Tagaya N, Kanehira E et al, Has laparoscopic surgery been accepted in Japan? The experience of a single surgeon, Obes Surg. 2008 Nov;18(11):1473-8
[29] Kuroe A, Fukushima M, Usami M, et al. Impaired beta-cell function and insulin sensitivity in Japanese subjects with normal glucose tolerance. Diabetes Res Clin Pract. 2003;59(1):71-77.
[30] Lakdawara M, Bhasker A, Asian Consensus meeting on Metabolic Surgery (ACMOMS), Report: Asian Consensus Meeting on Metabolic Surgery. Recommendations for the use of Bariatric and Gastrointestinal Metabolic Surgery for Treatment of Obesity and Type II Diabetes Mellitus in the Asian Population: August 9th and 10th, 2008, Trivandrum, India. Obes Surg. 2010 Jul;20(7):929-36.
[31] Le DS, Kusama K, Yamamoto S. A community- based picture of type 2 diabetes mellitus in Vietnam. J Atheroscler Thromb. 2006; 13(1):16-20. 73. 44. Stolk RP, Suriyawongpaisal P, Aekplakorn W, Woodward M, Neal B; InterASIA Collaborative Group. Fat distribution is strongly associated with plasma glucose levels and diabetes in Thai adults—the InterASIA study. Diabetologia. 2005; 48(4):657-660.
[32] Lear SA, Humphries KH, Kohli S, Chockalingam A, Frohlich JJ, Birmingham CL. Visceral adipose tissue accumulation differs according to ethnic back- ground: results of the Multicultural Community Health Assessment Trial (M-CHAT). Am J Clin Nutr. 2007; 86(2):353-359.
[33] Lee WJ, Chong K, Ser KH et al. Gastric bypass vs Sleeve gastrectomy for type 2 diabetes mellitus A randomized controlled trial. Arch Surg. 146(2),143-148, 2011
[34] Lee WJ, Huang MT, Lai IR et al. Laparoscopic vertical banded gastric partition. Formos J of Surg 1999; 32: 165-171.
[35] Lee WJ, Huang MT, Yu PY et al. Laparoscopic vertical banded gastroplasty and laparoscopic gastric bypass: A comparison. Obes Surg 2004; 14: 626-34.

[36] Lee WJ, Ser KH, Chong K et al. Laparoscopic sleeve gastrectomy for diabetes treatment in nonmorbidly obese patients: efficacy and change of insulin secretion, Surgery. 2010 May;147(5):664-9.

[37] Liu KH, Chan Y, Chan W, Chan J, Chu W. Mesenteric fat thickness is an independent determinant of metabolic syndrome and identifies subjects with increased carotid intimamedia thickness. Diabetes Care. 2006; 29(2):379-384.

[38] M. Chandalia, N. Abate, A. Garg, J. Stray-Gundersen, and S. M. Grundy, "Relationship between generalized and upper body obesity to insulin resistance in Asian Indian men," Journal of Clinical Endocrinology and Metabolism, vol. 84, no. 7, pp. 2329–2335, 1999.

[39] M. Prentice, "The emerging epidemic of obesity in developing countries," International Journal of Epidemiology, vol. 35, no. 1, pp. 93–99, 2006.

[40] Ma RCW, Ko GT, Chan JC. Health hazards of obesity—an overview. In: Williams G, Frubeck G, eds. Obesity: Science to Practice. Hoboken, NJ: John Wiley & Sons; 2009:215-236.

[41] Mak KH, Ma S, Heng D, et al. Impact of sex, metabolic syndrome, and diabetes mellitus on cardiovascular events. Am J Cardiol. 2007; 100(2):227-233.

[42] Misra, R. M. Pandey, J. R. Devi, R. Sharma, N. K. Vikram, and N. Khanna, "High prevalence of diabetes, obesity and dyslipidaemia in urban slum population in northern India," International Journal of Obesity, vol. 25, no. 11, pp. 1722–1729, 2001.

[43] Moon Han S, Kim WW, Oh JH. Result of laparoscopic sleeve gastrectomy (LSG) at 1 year in Korean morbid obese patients. Obes Surg. 2005 Nov-Dec;15(10):1469-75.

[44] Nakagami T, Qiao Q, Carstensen B, et al; The DECODE-DECODA Study Group. Age, body mass index and type 2 diabetes—associations modified by ethnicity. Diabetologia. 2003; 46(8):1063-1070.

[45] NIH conference. Gastrointestinal surgery for severe obesity. Consensus Development Conference Panel.

[46] Nocca D, Guillaume F, Noel P, Impact of laparoscopic sleeve gastrectomy and laparoscopic gastric bypass on HbA1c blood level and pharmacological treatment of type 2 diabetes mellitus in severe or morbidly obese patients. Results of a multicenter prospective study at 1 year. Obes Surg. ;21(6):738-43 2011

[47] P. L. Griffiths and M. E. Bentley, "The nutrition transition is underway in India," Journal of Nutrition, vol. 131, no. 10, pp. 2692–2700, 2001.

[48] Raji, E. W. Seely, R. A. Arky, and D. C. Simonson, "Body fat distribution and insulin resistance in healthy Asian Indians and Caucasians," Journal of Clinical Endocrinology and Metabolism, vol. 86, no. 11, pp. 5366–5371, 2001.

[49] Ramachandran A, Mary S, Yamuna A, Murugesan N, Snehalatha C. High prevalence of diabetes and cardiovascular risk factors associated with urbanization in India. Diabetes Care. 2008; 31(5):893-898.

[50] Ramachandran and C. Snehalatha, "Current scenario of diabetes in India," Journal of Diabetes, vol. 1, pp. 18–28, 2009.

[51] Ramachandran and C. Snehalatha, Rising burden of obesity in Asia. Journal of Obesity Vol. 2010 1-8 2010

[52] Ramachandran, C. Snehalatha, A. Kapur et al., "High prevalence of diabetes and impaired glucose tolerance in India: National Urban Diabetes Survey," Diabetologia, vol. 44, no. 9, pp. 1094–1101, 2001.
[53] Ramachandran, C. Snehalatha, A. Yamuna, N. Murugesan, and K. M. V. Narayan, "Insulin resistance and clustering of cardiometabolic risk factors in urban teenagers in Southern India," Diabetes Care, vol. 30, no. 7, pp. 1828–1833, 2007.
[54] Ramachandran, C. Snehalatha, and V. Vijay, "Temporal changes in prevalence of type 2 diabetes and impaired glucose tolerance in urban southern India," Diabetes Research and Clinical Practice, vol. 58, no. 1, pp. 55–60, 2002.
[55] Ramachandran, S. Mary, A. Yamuna, N. Murugesan, and C. Snehalatha, "High prevalence of diabetes and cardiovascular risk factors associated with urbanization in India," Diabetes Care, vol. 31, no. 5, pp. 893–898, 2008.
[56] RamachandranA. Epidemiology of diabetes in India—three decades of research. J Assoc Physicians India. 2005; 53:34-38.
[57] Report of WHO Consultation, "Obesity: preventing and managing the global epidemic," World Health Organization— Technical Report Series, no. 894, pp. 1-253, 2000.
[58] Reynolds K, Gu D, Whelton PK, et al; InterASIA Collaborative Group. Prevalence and risk factors of overweight and obesity in China. Obesity (Silver Spring). 2007; 15(1):10-18.
[59] Rubino F, Kaplan LM, Schauer PR et al. The Diabetes Surgery Summit consensus conference: recommendations for the evaluation and use of gastrointestinal surgery to treat type 2 diabetes mellitus. Ann Surg. 2010 Mar;251(3):399-405.
[60] S. Yajnik, H. G. Lubree, S. S. Rege et al., "Adiposity and hyperinsulinemia in Indians are present at birth," Journal of Clinical Endocrinology and Metabolism, vol. 87, no. 12, pp. 5575–5580, 2002.
[61] Snehalatha, V. Viswanathan, and A. Ramachandran, "Cut- off values for normal anthropometric variables in Asian Indian adults," Diabetes Care, vol. 26, no. 5, pp. 1380–1384, 2003.
[62] T. Gill, "Young people with diabetes and obesity in Asia: a growing epidemic," Diabetes Voice, vol. 52, pp. 20–22, 2007.
[63] Thomas GN, Schooling CM, McGhee SM, et al; Hong Kong Cardiovascular Risk Factor Prevalence Study Steering Committee. Metabolic syndrome in- creases all-cause and vascular mortality: the Hong Kong Cardiovascular Risk Factor Study. Clin Endocrinol (Oxf). 2007;66(5):666-671.
[64] Ti TK. Singapore experience in obesity surgery. Obes Surg 2004; 14: 1103-7.
[65] Veena SR, Geetha S, Leary SD, et al. Relation- ships of maternal and paternal birthweights to features of the metabolic syndrome in adult offspring: an inter-generational study in South India. Diabetologia. 2007;50(1):43-54.
[66] W. Aekplakorn, Y. Chaiyapong, B. Neal et al., "Prevalence and determinants of overweight and obesity in Thai adults: results of the Second National Health Examination Survey," Journal of the Medical Association of Thailand, vol. 87, no. 6, pp. 685–693, 2004.
[67] W. Zheng, D.F. McLerran, B. Rolland et al., Association between Body- Mass Index and Risk of Death in more than 1 million Asians. , The New England Journal of Medicine, 364: 8 719-729, 2011

[68] W.J.Lee and W. Wang, Bariatric surgery: Asia-Pacific perspective, Obes. Surg. 15, 751-757, 2005

[69] Wang C, Hou X, Bao Y, et al. The metabolic syndrome increased risk of cardiovascular events in Chinese—a community based study [published on- line ahead of print November 27, 2008]. Int J Cardiol. doi:10.1016/j.ijcard.2008.10.012.

[70] Wang W, Huang MT, Lee WJ, et al. Laparoscopic Roux-en-Y gastric bypass for morbid obesity. Formos J Surg 2003; 36: 104-11.

[71] WHO Expert Consultation. Appropriate body-mass index for Asian populations and its implications for policy and intervention strategies. Lancet 2004;363: 157-63.

[72] WildS, Roglic G, Green a, Sicree R, King H. Global prevalence of diabetes: estimates for the year 2000 and projections for 2030. Diabetes Care. 2004; 27(5):1047-1053.

[73] Wong KC, Wang Z. Prevalence of type 2 diabetes mellitus of Chinese populations in Mainland China, Hong Kong, and Taiwan. Diabetes Res Clin Pract. 2006; 73(2):126-134.

[74] World Health Organization, "Report of a joint WHO/FAO Expert. Consultation. Diet, nutrition and the prevention of chronic diseases," WHO technical report series No. 916, http://whqlibdoc.who.int/trs/who TRS 916.pdf.

[75] Y. Wu, "Overweight and obesity in China," British Medical Journal, vol. 333, no. 7564, pp. 362–363, 2006.

[76] Yokoyama H, Okudaira M, Otani T, et al. High incidence of diabetic nephropathy in early onset Japanese NIDDM patients: risk analysis. Diabetes Care. 1998;21(7):1080-1085.

[77] Yoon KH, Lee JH, Kim JW, et al. Epidemic obesity and type 2 diabetes in Asia. Lancet. 2006; 368(9548):1681-1688.

[78] Zhang X, Shu XO, Yang G, et al. Abdominal adiposity and mortality in Chinese women. Arch Intern Med. 2007;167(9):886-892.

15

Robotic-Assisted Bariatric Surgery

Ulises Garza, Angela Echeverria and Carlos Galvani
Section of Minimally Invasive & Robotic Surgery, Department of Surgery, College of Medicine, University of Arizona, Tucson, USA

1. Introduction

Obesity is a serious public health problem in the United States. The prevalence of obesity is growing every year, not only in adults but also in the pediatric population (Ogden et al., 2002). Obesity is now the second leading cause of death in the United States after tobacco-related disease, and 400,000 Americans died of obesity-related causes in 2000 (Mokdad et al., 2004). It is well known that obesity contributes to such comorbidities as noninsulin- dependent diabetes mellitus, hypertension, and hypertri-glyceridemia or hypercholesterolemia. Surgical treatment of morbid obesity is recognized as long-term effective therapy, and its goal is to limit or eliminate these comorbidities (Dixon & O'Brien, 2002; Giusti et al., 2004).

Robotically-assisted surgery's most notable contributions are reflected in its ability to extend the already well-established benefits of minimally invasive surgery to procedures not routinely performed using minimal access techniques (i.e., total esophagectomies, coronary artery bypass grafting, and radical prostatectomies). This technology may ultimately increase the number of physicians who are able to provide the benefits of minimal access surgery to their patients without the increased risks of complications associated with initial learning curves. We believe that the progress and development of robotic surgery will eventually provide all bariatric surgeons with the option of a minimally invasive approach. As more patients become aware of the clinical outcomes from minimally invasive surgical treatment for morbid obesity, they will actively seek a bariatric surgeon skilled in these techniques. The additional advantages afforded by the use of minimally invasive surgical techniques, coupled with the desire to retain the natural ergonomics and visual advantages of open surgery, have propelled the development and progression of robot-assisted surgery. Current robotics systems have already begun to return the "natural feel" of open access afforded by laparotomy to minimally invasive surgeons.

A survey of surgeons in 2003 revealed that only few surgeons in the United States were currently using a robotic surgical system for bariatric surgery (Jacobsen et al., 2003). This statistic can be explained by the small number of bariatric cases performed laparoscopically and by the limited number of institutions with a robotics system available for use. The first robot-assisted adjustable gastric banding was reported in 1999 (Cadiere et al., 1999), and Horgan and collaborators performed the first robot-assisted gastric bypass in September 2000 (Horgan et al., 2001). Since that time there have been numerous publications detailing the use of robotic assistance in bariatric surgery.

Herein, we examine the current use of robotics in bariatric surgery as well as its potential advantages and disadvantages.

1.1 The da Vinci robotic system

Using robots to perform surgery once seemed a futuristic fantasy. Nonetheless, since the FDA approval in the year 2000, robotic surgery and the use of the da Vinci Surgical System™ (DVSS Intuitive Surgical Corporation, Sunnyvale, Calif) has widely extended. The DVSS became the first robotic surgical system cleared by the FDA for general laparoscopic surgery. In the following years, the FDA cleared the da Vinci Surgical System™ for thoracoscopic surgery, for cardiac procedures, urologic, and gynecologic procedures.

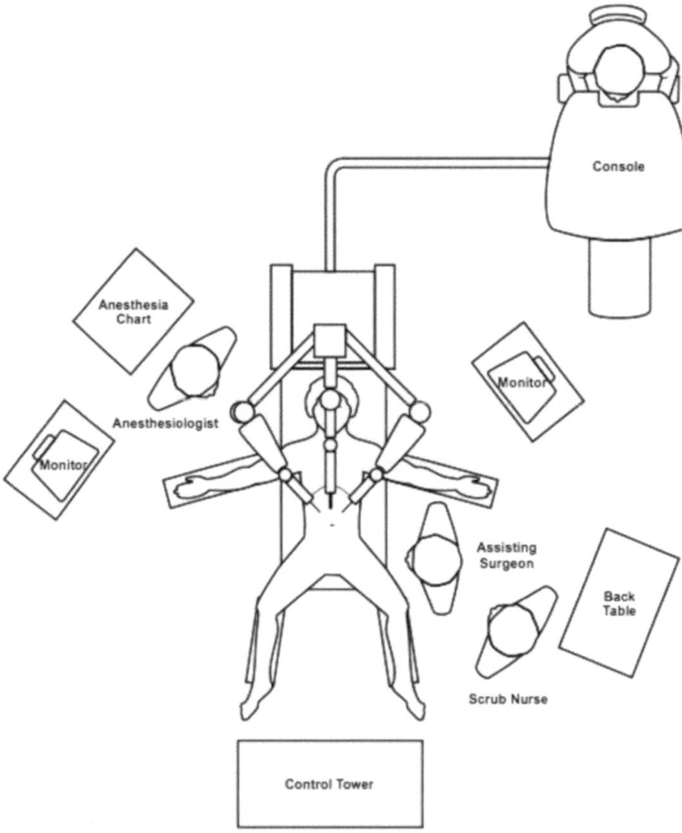

Fig. 1. Operating room setup for Robotic-Assisted Gastric Banding.

In the US, approximately 1,950 units are actually working, 347 in Europe, and 182 distributed throughout the rest of the world.

The equipment has three different components (1).

- **Surgeon Console**: At which the surgeon operates while comfortably seated, using four pedals, a set of console switches, and two master controls. The movements of the surgeon's fingers are transmitted by the master controls, to the tip of the instruments located inside the patient. A high-resolution three-dimensional view of the surgical field is obtained using a 12 mm scope, which contains two 5 mm three-chip video cameras that integrate images.

- **Control Tower:** monitor, light sources, and cord attachments for the cameras.
- **Patient side cart:** consisting of four robotic arms, one arm positions the laparoscope and the other three arms allow placement and manipulation of a variety of da Vinci-specific instruments.

The bariatric procedures performed vary from a simple laparoscopic adjustable gastric band up to the most complex biliopancreatic diversion/duodenal switch (BPD/DS).

2. Robotic gastric adjustable band placement

Laparoscopic adjustable gastric banding (LAGB) is one of the preferred methods for surgical treatment of morbid obesity (Muhlman et al., 2003). Excellent long-term results and postoperative improvement in quality of life have been reported (Cadiere et al., 2002; Dargent, 1999; Nehoda et al., 2001). The expanding use of the LAGB is probably driven by the encouraging data on its safety and effectiveness. LAGB is associated with a shorter learning curve and decreased perioperative complications compared to gastric bypass. For that reason, adoption of robotic technology for this procedure is scarce. Nevertheless, Cadiere et al., described the first robotic gastric band placement in 1999 (Cadiere et al., 1999). Later, several studies in the literature have reported the use of robotics for LAGB (Edelson et al., 2011; Moser & Horgan, 2004).

2.1 Surgical technique

The surgical technique was previously described Moser et al (Moser & Horgan, 2004). In brief, the patient is placed in the low lithotomy position with the legs and arms open. The surgeon operates between the patient's legs, with the assistant at the patient's left side (1).

Pneumoperitoneum can be achieved with the Veress needle technique or with the optiview assistance trocar up to 15 or 20 mm Hg. The first trocar used is a 10- to 12-mm trocar, which is inserted under direct vision or with an optiview trocar, 15 to 20 cm from the xyphoid process using a 10-mm, 0 or 30-degree scope, the rest of the trocars are introduced under direct vision. An 8-mm trocar (robotic arm) is placed immediately below the left rib cage in the mid clavicular line; also a 12-mm trocar is then placed on the left flank at the same level as the camera. Then, the patient is placed in the reverse Trendelenburg position, to allow a better visualization of the His Angle. A Nathanson liver retractor is inserted through a 5-mm incision placed below the xyphoid process. The last 8-mm trocar (robotic arm) is placed approximately 8 cm below the right rib cage. A Cadiere forceps or robotic grasper is used attached to the right arm and the harmonic scalpel to the left arm. The operation begins with detaching the phrenogastric ligament to expose the left crura. Then, the gastrohepatic ligament is opened to expose the caudate lobe of the liver, the inferior vena cava and the right crura. A retrogastric tunnel is created between the edge of the right crura and the posterior wall of the stomach until the articulated tip of the robotic instrument is visualized at the angle of His. The band is placed inside the abdomen, through the 12-mm trocar and the tip of the tubing is placed between the jaws of the Cadiere forceps, attached to the left arm, and the band is threaded around the stomach [2].

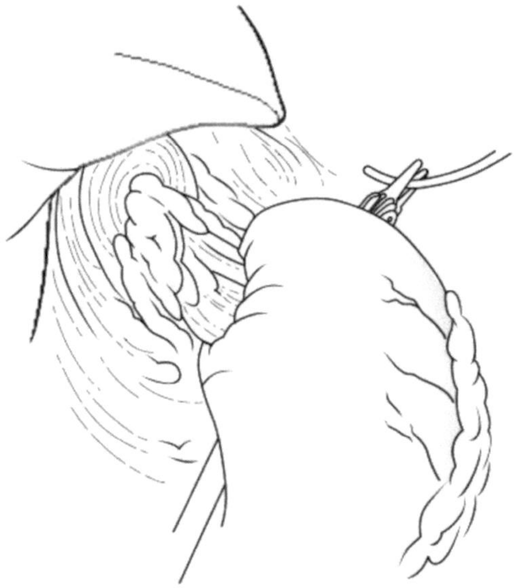

Fig. 2. The band is threaded around the stomach with Cadiere forceps.

The tip of the tubing is inserted into the band buckle and locked. After the band is in place, a wrap is fashioned out of the stomach to secure it using several nonabsorbable seromuscular sutures [3]. Finally, the port is then secured with nonabsorbable sutures or using built-in hooks.

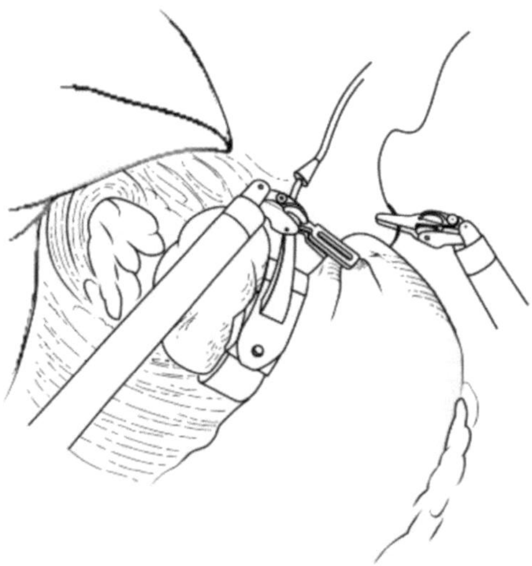

Fig. 3. A wrap is fashioned out of the stomach to secure the band in place.

3. Robotic-assisted Roux-en-Y gastric bypass

During the past 40 to 50 years, Roux-en-Y gastric bypass (RYGB) has been the preferred surgical procedure performed by bariatric surgeons in the United States. However, due to its complexity, this operation has always been challenged by alternative surgical procedures. Although gastric bypass has been shown to be safe and effective in maintaining long-lasting weight loss, it is associated with a steep learning curve and is not free from complications (Podnos et al., 2003; Schauer et al., 2003).

Robotic surgery is potentially ideal for the Roux-en-Y gastric bypass (RYGB), for a variety of reasons including: the shorter learning curve to perform advanced maneuvers such as suturing, precise dissection, and the ability to be used in patients with a high BMI (Kim & Buffington, 2011). For these reasons, currently gastric bypass is the fastest growing robotic-assisted bariatric procedure with a 50% growth in 2009.

3.1 Surgical technique

3.1.1 Robotic-assisted gastric bypass (Hybrid approach)

The patient is placed in the low lithotomy position with the legs and arms open; a beanbag is placed under the patient to support the steep reverse Trendelenburg position during the operation. Initially, the pneumoperitoneum is achieved by inserting a 12-mm trocar placed in the supraumbilical position using the Optiview system. Additional 12-mm trocars are placed in the left lower quadrant, right upper quadrant and left mid abdomen. Later, a 5-mm incision will be made below the xyphoid process to introduce a Nathanson liver retractor. Final configuration is shown in Figure 4.

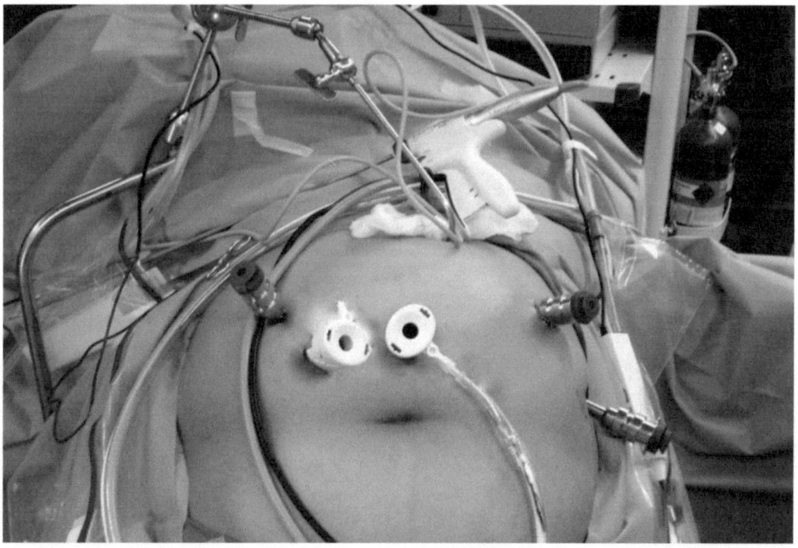

Fig. 4. Ports placement for Robotic-Assisted Gastric Bypass.

The next step consists in identifying the ligament of Treitz (LT) to run the small bowel distally 50 cm and dividing it using a vascular stapler; the mesentery of the bowel is divided using a vascular stapler or the harmonic scalpel. After creating a 100-cm jejunal limb (some authors used 150 cm [Moser & Horgan 2004]), a side-to-side jejunojejunal anastomosis is performed using a vascular stapler. The bowel opening can be closed using a needle holder with interrupted stitches of 3-0 silk or stapler. The defect between the mesentery is closed using a 2-0 Ethibond suture. The patient is then placed in a reverse Trendelenburg position (5).

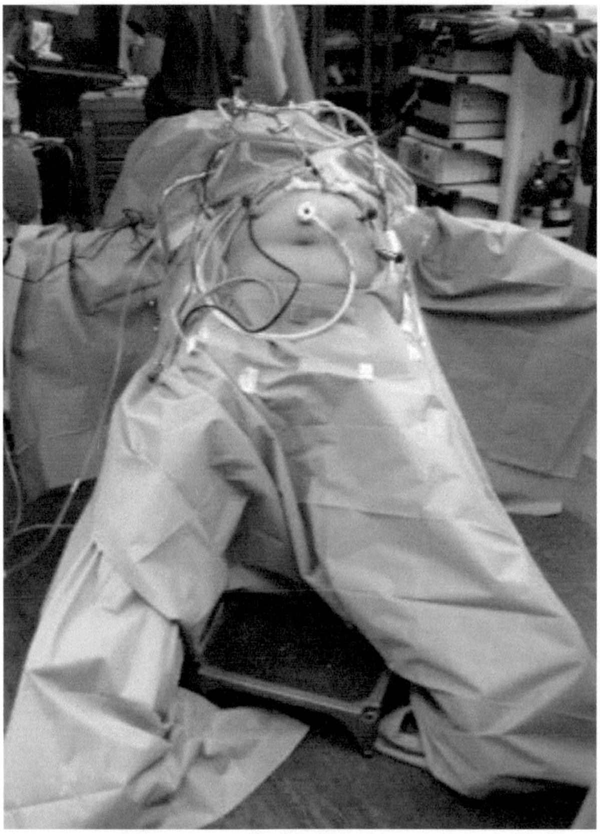

Fig. 5. Patient placed in reverse trendelenburg for Robotic-Assisted Gastric Bypass.

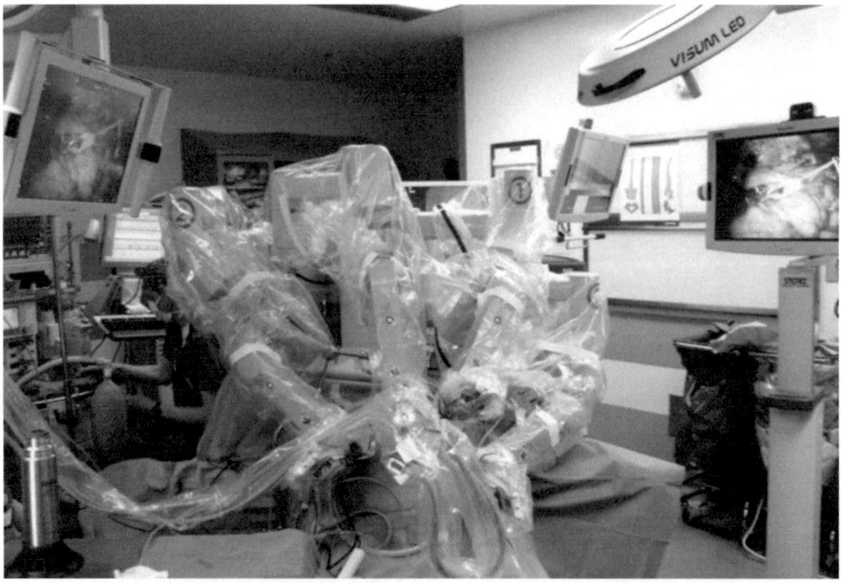

Fig. 6. da Vinci Surgical System™ positioned over the head of the patient.

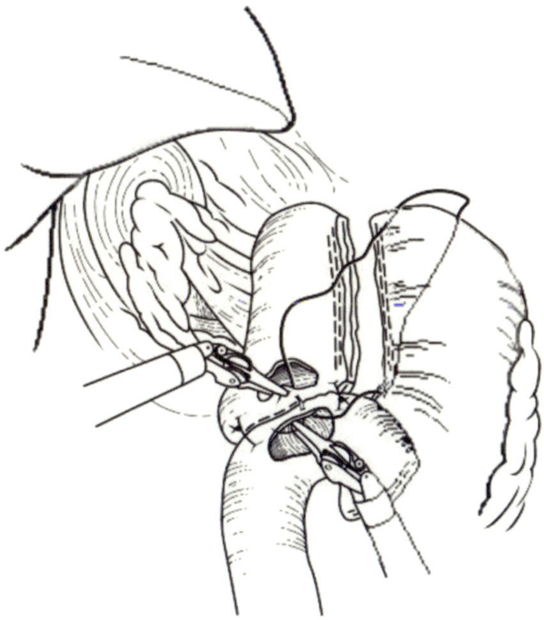

Fig. 7. Creation of the gastrojejunostomy.

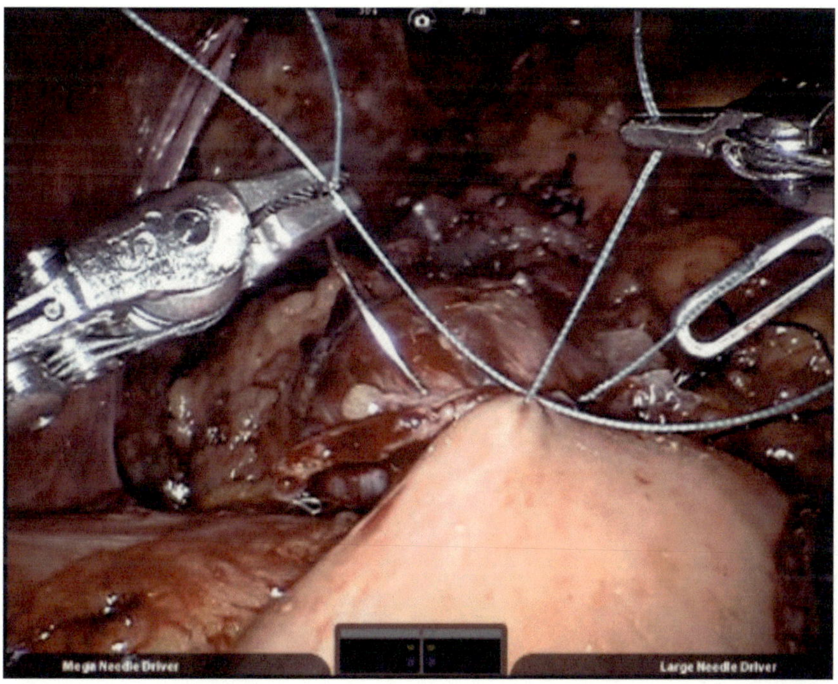

Fig. 8. Gastrojejunal anastomosis posterior running suture created.

As previously described, a 5-mm incision is made in the subxiphoid area to insert the Nathanson retractor for the anterior mobilization of the left liver lobe. The omentum is mobilized and sectioned using the harmonic scalpel. The retrogastric tunnel is created using the harmonic scalpel starting at the lesser curve approximately 5 cm from the gastroesophageal junction. Two or three fires (one perpendicular and one/two parallels) to the lesser curvature of the stomach are used to create the gastric pouch. The Roux limb is brought up antecolic for creation of the gastrojejunostomy. Horgan et al. (Horgan & Vanuno, 2001) first described the technique for the creation of the gastrojejunostomy in 2001.

The surgical arm cart of the da Vinci Surgical System™ (Intuitive Surgical, Inc., Sunnyvale, CA) is positioned over the head of the patient with the arms going through right upper quadrant and left upper quadrant ports (6).

The da Vinci ports are introduced into the 12-mm trocars. A Cadiere forceps is attached to the right arm and a needle holder to the left arm. The gastrojejunal (GJ) anastomosis (7, 8) is performed hand sewn in two layers using running 3-0 Ethibond for the posterior layer and 3-0 Vycril of the anterior layer [1].

Then, using a harmonic scalpel, a 1.5-cm opening is created in both the jejunum and the stomach (9, 10).

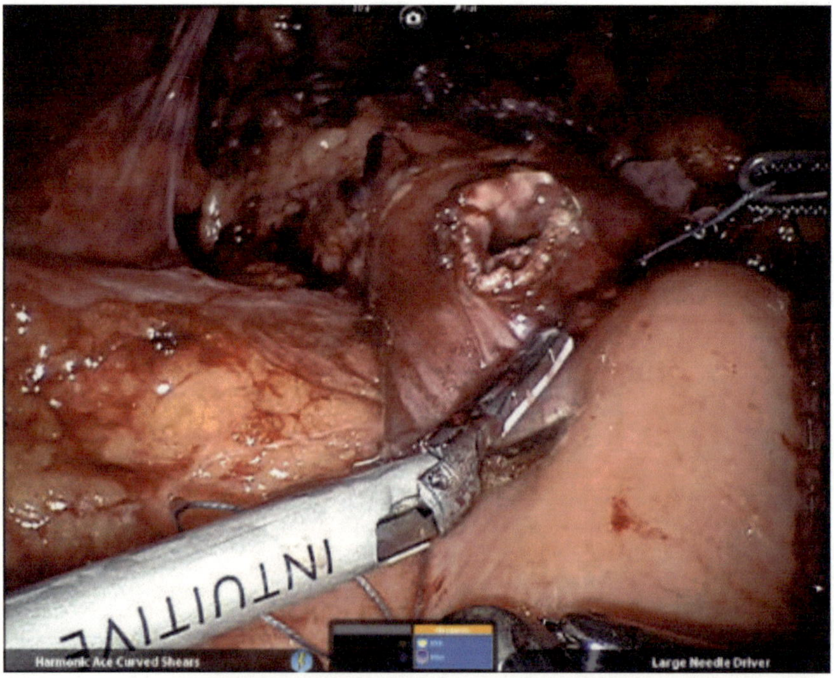

Fig 9. An opening is created in the jejunum limb with the harmonic scalpel.

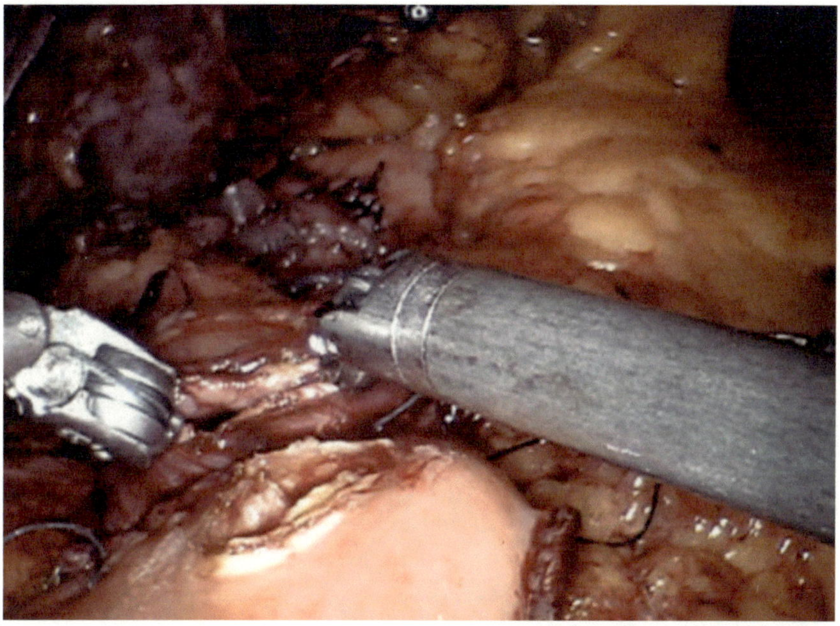

Fig. 10. An opening is created in both the jejunum and the stomach.

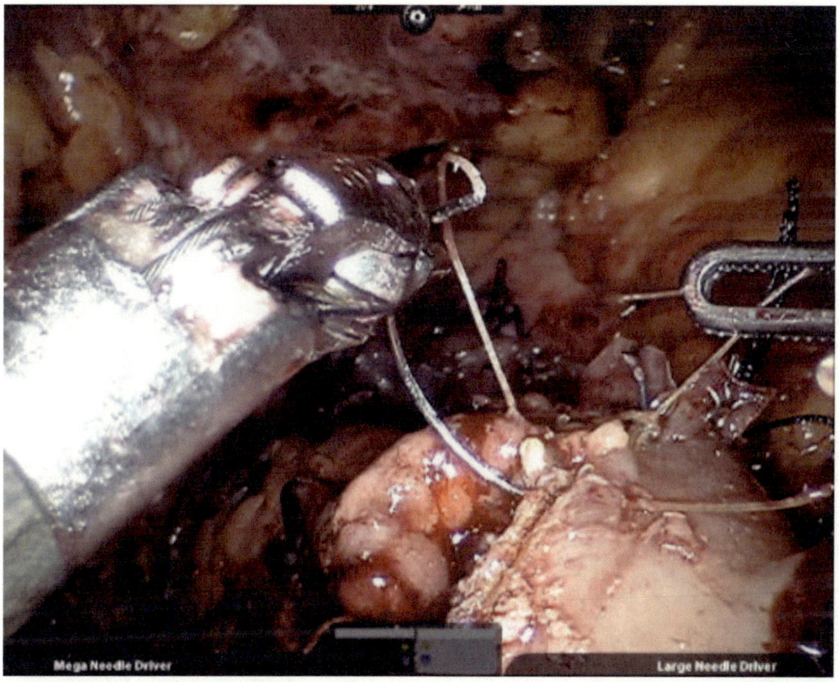

Fig. 11. Creation of the anterior layer of the GJ anastomosis using 3-0 Vycril on a running fashion.

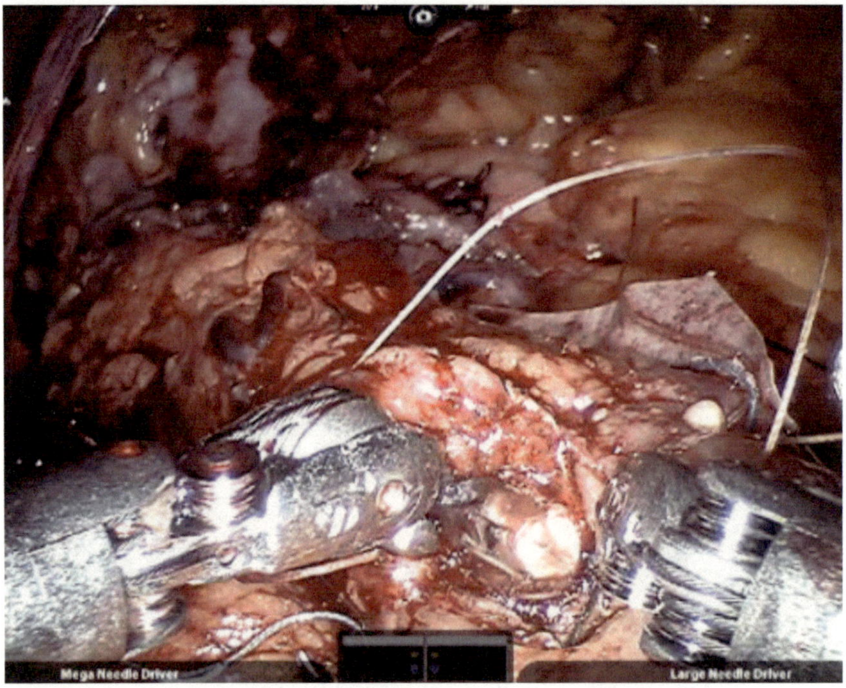

Fig. 12. An NGT is passed down to the gastric pouch and into the jejunum limb to maintain patency of the anastomosis.

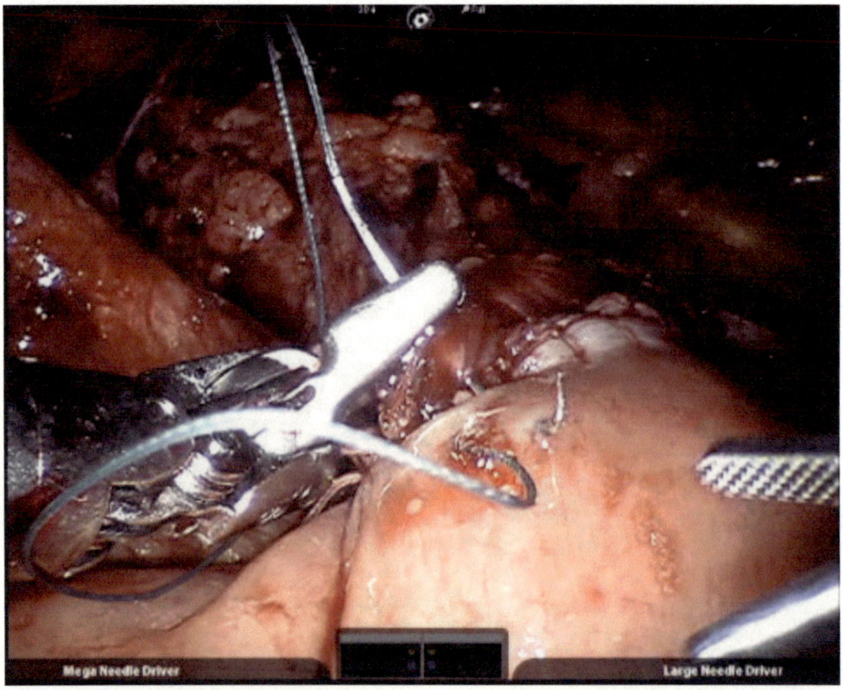

Fig. 13. Posterior layer of the GJ anastomosis using 3-0 Ethibond running suture.

Once gastrotomy and enterotomy are created the anterior layer of the anastomosis is started using 3-0 Vycril on a running fashion (11). A nasogastric tube (NGT) is passed down the gastric pouch and into the Roux limb to maintain the patency of the anastomosis (12). The posterior layer is then completed with running 3-0 Ethibon (13). Once the anastomosis is finished, using the NGT, the jejunum is clamped distally, and 60 mL of methylene blue is introduced to rule out the presence of leak. Peterson space is closed in a running fashion with non-reabsorbable suture.

3.1.2 Totally robotic gastric bypass

The orientation of the left and right robot arms reflects the console surgeon's and assistant's left and right (14).

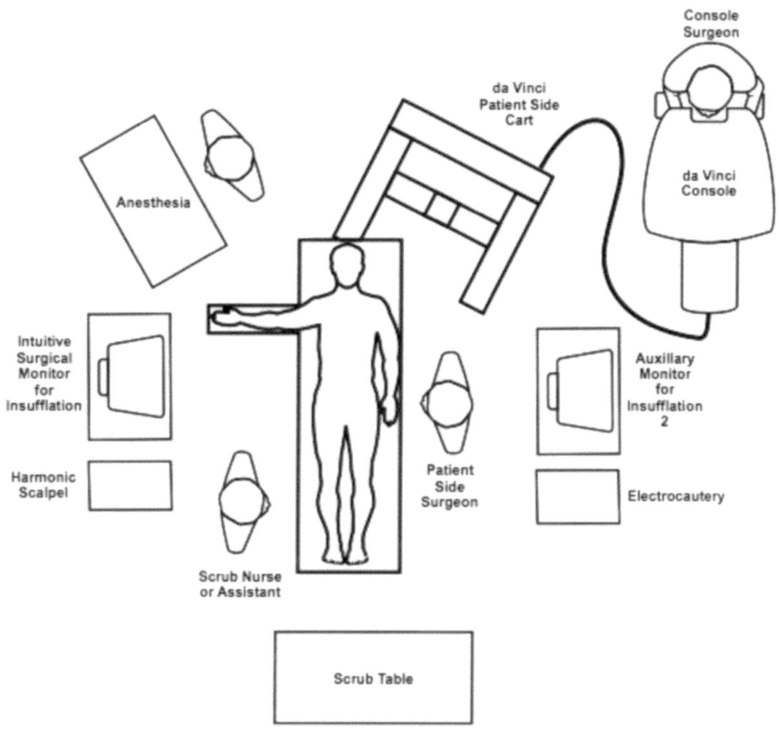

Fig. 14. Operating room setup. Totally robotic gastric bypass.

Mohr et al. (Mohr et al., 2005) describes the technique with six ports using a double cannulation of the Intuitive Surgical cannulas of 8 mm, which fitted inside a 10/12 mm port, this allows the robot arm to be removed from the port with the cannula still attached for a stapling tool and also, for the quick replacement of the robotic arm. Laparoscopy is started first placing the camera port using an Optiview nonbladed trocar and a 0° scope. Pneumoperitoneum is achieved. A total of 5 ports [a left subcostal port, two right trocars (one at the subcostal margin and one at the right flank), two trocars for the assistant (one at the left flank and one to the right of the supraumbilical midline)] are placed under direct visualization (15). The transverse mesocolon is retracted superiorly with a laparoscopic grasper allowing visualization of the ligament of Treitz.

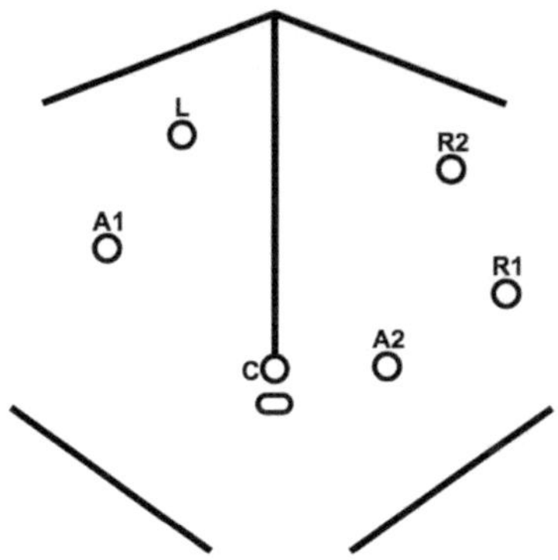

Fig. 15. Operative port placement. A, Port positions in a patient. B, Diagram of port placement. L indicates left; C,camera; A1, assistant1; A2, assistant2; R1, right 1; R2, right 2.

The robot is then docked in and it is positioned at the patient's left shoulder at a steep angle (15° - 30° off patient midline) and as close to the table as the base permits (16).

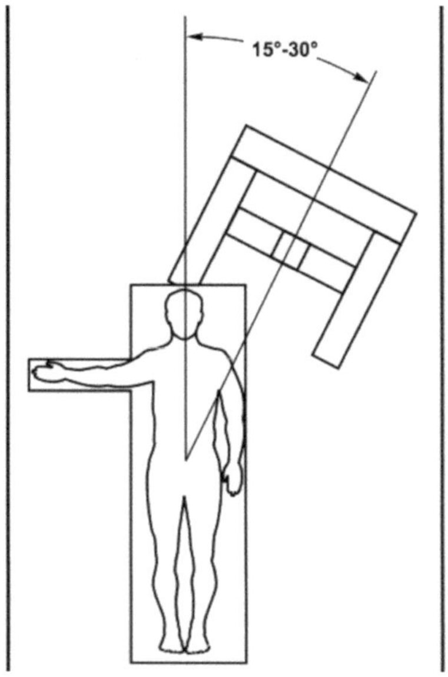

Fig. 16. Base position with respect to the operating room table.

The left arm is positioned such that the external yaw axis is as close to vertical as possible. The right arm should be brought in relatively low, and the setup joints tucked close to the base so that the tool holder is in the middle of its range of motion in the pitch axis (17).

The jejunojejunostomy is made first, but some authors prefer to make the gastric pouch first (Kim & Buffington, 2011). The surgeon manipulates the bowel with Cadiere graspers or bowel graspers at the robotic console, aided by the surgeon's assistant who also transects the bowel 20 to 40 cm from the LT using a white stapler through the left flank assistant's port (15). The jejunal mesentery is further divided by the surgeon's assistant using a LigaSure Atlas, da Vinci ultrasonic shears or stapler (Galvani et al., 2006; Horgan & Vanuno, 2001; Moser & Horgan, 2004).

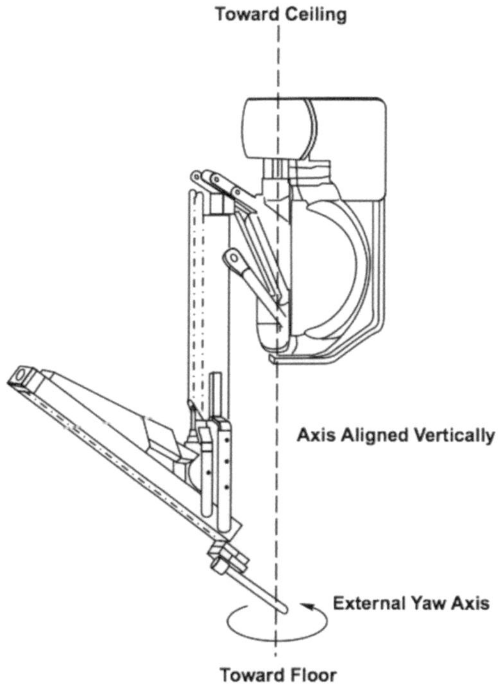

Fig. 17. The external yaw axis.

The assistant and the console surgeon then measure 100 to 150 cm of bowel for the Roux limb and align the Roux and biliopancreatic limbs joined by a 7-inch 3-0 Ethibond stay stitch placed by the console surgeon, aligning the bowel for the jejunojejunostomy using a needle driver and Debakey forceps and also creates the enterotomies with the Endowrist Permanent Hook below the stay stitch.

The stay stitch is used to provide counter traction for the assistant to complete the internal portion of the jejunojejunostomy with the linear stapler. The console surgeon closes the enterotomy with a running 3-0 Ethibond single-layer suture. The mesenteric defect is then closed with interrupted or running non-absorbable sutures. The surgeon's assistant with a Ligasure Atlas divides the omentum and the Roux limb is brought up antecolic. The next step is to work at the gastroesophageal (GE) area that involves removing the right robot arm from the right flank double cannulated port, inserting the Intuitive Surgical port at the right subcostal port position (15), and redocking the arm.

The liver is retracted using a 5-mm liver retractor through the assistant's right supraumbilcal port and held in place with a laparoscopic instrument holder. The console surgeon is then ready to work at the GE junction after repositioning the surgical instruments and camera visualizing the angle of His which is dissected with the electrocautery hook.

When completed, dissection of the gastric pouch begins. Dissection initiates 5 cm along the lesser curve and with the electrocautery hook into the retrogastric space. The assistant removes the left robotic arm from the double cannulated left subcostal margin port, introduces the stapler, and creates the lower border of the gastric pouch with a blue cartridge (3.5 mm).

The left robot arm is replaced, and the console surgeon provides traction for the surgeon's assistant to staple the lateral border of the pouch, which is sized using a transoral 36F tube, aided by an esophageal retractor.

The console surgeon then creates the enterotomies and a 2-layer sutured anastomosis. The outer and inner layers are sutured with running 7-in and 6-in 3-0 Ethibond sutures, respectively, with the 36F tube used to stent the anastomosis open while completing the anastomosis. A leak test is then performed insufflating it underwater; or using the methylene blue leak test (Galvani et al., 2006; Kim & Buffington, 2011; Moser & Horgan, 2004). The robot and all ports are removed and the skin incisions closed.

4. Robotic sleeve gastrectomy

The laparoscopic sleeve gastrectomy was initially reported by Ren et al. (Ren et al., 2000) in 2000 as part of the duodenal switch for super-super morbidly obese patients and later described by Regan (Regan et al., 2003) as a staged operation for morbid obesity in 2003. The rationale for sleeve gastrectomy was initially to lower the morbidity of this complex surgical procedure by offering a less challenging operation, decreasing operative time, and allowing patients to lose weight before proceeding with the second stage. Because of the excellent results in these patients, several studies (Lee et al., 2007) have supported the use of the sleeve gastrectomy as a primary bariatric operation. The main advantages of this operation are that it is not as technically challenging as gastric bypass or biliopancreatic diversion-duodenal switch (BPD-DS), thereby decreasing operative times and morbidity. As a result, robotic technology for sleeve gastrectomy has not been widely adopted amongst bariatric surgeons. The use of the robot for this procedure is still debated. However, few series have been reported in the literature (Ayloo et al., 2011; Diamantis et al., 2011).

4.1 Surgical technique

The surgical technique is described by Diamantis et al. in their first clinical experience series (Ayloo et al., 2011; Diamantis et al., 2011), which is similar to a Standard Laparoscopic Sleeve Gastrectomy (LSG). The first step is achieving pneumoperitoneum. Then, a 12-mm port 8 cm above the umbilicus for the camera, a right 12-mm trocar is positioned at the epigastrium, 5 cm towards the left of the midline, and a left 12-mm trocar placed at least 8 cm far away from the camera port, in order to avoid collision of the robotic arms that would hamper the advancement of the procedure. A double cannulation technique is used inserting the 8-mm metallic robotic ports through the standard 12-mm trocars. Two further 12-mm trocars are inserted, one at the right anterior axillary line, 2 cm below the subcostal arch for liver retraction and one at the symmetrical site on the left side to retract the gastrosplenic ligament (18).

All the trocars and robotic cannulas are inserted under the guidance of the standard laparoscopic camera and the robotic system approached the patient and is installed ("docked") afterwards. The robotic camera is docked last, and the robotic cart is positioned over the patient's left shoulder.

Only three arms of the da Vinci S Surgical System™ are used (camera and two working arms). Once the general setup is ready, the procedure begin with the console surgeon grasping with a Cadiere forceps, the greater curvature of the stomach at its lowest part and the gastrocolic ligament is cut with the da Vinci harmonic scalpel. The division of the gastrocolic and gastrosplenic ligament continues exactly like in a standard LSG. Once the angle of His is clearly visible and mobilized from the left crus, division of the gastrocolic ligament ends 4-6 cm proximally from the pylorus. At this point instead of a bougie preferred by some surgeons, an intra-operative endoscopy can be used for the calibration of the gastric sleeve. Once the endoscope lies across the lesser gastric curvature will taylor the gastrectomy. The console surgeon holds and abducts the mobilized greater gastric curvature with a Cadiere forceps through the right working trocar and the left robotic arm is undocked. The table surgeon inserts the stapler, loaded with a green cartridge, through the working port at the right site of the patient and divides the stomach in a direction from the lowest tip of the greater gastric curvature, 4 cm proximally to the pylorus, towards the lateral edge of the endoscope.

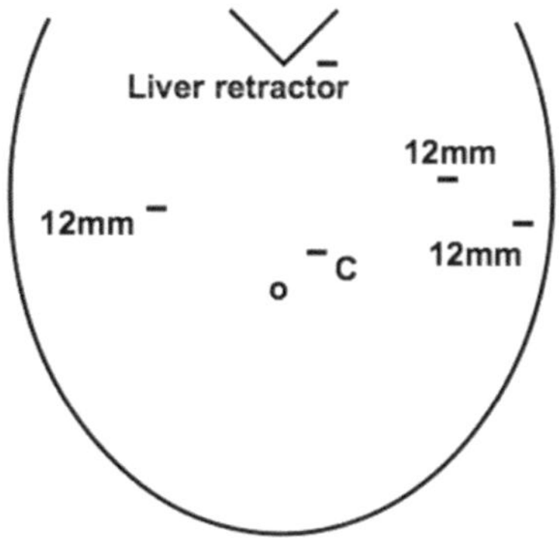

Fig. 18. Port Placement. C = camera.

All staple lines are regularly reinforced with prosthetic material (GORE SEAMGUARD bioabsorbable staple line reinforcement, W. L. GORE and Associates Inc.). The left robotic arm is docked once again after the first two fires. The stapling continues in a cephalad direction with the traction of the gastric sleeve using the Cadiere forceps, while the right arm is undocked for the insertion of the stapler, and division of the stomach; also the laparoscopic could be used to mobilize the greater gastric curvature. The stomach is divided till the angle of His, then the endoscope is smoothly withdrawn. Ayloo et al. (Ayloo, et al., 2011) also describes the assistance of the robot to invert the stapling line by placing sero-serosal sutures of 2-0 PDS (Ethicon) beginning at the angle of His. The staple line is then inspected from inside bleeding and air leak. A leak test is also performed filled with diluted Povidone 10% solution or methylene blue by some other authors (Galvani et al., 2006; Moser & Horgan, 2004). Finally, the transected, redundant part of the stomach is removed through the left lateral port site mainly through a fascial digital dilation.

5. Robotic-assisted biliopancreatic diversion and duodenal switch

The duodenal switch (DS) operation for bariatric surgery was initially described by Hess as a modification of the Scopinaro biliary pancreatic diversion (BPD). Today, it is accepted as the most effective weight reduction procedure (Anthone et al., 2003). In spite of this, the operation represents only about 0.89% of the bariatric procedures performed in the US (DeMaria et al., 2010). This is probably due to the technical challenges that surgeons are faced with BPD-DS. Consequently, the vast majority of procedures are done primarily open. However, the introduction of laparoscopy has decreased its morbidity (Kim et al., 2003). The addition of robotics could potentially increase the number of minimally invasive BPD-DS procedures performed. Conversely, there are only two reports in the literature describing the use of robotic technology for BPD-DS (Sudan et al., 2007).

5.1 Surgical technique

Sudan et al. (Sudan et al., 2007) describes the surgical technique placing the patient in a supine position. After achieving pneumoperitoneum, a 12-mm port with a 0° camera is used to enter the abdominal cavity. Four additional 12-mm ports are placed, and the Nathanson liver retractor is placed intraoperatively through an epigastric 5-mm incision (19).

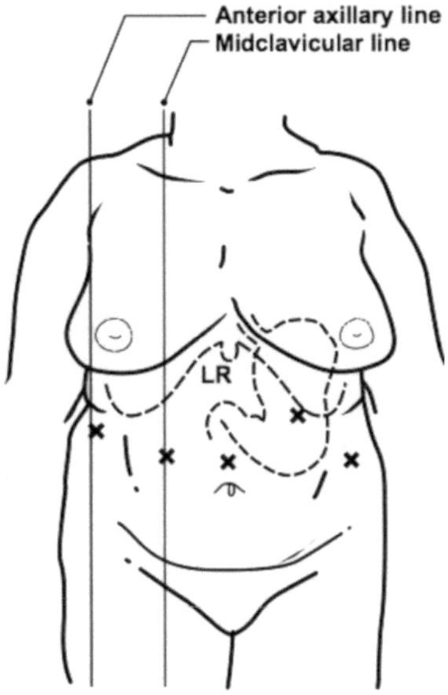

Fig. 19. Port sites. The midclavicular line ports are used for robotic arms. LR, site for Nathanson liver retractor placement.

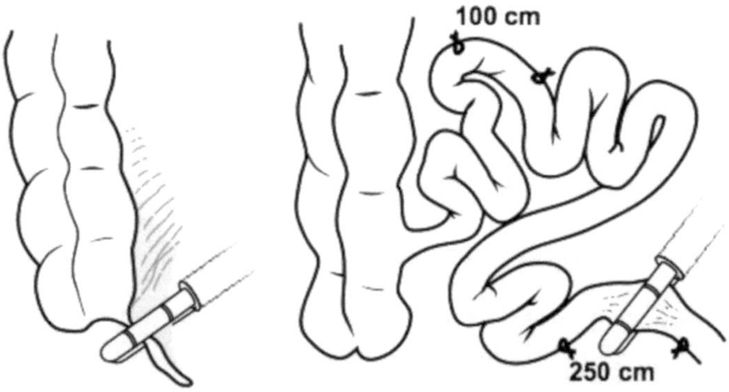

Fig. 20. Appendectomy followed by placement of marking stitches at points 100 and 250 cm proximal to the ileocecal valve. Bowel is transected 250 cm proximal to the ileocecal valve.

Midclavicular ports are used for the da Vinci arms when the duodeno-ileal (proximal alimentary limb) anastomosis is performed. Standard laparoscopic procedure is made first by positioning the patient in the Trendelenberg position and tilted to the left and an appendectomy is performed, as practiced by open BPD/DS surgeons. Marking sutures are placed 100 and 250 cm from the ileocecal junction, and the bowel is divided at the 250-cm mark using an endolinear cutter stapler (20).

The mesentery of the alimentary limb of small bowel is divided using the Harmonic Scalpel for a tension-free anastomosis to the duodenum. The biliary limb then is anastomosed to the common channel at the 100-cm mark using two applications of the 45-mm vascular endolinear cutter staplers (21).

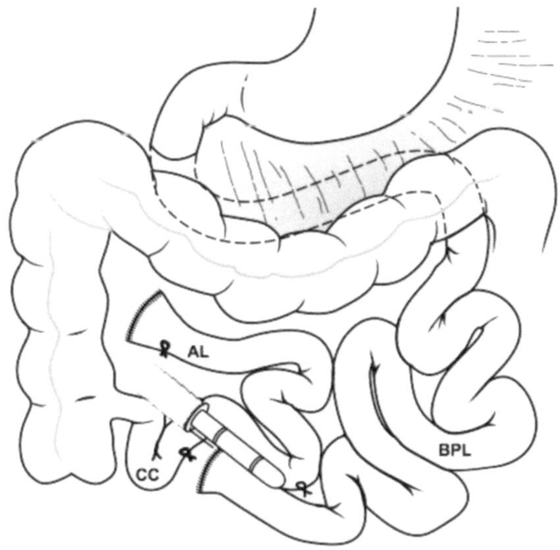

Fig. 21. The distal enteroenteric anastomosis is performed using a 45-mm vascular load endoscopic stapler. The 100-cm-long common channel (CC) is shown. AL, eventual alimentary limb; BPL, eventual biliopancreatic limb.

The enterotomy for the staplers is closed transversely using hand sewn intracorporeal suturing. The mesenteric defect between the biliary limb and the common channel is closed with running nonabsorbable suture, and the distal anastomosis is marked with three large radio-opaque hemoclips for future identification purposes. After performance of a cholecystectomy, the greater curvature of the stomach is mobilized using the Harmonic Scalpel, beginning 4 cm distal to the pylorus and working proximally to the angle of His. The duodenum is divided using the endolinear cutter stapler, and a sleeve gastrectomy is performed to reduce the capacity of the stomach to 150 ml (22). Methylene blue is used to ensure absence of leaks in the gastric staple line. The stapled edge of the alimentary limb is next positioned in a retrocolic fashion, and the da Vinci system is docked by bringing it over the patient´s right shoulder.

After setting up the robot, a two-layer sutured anastomosis is then created using 2-0 Surgilon and 2-0 Vicryl in a running fashion (23).

The mesenteric defect between the alimentary limb and the retroperitoneum and transverse mesocolon is closed. The duodenoileal anastomosis then is checked with methylene blue to exclude a leak. All the specimens that had been resected (i.e., gallbladder, resected stomach, appendix) are placed in endobags and retrieved through the umbilical port site. After removal of the ports, the incisions are closed with skin staples. Final configuration is shown in Figure 24.

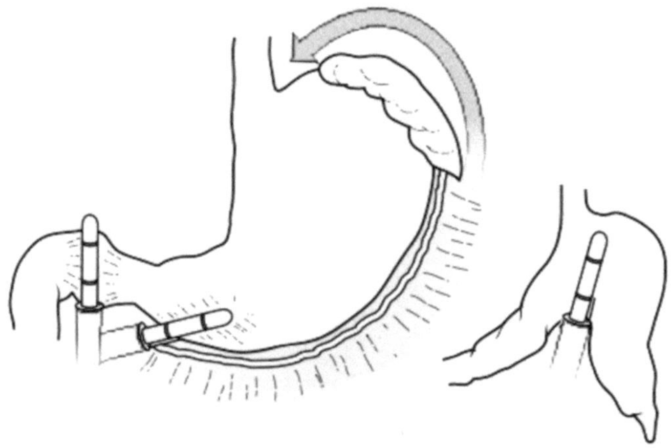

Fig. 22. Mobilization of the proximal 4 cm of the duodenum and the greater curvature of stomach is followed by transection of the duodenum and resection of the greater curvature of the stomach to result in a gastric remnant with a capacity of 150 ml.

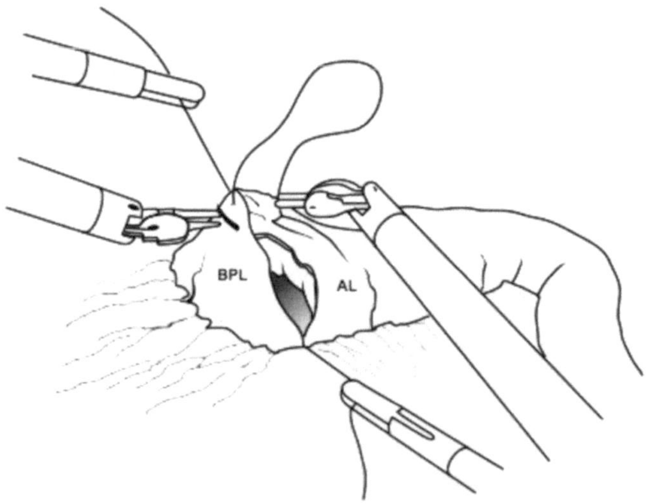

Fig. 23. A two-layered anastomosis is performed between the duodenum (Duo) and the alimentary limb (AL), which is brought up in retrocolic fashion. The robotic arms are used for suturing. The laparoscopic instruments handled by the bedside surgeon provide exposure and traction with stay sutures.

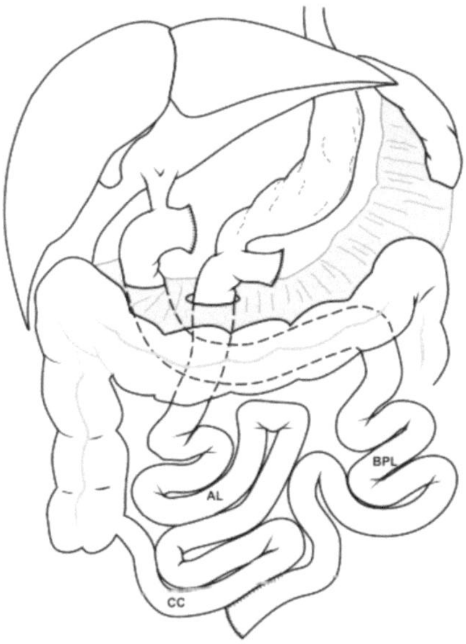

Fig. 24. The final configuration results in a 100-cm-long common channel (CC). The alimentary limb (AL) and the biliopancreatic limb (BPL) are demonstrated. The length of the AL is 250 cm.

6. Discussion

6.1 Laparoscopic adjustable gastric band vs. robotic adjustable gastric band (RAGB)

There are two series that compared LAGB vs. RAGB in the literature. Both of them demonstrated no advantages in using robotic surgery in terms of hospital stay, complications and postoperative weight loss (Edelson et al., 2011; Moser & Horgan, 2004). However, both series noticed benefits in the super obese patients such as those BMI $\geq$ 50 kg/m^2. In this particular group of patients the thickness of the abdominal wall increases the torque of standard bariatric instruments. The authors attributed these findings to the characteristics of the robotic system such as longer and stiffer instrumentation, and mechanical power (Edelson et al., 2011; Jacobsen et al., 2003). Specifically, operative time in these patients is reported to be shorter than the LAGB counterparts (Edelson et al., 2011). In addition, gastric banding seems to be an acceptable training platform for the novice robotic surgeon. The increased procedural cost is another mayor disadvantage for the widespread implementation of robotics (Gill et al., 2011).

6.2 Laparoscopic gastric bypass vs. robotic assisted gastric bypass (RYGB) and totally robotic gastric bypass (TRYGB)

Robotic RYGB is increasingly accepted as a safe alternative to laparoscopic RYGB (Gill et al., 2011; Jacobsen et al., 2003; Moser & Horgan 2004). Evidence shows that both offer the same long-term postoperative benefits like excess weight loss and resolution of comorbidities (Snyder et al., 2008). Several authors have described a decreased gastrojejunostomy leak rate while using the robotic system (Galvani et al, 2006; Gill et al., 2011; Moser & Horgan, 2004; Snyder et al., 2008; Wilson et al., 2008). Therefore, lowering the overall complications rate of the procedure and potentially decreasing costs (Snyder et al, 2008). An additional advantage is the shortening of the learning curve, since it has been suggested that the learning curve for laparoscopic RYGB is about a 100 cases (Schauer et al., 2003). Our experience suggested that the learning curve for achieving optimal outcomes and low complication rate plateau after the first 20 cases, indicating a shorter learning curve than conventional laparoscopy. These advantages of the robotic RYGB include the limited possibility to access different areas of the abdomen after the system is docked (Jacobsen et al., 2003; Moser & Horgan, 2004; Snyder et al., 2008). For that reason, surgeons have opted to go either the hybrid or the totally robotic approach. It is worth mentioning, that in the so-called "Totally robotic gastric bypass" a qualified bedside assistant is necessary to perform stapling of the stomach and small bowel. Making obvious also the need of further instrumentation. For these reasons, in spite of a shorter learning curve, the totally robotic gastric bypass is not widely accepted.

6.3 Laparoscopic sleeve gastrectomy (LSG) vs. robotic sleeve gastrectomy (RSG)

The reported experience in RSG is scarce (Ayloo et al., 2011; Diamantis et al., 2011). Available evidence demonstrates that the procedure is safe and feasible. No clinical advantages have been shown when using RSG in terms of hospitalization, morbidity, mortality and 1-year weight loss. The use of the robot can be of benefit in the super obese with the mechanical force needed to overcome the torque of a thick abdominal wall. Obviously the precision of the system is a key advantage for surgeons that routinely oversaw the staple line. Additionally, it is also helpful as a training model for fellows and residents.

An important point to keep in mind at the time of making the decision to perform a RSG is to consider the added cost of the procedure. The routine use of the Robot for Sleeve Gastrectomy has yet to be defined.

6.4 Robotic assisted biliopancreatic diversion and duodenal switch (RABPD)

The operation represents only about 0.89% of the bariatric procedures performed in the US (DeMaria et al., 2010). Since most of the BPD/DS are done open, the introduction of the robotics could potentially increase the number of minimally invasive cases performed. Conversely, the experience with RABPD is very limited. Today, there are only two studies in the literature about the use of the RABPD (Sudan et al., 2007; Wilson et al., 2008). The authors described that the main advantages include accurate suturing, better control over the size of the anastomosis, elimination of the potential for oropharyngeal and esophageal trauma while inserting the anvil of the circular stapler. The impossibility to work in different areas of the abdomen after setup it is also a disadvantage. The precision of the robot has shown low complication rates.

7. Conclusion

The advantages of the robotic surgery are more obvious in more technically demanding procedures that require the creation of gastrointestinal anastomosis. The mechanical power offered by the robotic system makes this approach the attractive alternative for super obese patients.

The learning curve of the robotic system is shorter than for the standard laparoscopic approach, allowing more surgeons to offer patients the same safety and successful outcomes currently available through open surgical techniques but without the significant morbidities of large surgical wounds.

The limitation of the robotic system still remains the high operational and acquisitional cost of the system. Moreover, for certain bariatric procedures like RAGB, RSG, and the RABPD its benefits have yet to be defined.

The development of new robotic instruments, minimization of the robotic systems and cost reduction will potentially encourage bariatric surgeons to adopt this technology.

8. References

Anthone, G.J., et al., *The duodenal switch operation for the treatment of morbid obesity.* Ann Surg, 2003. 238(4): p. 618-27; discussion 627-8.

Ayloo, S., et al., *Robot-assisted sleeve gastrectomy for super-morbidly obese patients.* J Laparoendosc Adv Surg Tech A, 2011. 21(4): p. 295-9.

Cadiere, G.B., et al., *The world's first obesity surgery performed by a surgeon at a distance.* Obes Surg, 1999. 9(2): p. 206-9.

Cadiere, G.B., et al., *Laparoscopic adjustable gastric banding.* Semin Laparosc Surg, 2002. 9(2): p. 105-14.

Dargent, J., *Laparoscopic adjustable gastric banding: lessons from the first 500 patients in a single institution.* Obes Surg, 1999. 9(5): p. 446-52.

DeMaria, E.J., et al., *Baseline data from American Society for Metabolic and Bariatric Surgery-designated Bariatric Surgery Centers of Excellence using the Bariatric Outcomes Longitudinal Database.* Surg Obes Relat Dis, 2010. 6(4): p. 347-55.

Diamantis, T., et al., *Initial experience with robotic sleeve gastrectomy for morbid obesity.* Obes Surg, 2011. 21(8): p. 1172-9.

Dixon, J.B. and P.E. O'Brien, *Changes in comorbidities and improvements in quality of life after LAP-BAND placement.* Am J Surg, 2002. 184(6B): p. 51S-54S.

Edelson, P.K., et al., *Robotic vs. conventional laparoscopic gastric banding: a comparison of 407 cases.* Surg Endosc, 2011. 25(5): p. 1402-8.

Galvani, C. and S. Horgan, *[Robots in general surgery: present and future].* Cir Esp, 2005. 78(3): p. 138-47.

Galvani, C., et al., *Laparoscopic adjustable gastric band versus laparoscopic Roux-en-Y gastric bypass: ends justify the means?* Surg Endosc, 2006. 20(6): p. 934-41.

Gill, R.S., et al., *Robotic-assisted bariatric surgery: a systematic review.* Int J Med Robot, 2011.

Giusti, V., et al., *Effects of laparoscopic gastric banding on body composition, metabolic profile and nutritional status of obese women: 12-months follow-up.* Obes Surg, 2004. 14(2): p. 239-45.

Horgan, A.F., et al., *Atypical diverticular disease: surgical results.* Dis Colon Rectum, 2001. 44(9): p. 1315-8.

Horgan, S. and D. Vanuno, *Robots in laparoscopic surgery.* J Laparoendosc Adv Surg Tech A, 2001. 11(6): p. 415-9.

Jacobsen, G., R. Berger, and S. Horgan, *The role of robotic surgery in morbid obesity.* J Laparoendosc Adv Surg Tech A, 2003. 13(4): p. 279-83.

Kim, W.W., et al., *Laparoscopic vs. open biliopancreatic diversion with duodenal switch: a comparative study.* J Gastrointest Surg, 2003. 7(4): p. 552-7.

Kim, K. and C. Buffington, *Totally robotic gastric bypass: approach and technique.* J Robotic Surg, 2011. 5(1): p. 47-50.

Lee, C.M., P.T. Cirangle, and G.H. Jossart, *Vertical gastrectomy for morbid obesity in 216 patients: report of two-year results.* Surg Endosc, 2007. 21(10): p. 1810-6.

Mohr, C.J., G.S. Nadzam, and M.J. Curet, *Totally robotic Roux-en-Y gastric bypass.* Arch Surg, 2005. 140(8): p. 779-86.

Mokdad, A.H., et al., *Actual causes of death in the United States, 2000.* JAMA, 2004. 291(10): p. 1238-45.

Moser, F. and S. Horgan, *Robotically assisted bariatric surgery.* Am J Surg, 2004. 188(4A Suppl): p. 38S-44S.

Muhlmann, G., et al., *DaVinci robotic-assisted laparoscopic bariatric surgery: is it justified in a routine setting?* Obes Surg, 2003. 13(6): p. 848-54.

Nehoda, H., et al., *Results and complications after adjustable gastric banding in a series of 250 patients.* Am J Surg, 2001. 181(1): p. 12-5.

Ogden, C.L., et al., *Prevalence and trends in overweight among US children and adolescents, 1999-2000.* JAMA, 2002. 288(14): p. 1728-32.

Podnos, Y.D., et al., *Complications after laparoscopic gastric bypass: a review of 3464 cases.* Arch Surg, 2003. 138(9): p. 957-61.

Regan, J.P., et al., *Early experience with two-stage laparoscopic Roux-en-Y gastric bypass as an alternative in the super-super obese patient.* Obes Surg, 2003. 13(6): p. 861-4.

Ren, C.J., E. Patterson, and M. Gagner, *Early results of laparoscopic biliopancreatic diversion with duodenal switch: a case series of 40 consecutive patients.* Obes Surg, 2000. 10(6): p. 514-23; discussion 524.

Schauer, P., et al., *The learning curve for laparoscopic Roux-en-Y gastric bypass is 100 cases.* Surg Endosc, 2003. 17(2): p. 212-5.

Snyder, B. and e. al., *Lowering gastrointestinal leak rates: a comparative analysis of robotic and laparoscopic gastric bypass.* J Robotic Surg, 2008. 2: p. 159-163.

Snyder, B.E., et al., *Robotic-assisted Roux-en-Y Gastric bypass: minimizing morbidity and mortality.* Obes Surg, 2010. 20(3): p. 265-70.

Sudan, R., V. Puri, and D. Sudan, *Robotically assisted biliary pancreatic diversion with a duodenal switch: a new technique.* Surg Endosc, 2007. 21(5): p. 729-33.

Wilson, E.B., et al., *Robotic Bariatric Surgery: Outcomes of Laparoscopic Biliopancreatic Diversion and Gastric Bypass.* Surg Obes Relat Dis, 2008. 4: p. 312-357.

16

Scarless Bariatric Surgery

Chih-Kun Huang, Rajat Goel and Satish Pattanshetti
Bariatric & Metabolic International (B.M.I) Surgery Center/E-Da Hospital, Taiwan, ROC

1. Introduction

Bariatric surgery has been established as the best and most effective treatment for morbid obesity. It leads to sustained weight loss, life style changes and improves quality of life. Since Wittgrove et al. introduced the laparoscopic Roux-en-Y gastric bypass technique in 1994, the number of operations performed has grown rapidly, and there has been a rapid reduction in the number of complications with quicker recovery. At present, the laparoscopic approach has become the most popular technique in performing bariatric surgery in the world. However laparoscopic technique requires five to seven abdominal incisions to facilitate placement of the multiple trocars. Because of the need for the numerous ports, the cosmetic results are unacceptable to some patient subgroup, like young females. These visible scars may fade over time; however, the healing process is highly individualistic, and the cosmetic outcome may not be appealing to all patients. In recent years, concept of "No scar surgery" is quickly expanding in various surgical fields, including weight loss surgery.

Newer techniques have eliminated the need for multiple ports and the inevitable scarring that follows. Natural orifice transluminal endoscopic surgery (NOTES), which produces no scarring, has been considered to be a landmark in the advancement of laparoscopy. Recently, another emerging procedure, single-incision laparoscopic surgery (SILS), has been used for appendectomy, cholecystectomy and colectomy. This new approach minimizes the scars and is considered minimally invasive. In bariatric surgeries, the SILS technique has been employed to perform adjustable banding , sleeve gastrectomy, Roux-en -Y gastric bypass and biliopancreatic diversion procedures. Here we will review the surgical techniques and results of various scarless bariatric surgery, including NOTES and SILS.

2. NOTES bariatric surgery

Since the introduction of NOTES in 2004, researchers have used it for various surgical interventions [1-3]. This new approach minimizes the scars and is considered minimally invasive. Even with the worldwide popularity of NOTES, the present techniques and instruments used are still under-developed before making it really applicable in clinical employment. There is also ethical concern because of transvaginal or transrectal approach, sacrificing the integrity of organ. There is also technical difficulty due to the long distance between vagina/rectum and stomach making instrument handling and tissue manipulation more complicated with present technology, and there is also concern about the closure of orifice. The implication on bariatric surgery was only reported in sleeve gastrectomy and adjustable gastric banding with hybrid method, combining laparoscopic and endoscopic approach [4-6]. For more complicated procedures, such as gastric bypass are still at experimental stage [7].

3. SILS bariatric surgery

Single-incision laparoscopic surgery (SILS) was first described as early as 1992 by Pelosi et al. performed single-puncture laparoscopic appendectomy and hysterectomy [8, 9]. Currently SILS is considered to be a bridging technique to natural orifice transluminal endoscopic surgery (NOTES). It has emerged as another modality of carrying out the bariatric procedures. SILS can be performed using refinements of existing technology and experienced surgeons can perform SILS even with traditional laparoscopic instruments. Applications of SILS have expanded rapidly and various procedures including bariatric surgery have been carried out with this technique. Initially, SILS was used in bariatric procedures such as adjustable gastric banding (AGB) and sleeve gastrectomy because these procedures require the extension of a trocar incision for the placement of a subcutaneous port or for extracting the resected gastric specimen [10-12]. The incision was mainly in the upper abdomen in the beginning in this single-incision transabdominal (SITA) laparoscopic approach. It was felt that the patients would have a better cosmetic outcome if the SILS could be performed via a transumbilical incision as the umbilicus can hide the surgical wound, leaving no visible abdominal scars. Single incision transumbilical (SITU) laparoscopic procedures seem to attract more surgeons because of the higher satisfaction from patients. Recently surgeons started to perform SILS in more complex bariatric procedures such as gastric bypass and biliopancreatic diversion procedures that require gastrointestinal anastomosis [13-14]. Here we review the surgical technique of SITA and SITU bariatric surgery.

3.1 Liver retraction in SILS bariatric surgery

For upper gastrointestinal laparoscopic surgery, liver retraction is necessary to ensure adequate working space. In morbidly obese patients, the hypertrophic left lobe of liver invariably hinders the surgeon's view of the entire stomach. In multi-port bariatric procedures, most surgeons use a Nathanson's liver retractor via a subxiphoid incision to retract liver. To avoid the incision in SILS, retraction of the liver is a major challenge. Sakaguchi et al [15] invented a device for the retraction of the liver during conventional laparoscopic gastrectomy. However, in morbidly obese patients, the technique, which involves the dissection of the left triangular ligament of the left liver lobe, is more difficult to employ because most of these patients have a hypertrophic left liver lobe. Tacchino *et al.* used a transfixation suture, applied on the right crus and suspended outside as a liver retractor suture [14, 16-17]. We have invented a new liver suspension tape technique via puncturing liver at peripheral area that can be used to lift even massive livers in morbidly obese patients. [Figures 1-3] [13]. Another non-puncturing method with a penrose drain and endo-hernia stapler has also been reported by us [18]. These techniques have been proved to be a quick and safe method in SILS bariatric surgery.

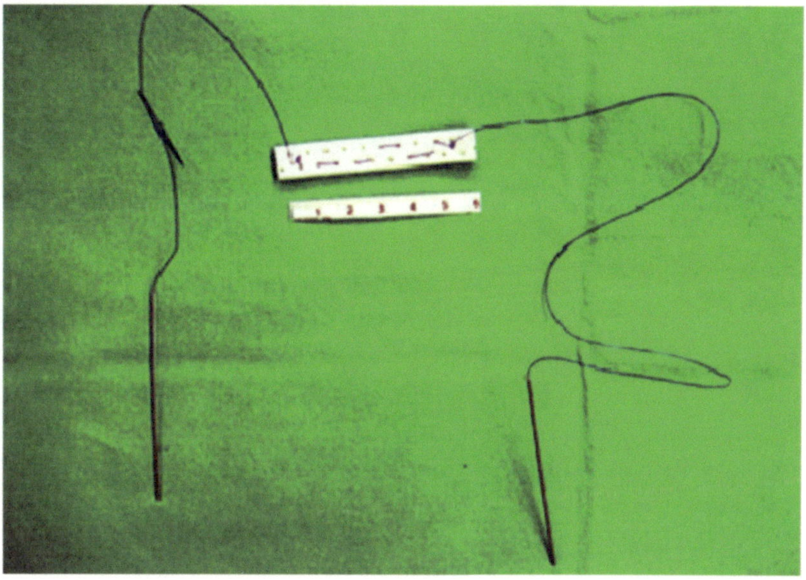

Fig. 1. Design of liver suspension tape developed by Huang et al.

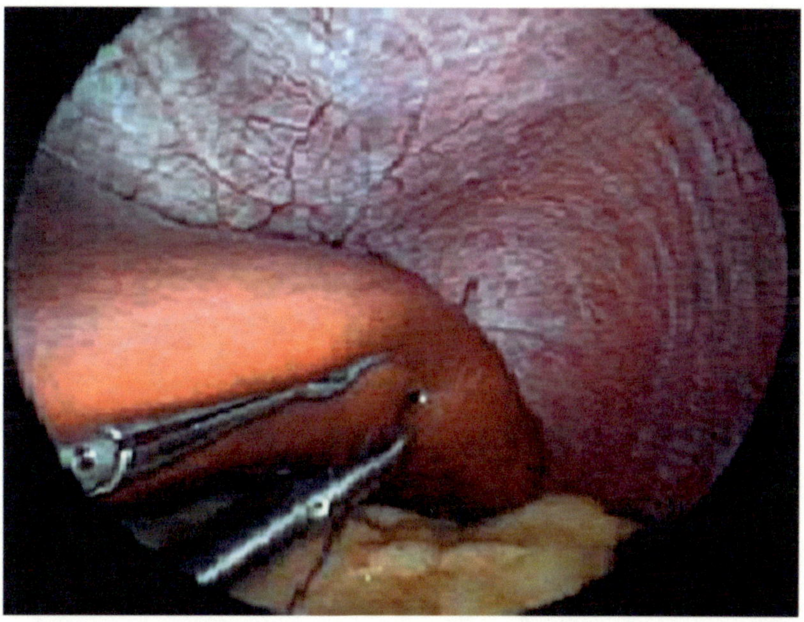

Fig. 2. We measure a 6-cm length of a Jackson-Pratt drain, cut it and fix a with 2-0 polypropylene suture on either side.

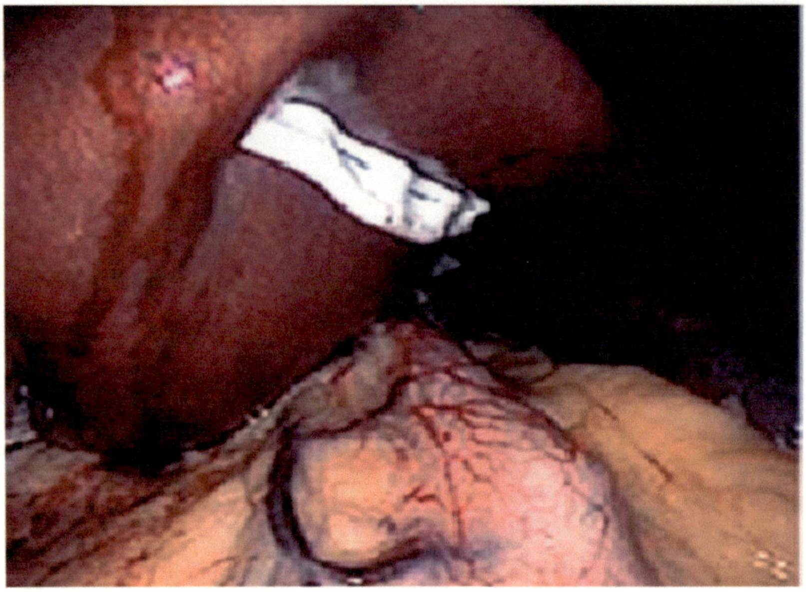

Fig. 3. The lateral segment of the left liver is suspended by passing the suture through it.

3.2 Adjustable gastric bading

Laparoscopic AGB (LAGB) is considered to be the most physiological and safe bariatric surgery, not involving cutting and anastomosis of gastrointestinal tract [19]. Although the weight loss observed is slower, the procedure is popular. In AGB, the surgeons utilize the pars flaccida approach to place a band and then place 2-3 gastro-gastric sutures to hold it in place. It was believed that LAGB is a good surgery for bariatric surgeons to start the SILS bariatric

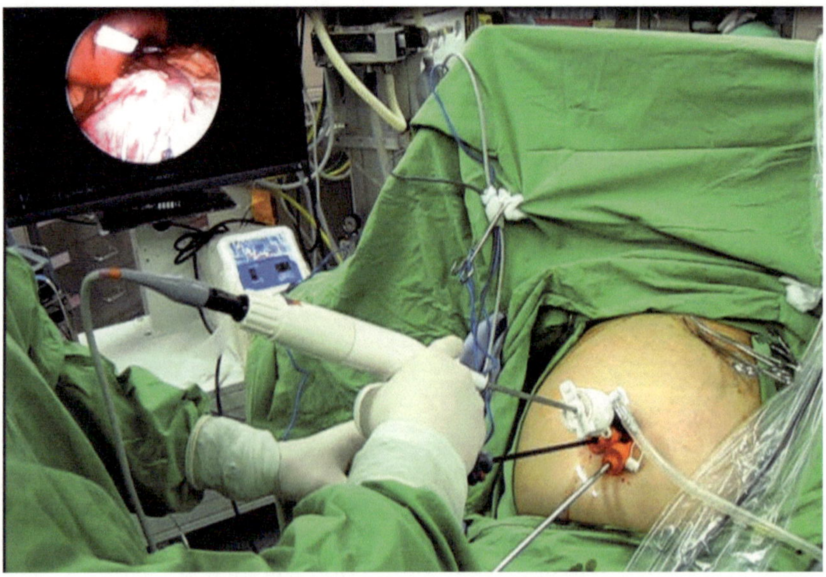

Fig. 4. Port positioning for SITU procedure.

procedure because it is a technically less demanding procedure and a 4-cm incision is required for placement of the port. Nguyen et al [10] reported the first case of single-incision laparoscopic AGB. This is also believed to be the first SILS bariatric surgery reported. Although the procedure was performed with a SITA method, it opened up the possibility of SILS in bariatric surgery. Keidar et al [20] also used the SITA method by adding a liver retractor incision and the operative time was about 60 minutes. SITU-LAGB was reported by Teixeira et al [21] and the patients included had neither hepatomegaly nor central obesity. Super-obese patients were also not considered for inclusion in this study. One conversion was observed in 22 reported patients. We also reported two cases with SITU method where through single transumbilical incision multiple fascial punctures were performed to carry out the procedure (Figure 4) [22]. Tacchino et al used SILS port for the procedure [16]. But till now, there are no reported series comparing the outcomes of SILS LAGB and multiple-port LAGB.

3.3 Sleeve gastrectomy

Sleeve gastrectomy is an emerging procedure for weight loss that provides rapid and satisfactory weight loss without any long-term vitamin deficiency. The procedure starts by mobilizing the greater curvature starting 4-6-cm from the pylorus till the angle of His. A vertical gastrectomy is then performed with endoscopic staplers. The resected stomach is extracted via an incision. The SILS approach was applied to sleeve gastrectomy as an incision was required for extraction of the resected gastric tube anyway. Saber et al reported both SITU and SITA combined with a single port or multiple trocars [23, 24]. They also compared the result of SILS and multiport sleeve gastrectomy. Single-incision laparoscopic sleeve gastrectomy was associated with less postoperative pain, a lower need for analgesics and a decreased length of hospital stay compared to the conventional multi-port laparoscopic sleeve gastrectomy [25]. In these studies, most patients were superobese and one patient developed wound infection that required drainage [26]. We are also doing SITU procedures for sleeve gastrectomy in selected patients and trocar positioning is similar as AGB.

3.4 Gastric bypass

Laparoscopic Roux-en-Y gastric bypass (LRYGB) has been considered as the gold standard of bariatric surgery. In the standard Roux-en-Y gastric bypass, a 25-ml pouch is constructed and anastomosed to a Roux loop of jejunum. This is followed by closure of the mesenteric and Peterson's defect. Till now only two authors have reported the results of the SILS approach for gastric bypass. Tacchino et al elongated the gastric pouch to 6 cm in length to speed up the dissection and decrease the tension on the gastrojejunal anastomosis. Two gastric bypass procedures were adopted - 16 patients receiving a single loop and two receiving a double loop. The single-loop gastric bypass involved only one anastomosis, and was thought to decrease the difficulties of technique [27]. We also developed a novel method using a SITU approach and subsequently performing an omega-umbilicoplasty for the Roux-en-Y gastric bypass [22, 28]. The increased space of manipulation in the 6-cm incision and subsequent umbilicoplasty design makes the procedure easier, saves time and is still scarless [Figures 5-6]. It could be offered as a bridge surgery in the early learning curve of performing SITU procedures, and then you can directly go to the 4 cm umbilical incision without need of umbilicoplasty. In fact, the procedures might need some modifications including use of an Endostich device for suturing and some stay sutures for counter traction. No complications were observed in these two reports.

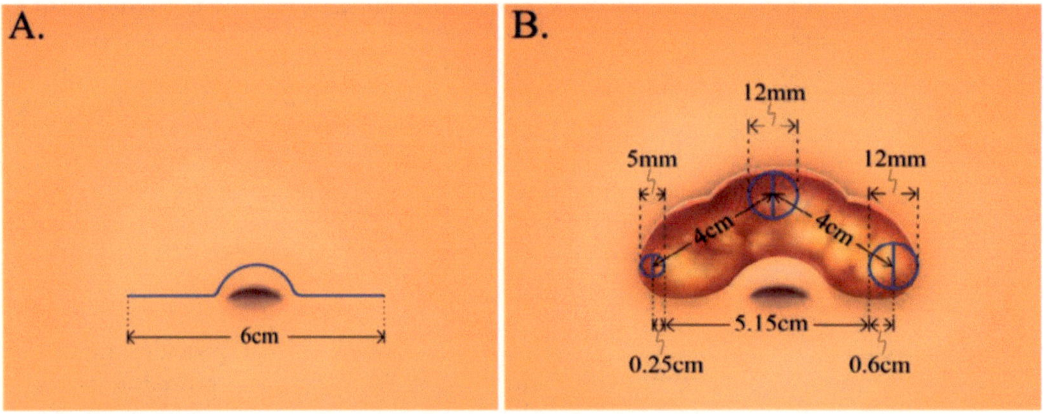

Fig. 5. Design of single-incision transumbilical laparoscopic bariatric surgery (multiple ports) by Huang et al. Schematic of a 4-6-cm ω-incision in the supra-umbilical area. (A) Schematic of the distance between the trocars (5 mm, 12 mm, 12 mm) that can reach (B) 4-cm more with this design thus increasing the space for manipulation.

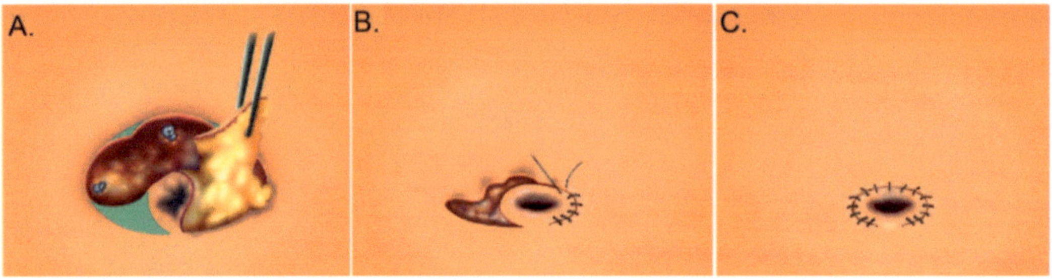

Fig. 6. Closure of the ω-incision (A) At the conclusion of the surgery the trocars are removed and the fascia is repaired. The subcutaneous fat and skin at the angle is removed (Green area). (B) An umbilicoplasty is performed. (C) The wound becomes circular and is buried in the umbilicus.

3.5 Biliopancreatic diversion

Biliopancreatic diversion is a malabsorptive technique of bariatric surgery that has gained wide acceptance especially in super-obesity. It is performed by carrying out a horizontal transaction of stomach combined with a gastroenterostomy and enteroenterostomy. The surgery is considered to be the most complex bariatric procedure. Tacchino et al reported the first case with SITU / single-port method [14] in a 57-year-old man with a body mass index of 43 kg/m2. The procedure took 130 minutes to finish and there were no complications.

4. Discussion

SILS has recently gained acceptance in bariatric surgery as the procedure has possible benefits. It is an alternative to NOTES - an experimental procedure whose feasibility is frequently debated. [21, 22] The surgical technique involved is almost identical to that required for conventional laparoscopic surgery. If the surgery is performed transumbilically, the surgical scar is almost completely hidden inside the belly button and the surgical site is scarless. Although some surgeons argue that very obese patients are not concerned about the scarring up to 70% of patients undergoing bariatric procedures are women and consider scarring to be an important factor. We have done a comparative study in SITU-LRYGB and 5-port LRYGB [29]. Also, though the operation times were longer, the recovery and hospitalization was similar in both groups. The promising result showed better patient satisfaction regarding the cosmesis in the SITU group (Figure 7). Despite its advantages in SILS bariatric surgery, the small umbilical incision tends to "crowd" the trocars in a very limited surgical field. The resulting reduced instrument triangulation and inability to retract tissue by the assistant make this procedure more arduous. At first, it is essential to use a 30° 5-mm laparoscope to avoid conflict with other surgical instruments. Some surgeons have used a semi-flexible endoscopic camera system to make the procedure more comfortable. Second, handling a hypertrophic liver and abundant visceral fat is also critical in morbidly obese patients. Third, longer endoscope, longer graspers and longer linear staplers are also highly recommended. In addition, patient selection is important for this surgery and some patients are not well-suited for these procedure. Most authors do not recommend this procedure for those with a BMI greater than 50 kg/m^2. Not only because of abundant abdominal fat that makes surgery very difficult, especially for a LRYGB, which needs anastomosis technique, also mostly postoperative abdomino-plasty is inevitable in super-obese patients after gravid weight loss. Due to the longer-than-normal working distance between the angle of His and the umbilicus in the SILS procedure, it should be avoided in tall patients (height >180 cm). As this procedure requires far more skill than a conventional 5-port surgery, it should only be undertaken by very experienced bariatric surgeons.

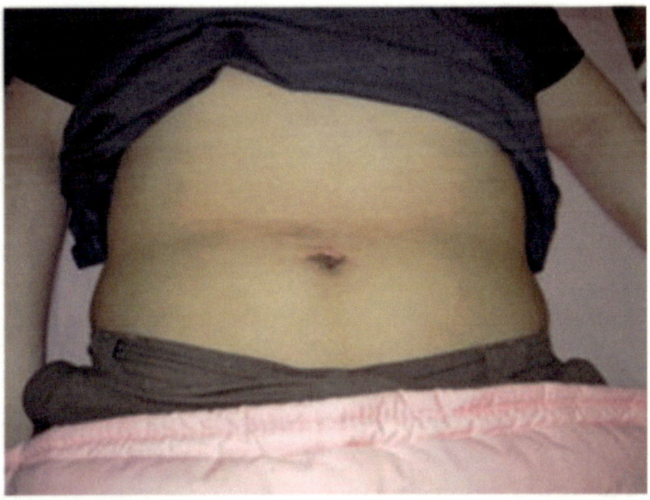

Fig. 7. Scar of SITU LRYGB in follow up.

To start with the 3-ports surgery could make surgeons more familiar with the surgcial setting without assistant's counter-traction and could bring you steady to the success of SILS procedure.

5. Conclusions

In conclusion, no scar bariatric surgery is a new unavoidable trend because of concern about the privacy and quality of life. At present, SILS bariatric has been shown to be a technically more feasible and reproducible procedure for a select group of morbidly obese patients than NOTES. Because of the abundant visceral and subcutaneous fat and multiple co-morbidities in morbid obesity, it is more challenging for surgeons to perform the procedures with SILS. It is clear that extensive development of new instruments and technology will make these procedures easier to perform. Careful selection of candidate is a key for the success of this surgery. Nevertheless, randomized studies to compare the SILS bariatric procedures with traditional multi-port surgery are essential to further develop this highly technique-dependent surgery.

6. References

[1] de la Fuente SG, Demaria EJ, Reynolds JD, Portenier DD, Pryor AD. New developments in surgery: Natural Orifice Transluminal Endoscopic Surgery (NOTES). Arch Surg 2007;142:295-7.

[2] McGee MF, Rosen MJ, Marks J, Onders RP, Chak A, Faulx A, et al. A primer on natural orifice transluminal endoscopic surgery: Building a new paradigm. Surg Innov 2006;13:86-93.

[3] Flora ED, Wilson TG, Martin IJ, O'Rourke NA, Maddern GJ. A review of natural orifice translumenal endoscopic surgery (NOTES) for intra-abdominal surgery: Experimental models, techniques, and applicability to the clinical setting. Ann Surg 2008;247:583-602.

[4] Ramos AC, Zundel N, Neto MG, Maalouf M. Human hybrid NOTES transvaginal sleeve gastrectomy: initial experience. Surg Obes Relat Dis. 2008 Sep-Oct;4(5):660-3. Epub 2008 Jul 15.

[5] Michalik M, Orlowski M, Bobowicz M, Frask A, Trybull A. The first report on hybrid NOTES adjustable gastric banding in human. Obes Surg. 2011 Apr;21(4):524-7.

[6] Buesing M, Utech M, Halter J, Riege R, Saada G, Knapp A. Sleeve gastrectomy in the treatment of morbid obesity : Study results and first experiences with the transvaginal hybrid NOTES technique. Chirurg. 2011 Aug;82(8):675-83. German.

[7] Hagen ME, Wagner OJ, Swain P, Pugin F, Buchs N, Caddedu M, Jamidar P, Fasel J, Morel P. Hybrid natural orifice transluminal endoscopic surgery (NOTES) for Roux-en-Y gastric bypass: an experimental surgical study in human cadavers. Endoscopy. 2008 Nov;40(11):918-24

[8] Pelosi MA, Pelosi MA 3rd. Laparoscopic appendectomy using a single umbilical puncture (minilaparoscopy). J Reprod Med 1992;37:588-94.

[9] Pelosi MA, Pelosi MA 3rd. Laparoscopic supracervical hysterectomy using a single-umbilical puncture(mini-laparoscopy). J Reprod Med 1992;37:777-84.

[10] Nguyen NT, Hinojosa MW, Smith BR, Reavis KM. Single laparoscopic incision transabdominal (SLIT) surgery-adjustable gastric banding: A novel minimally invasive surgical approach. Obes Surg 2008;18:1628-31.
[11] Saber AA, Elgamal MH, Itawi EA, Rao AJ. Single-incision laparoscopic sleeve gastrectomy (SILS): A novel technique. Obes Surg 2008;18:1338-42.
[12] Reavis KM, Hinojosa MW, Smith BR, Nguyen NT. Single-laparoscopic incision transabdominal surgery sleeve gastrectomy. Obes Surg 2008;18:1492-4.
[13] Huang CK, Houng JY, Chiang CJ, Chen YS, Lee PH. Single-incision transumbilical laparoscopic Roux-en-Y gastric bypass: A first case report.Obes Surg 2009;19:1711-5.
[14] Tacchino RM, Greco F, Matera D. Single-incision laparoscopic biliopancreatic diversion. Surg Obes Relat Dis 2010;6:444-5.
[15] Sakaguchi Y, Ikeda O, Toh Y, Aoki Y, Harimoto N, Taomoto J, et al. New technique for the retraction of the liver in laparoscopic gastrectomy. Surg Endosc 2008;22:2532-4.
[16] Tacchino RM, Greco F, Matera D. Laparoscopic gastric banding without visible scar: A short series with intraumbilical SILS. Obes Surg 2010;20:236-9.
[17] de la Torre RA, Satgunam S, Morales MP, Dwyer CL, Scott JS. Transumbilical single-port laparoscopic adjustable gastric band placement with liver suture retractor. Obes Surg 2009;19:1707-10.
[18] Huang CK, Lo CH, Asim S, Houng JY, Huang SF. A Novel Technique for Liver Retraction in Laparoscopic Bariatric Surgery. Obes Surg. 2010.
[19] Nguyen NT, Slone JA, Nguyen XM, Hartman JS, Hoyt DB. A Prospective Randomized Trial of Laparoscopic Gastric Bypass Versus Laparoscopic Adjustable Gastric Banding for the Treatment of Morbid Obesity: Outcomes, Qualityof Life, and Costs. Ann Surg. 2009.
[20] Keidar A, Shussman N, Elazary R, Rivkind AI, Mintz Y. Right-sided upper abdomen single-incision laparoscopic gastric banding. Obes Surg 2010;20:757-60.
[21] Teixeira J, McGill K, Koshy N, McGinty J, Todd G. Laparoscopic single-site surgery for placement of adjustable gastric band--a series of 22 cases. Surg Obes Relat Dis 2010;6:41-5.
[22] Huang CK, Tsai JC, Lo CH, Houng JY, Chen YS, Chi SC, Lee PH. Preliminary Surgical Results of Single-Incision Transumbilical Laparoscopic Bariatric Surgery. Obes Surg.2010.
[23] Saber AA, El-Ghazaly TH. Early experience with single-access transumbilical adjustable laparoscopic gastric banding. Obes Surg 2009;19:1442-6.
[24] Saber AA, El-Ghazaly TH, Elian A. Single-incision transumbilical laparoscopic sleeve gastrectomy. J Laparoendosc Adv Surg Tech A 2009;19:755-8.
[25] Saber AA, El-Ghazaly TH, Dewoolkar AV, Slayton SA. Single-incision laparoscopic sleeve gastrectomy versus conventional multiport laparoscopic sleeve gastrectomy: Technical considerations and strategic modifications. Surg Obes Relat Dis.2010.
[26] Gentileschi P, Camperchioli I, Benavoli D, Lorenzo ND, Sica G, Gaspari AL. Laparoscopic single-port sleeve gastrectomy for morbid obesity: Preliminary series. Surg Obes Relat Dis.2010.
[27] Tacchino RM, Greco F, Matera D, Diflumeri G. Single-incision laparoscopic gastric bypass for morbid obesity. Obes Surg 2010;20:1154-60.

[28] Huang CK, Yao SF, Lo CH, Houng JY, Chen YS, Lee PH. A Novel Surgical Technique: Single-Incision Transumbilical Laparoscopic Roux-en-Y Gastric Bypass. Obes Surg. 2010 Oct;20(10):1429-35.
[29] Huang CK, Lo CH, Houng JY, Chen YS, Lee PH. Surgical results of single-incision transumbilical laparoscopic Roux-en-Y gastric bypass. Surg Obes Relat Dis. 2010 Dec 25.